Class: 306.
Accession No: 1
Type: 3wk .

KU-184-320

Unequal Health

How Inequality Contributes to Health or Illness

Second Edition

Grace Budrys

THE LIBRARY
TOWER HAMLETS COLLEGE
POPLAR HIGH STREET
LONDON E14 0AF
Tel: 0207 510 7763

ROWMAN & LITTLEFIELD PUBLISHERS, INC.
Lanham • Boulder • New York • Toronto • Plymouth, UK

Published by Rowman & Littlefield Publishers, Inc.
A wholly owned subsidary of The Rowman & Littlefield Publishing Group, Inc.
4501 Forbes Boulevard, Suite 200, Lanham, Maryland 20706
http://www.rowmanlittlefield.com

Estover Road, Plymouth PL6 7PY, United Kingdom

Copyright © 2010 by Rowman & Littlefield Publishers, Inc.

All rights reserved. No part of this book may be reproduced in any form or by any
electronic or mechanical means, including information storage and retrieval systems,
without written permission from the publisher, except by a reviewer who may quote
passages in a review.

British Library Cataloguing in Publication Information Available

Library of Congress Cataloging-in-Publication Data
Budrys, Grace, 1943–
 Unequal health : how inequality contributes to health or illness / Grace Budrys.
 — 2nd ed.
  p. ; cm.
 Includes bibliographical references and index.
 ISBN 978-0-7425-6506-7 (cloth : alk. paper) — ISBN 978-0-7425-6507-4 (pbk. : alk.
paper)
 1. Social medicine. 2. Medical statistics. 3. Health behavior. 4. Health status
indicators. I. Title.
 [DNLM: 1. Health Status Indicators—United States. 2. Socioeconomic Factors—
United States. WA 900 AA1 B8995u 2010]
 RA418.B83 2010
 362.1'042—dc22
                                                                    2009029774

♾ ™ The paper used in this publication meets the minimum requirements of
American National Standard for Information Sciences—Permanence of Paper
for Printed Library Materials, ANSI/NISO Z39.48-1992.

Printed in the United States of America

Contents

~

Acronyms

AARP	American Association of Retired Persons
ACS	American Cancer Society
AFDC	Aid to Families with Dependent Children
AHA	American Heart Association
AHRQ	Agency for Healthcare Research and Quality
AIDS	acquired immunodeficiency syndrome
BMI	Body Mass Index
CDC	Centers for Disease Control
CEO	chief operating officer
CHIP	Children's Health Insurance Program
CIA	Central Intelligence Agency
COT	Congressional Office of Technology Assessment
CPI	(National) Consumer Price Index
DASH	Dietary Approaches to Stop Hypertension
GAO	government accountability office
GNP	gross national product
HEDIS	healthcare effectiveness data and information set
HIV	human immunodeficiency virus
HMO	health maintenance organization
HSA	health savings account
IMF	International Monetary Fund
IOM	Institute of Medicine
MI	myocardial infarction

MRSA	methicillin-resistant Staphylococcus aureus
NCHS	National Center for Health Statistics
NCQA	National Committee for Quality Assurance
NHANES	National Health and Nutrition Examination Survey
NHIS	National Health Interview Survey
NHLBI	National Heart, Lung, and Blood Institute
NIDA	National Institute on Drug Abuse
NIH	National Institutes of Health
OECD	Organisation for Economic Cooperation and Development
OMB	U.S. Office of Management and Budget
ORWH	Office of Research on Women's Health
PTSD	posttraumatic stress disorder
SARS	severe acute respiratory syndrome
S-CHIP	State Children's Health Insurance Program
SSI	supplemental social security insurance
TANF	Temporary Assistance to Needy Families
VA	Veterans Administration
WHO	World Health Organisation
WIC	(supplemental food assistance for) women, infants, and children
XDR TB	extensive resistant tuberculosis
YPLL	years of potential life lost

CHAPTER ONE

~

Introduction

Have you noticed how many stories dealing with health problems are being featured by the news media? At one level the explanation is obvious—people want information that promises to provide relief from any pain they are experiencing as well as from the inconvenience and emotional upset that illness brings. Why the level of interest seems to be escalating is more complicated.

One part of the explanation is that researchers really are coming up with more findings on diagnostics, treatments, and disease trajectories and they are publishing their findings in the growing number of scientific journals at an unprecedented rate. Reporters, who realize that their readers are interested in hearing about medical advances, regularly check out articles in these journals to see what might be newsworthy. The stories they write invariably present whatever scientific findings catch their attention as important breakthroughs. Many are. In other cases, researchers are publishing their results because their findings confirm the results of previous studies, which is not nearly as attention-grabbing as saying the findings constitute a major breakthrough. So, such disclaimers are not always mentioned in the news stories. Admittedly, some researchers don't bother to mention that either. In point of fact, it is not always easy to tell what is and what is not groundbreaking. What is indisputably clear is that we are being exposed to a steady stream of news stories about topics related in some way to our health and advice on what we should be doing to improve our health.

Advances in technology have also made it possible for researchers to publish their findings in electronic versions of scientific journals, which do

1

not take nearly as long to appear as articles in print journals. Some journals now use both formats, which has the effect of increasing exponentially both the volume and speed at which information is being disseminated. The Internet has revolutionized research—not only because it makes the findings available to a wider audience more quickly, but because it makes volumes of statistics on health collected by government agencies available at the click of a button to researchers and anyone else interested in tracking who is sick and dying from what cause.

Not to be dismissed as a factor that contributes to the level of attention health issues are attracting is the continuous barrage of pharmaceutical ads telling us that we should check out our "symptoms" with our doctors because those symptoms might be indicative of a disease for which the pharmaceutical company has developed medications that will certainly bring us relief (if not a cure). Why people are so intensely interested in what pharmaceuticals can do for them is due to something that goes beyond the effectiveness of pharmaceutical advertising. Increasing numbers of Americans, as is true of people in all industrially advanced societies, are suffering from and dying of chronic illnesses. There are only two responses available to us to ameliorate the effects of chronic illness once we are affected. The first is altering our behavior, and the second is signing up for a regimen of pill consumption. Taking medications may be tedious and costly, but most people think that it is a lot easier to do that than changing one's lifestyle. We really don't want to hear that we should watch our diets, exercise, stop engaging in all those health-damaging behaviors—we have heard all that already! Knowing very well what we should be doing doesn't make it any easier. So, increasing numbers of us are consuming more pills and many of us are eager to hear about new and improved versions of those pills, because once we take a closer look, we find that the pills we are taking may bring about a new set of worries related to the side effects they produce.

As if that were not enough, there are now companies offering to provide us with genetic testing kits that will allow us to know our risk level for contracting any number of diseases. The question that experts are raising is whether this is having an empowering or endangering effect on the public. Not only is there the issue of psychological threat associated with expecting to contract a life-threatening disease, but there are privacy concerns. Of course, this assumes that one can be sure that the test results are accurate, which is not always so clear.

The flood of articles reporting research findings and accompanying commentary means that we will only be able to sample some of the findings related to the topics we will be discussing in the chapters to follow; and you can certainly expect to be confronted with more recent results after you finish reading this book. I am warning you to be prepared for loads of facts coming at you now and, once you start paying closer attention, for the foreseeable future. The aim, as far as I am concerned, is learning to sort it all out. Once you finish reading this book, you will be much better prepared to determine which news stories are presenting information that extends existing understandings, those that challenge prevailing understandings, and those that offer information that is truly revolutionary.

Purpose of the Book

After noting that there is a great deal of information out there, I would like to clarify the basic objective of this book. My aim is to address the question of why some people are healthier and live longer than others. We will do this by looking at it from the other end of the spectrum—finding out why some people get sick and die so much earlier than others. This topic has become known as the study of *health disparities*. As we become more closely involved in this pursuit, you will find that the risk of illness and premature death is not evenly distributed. Explaining why that is the case is the central objective of the chapters to follow.

The Conventional Wisdom

Of course, many Americans are convinced that they already know why some people are healthier and live longer than others. Don't most of the people you know think that a person's health depends on diet, exercise, not smoking, learning to overcome stress, and getting good medical care? When someone lives to a ripe old age after happily violating all this good advice, we smile and say it's genetic. Similarly, when someone dies before what we think is "their time" while following all of these rules, we all nod knowingly, shake our heads, and again say that it must be genetic. And that settles that!

That is known as *conventional wisdom*. What is so satisfying about this explanation for longevity is that it is widely shared, which makes us all feel that we are really "with it" because we are tuned in to what everyone around us knows to be true. In other words, what makes conventional wisdom explanations so popular is that they are grounded in a much bigger belief system that unites all of us as Americans. The American cultural value system has well-developed views about what foods are most tasty; what kinds of leisure activities are most enjoyable; which celebrities' antics we need to know about at the moment, and, of course, what explains why some people live longer than others.

To get past conventional wisdom explanations and discuss the topics that come up based on actual facts, we will be looking at a lot of tables, especially in the first few chapters. I know that statistics are sometimes intimidating. But I expect that you will overcome that feeling pretty soon and find the tables really interesting, because the realities they reveal are not only surprising—they are shocking.

You should expect to encounter fewer tables as we move through the book. Instead, you will see a steady increase in the number of references to the interpretations of the data offered by experts. The shift is logical. The tables in the early chapters present factual information that you can interpret yourself. As we move through the chapters, the interpretations of the data become more complicated and arguable. That happens because the subject matter becomes increasingly harder to capture, that is, to define and measure. Furthermore, as we move on in our discussion you will find fewer tables reporting on information gathered by the government on the population as a whole. The government does not collect data on such things as how much stress people experience. The topic is, however, clearly important and of interest to many people, so researchers study this and other similarly nebulous topics by designing their own studies, gathering their own statistics, and reporting the conclusions they reach. We will devote most attention to the health of the U.S. population but we will consider the health of people in other societies as well.

Because researchers are always trying to find better ways to collect data, there is constant innovation in how this kind of research is conducted, which means that new measures are continuously being introduced. Whether they end up being regarded as improvements over older, more established measures is resolved through discussion and debate. More information means that there is more to disagree about. Rather than becoming clearer, the picture keeps getting more complex. That helps to explain why conventional wisdom explanations are so much more satisfying to those people who have a low tolerance for complexity.

The pervasiveness of conventional wisdom explanations is attributable to the fact that the media never cease to remind us of the beliefs we are supposed to share as Americans. Not only is there the chatter coming from "talking heads" on the TV screen, but, as we noted already, there are all those commercials. As I am sure you will agree, there is an endless parade of products and services aimed at helping us attain not only better health, but a higher level of physical performance and great looks to boot. There are products to help us quit smoking, pills that insure sexual readiness, exercise machines and clubs that promise "buns of steel," and if all else fails, medical treatments like liposuction, which might be very useful after we consume those enormous portions of fried, fatty food we are being encouraged to eat by so many of the other ads. In short, the vast amount of media attention devoted to health issues means that it is hard to ignore hearing what we should and should not be doing to stay healthy.

It is also hard to avoid hearing about the negative health consequences associated with eating too much fatty food, smoking, abusing drugs, and engaging in risky sex. So why do people who engage in ill-advised behaviors do it? That is a crucial question. If we knew the answer, then changing people's behavior to make them healthier would be a lot easier. Of course, we would have to be convinced that the answer is accurate. As it is, there is little consensus about how we might go about helping anyone change their behavior. And, in the opinion of some, there is no need for the rest of us to be involved anyway—it is, after all, a matter of personal choice—isn't it? Of course, there are also those who point out that the rest of us will end up footing the bill for the medical care that people who engage in all those unhealthy behaviors will very likely require. Looking at it from that perspective means that there are consequential and practical reasons for figuring out what the solution is to achieving better health for many more members of our society. This is not to say that we have less reason to be concerned about the health of others if we do not bear a financial burden for it.

Maybe if we knew more about the kinds of people who engage in particular kinds of behavior we could target the message more accurately and get better results. Unfortunately, as most of us already know, targeted messages seem to be highly successful when used to market all those health-damaging products and completely unsuccessful when used to promote public health messages, but that's an entirely different topic. Why people behave the way they do, especially why they indulge in self-destructive behavior, is a complex issue, but an important one. We will discuss some very convincing answers that keep accumulating as we move forward in the book.

We will compare the behavior of groups of people according to age, sex, and race/ethnicity to see if we can find any patterns. Those who conduct market research to create advertising campaigns that are so successful in promoting all those negative behaviors know how to do this very well. To illustrate, we know that cigarette companies have spent a lot of money over the years finding out who is and who is not smoking their brand: young/old, rich/poor, women/men, and so on. We will do something like that by establishing demographic profiles to project who, for example, is becoming overweight, which we know is associated with a number of more serious health problems. We can see who is getting appropriate medical care, who is not getting it, and why not. In fact, once you start thinking about it, the basic information we need to plan effective interventions goes beyond simply documenting how many people are less healthy and at greater risk of dying. We need to determine whether these things are randomly distributed or if there is some kind of identifiable pattern. Does life expectancy vary by sex? Race? Then there are all those factors that matter but are not always easy to measure, such as stress, medical care, and genetic inheritance.

Just in case the thought has crossed your mind that all this could be interesting in the abstract, but it is pretty far off from anything that might be of primary interest to you and you are wondering why you should expend time and energy trying to understand any of it, you will surely be surprised at the answer. It will not take long for you to see that the questions we will be exploring regarding variations in death rates are related to a far greater range of issues than you might think at first glance. There is strong evidence to indicate that the rate of violent crime—but not theft—is directly correlated with mortality rates on a state-by-state basis. The distribution of income, voting behavior, and women's rights are associated with variations in mortality rates. Curiously, while the public may not be aware of the existence of such linkages on the domestic front, a growing number of entities that focus on international policy issues are quite concerned about the implications revealed by this kind of material for foreign policy. A particularly graphic example of this point comes from research carried out on behalf of the Central Intelligence Agency (CIA), which finds that political instability in developing countries is not a matter of chance—it is predictable. A country's infant mortality rate is the single best predictor. We will review the evidence on this topic in addition to many others. In short, expect to find the ramifications of what we discuss to go well beyond an exclusive focus on health.

So now you know where this discussion is going. Prepare yourself for our pursuit to identify the factors that enhance some people's chances of having a healthier, longer life and those that doom others to a greater chance of illness and early death. We will approach this quest using a systematic approach. We will address each of the topics that we have already touched on here in the following sequence: age, sex, race, poverty, lifestyle or health-related behaviors, medical care, genetics, and stress, and end with a topic that has been receiving a great deal of attention in recent years, namely, social inequality. As is clear from this list, there are a number of other topics we might have considered—environmental pollutants, for example, or mental illness. However, I had to draw the line somewhere and decided that there is more than enough material to digest if we limit ourselves to the topics I have identified so far.

We will start by assembling the information that is already available on health status and life expectancy. In an effort to interpret this information, we will consider as much of the relevant research and analysis by experts as we can accommodate in this relatively short book. Because the measures used by researchers are always being critiqued and debated, we will stop regularly to reflect on those measures and discuss the pros and cons of any alternative approaches we might think of. We will end with a summation of what we have learned—with the understanding that the search for conclusive and definitive answers to all the questions that researchers pose, plus those that you and I come up with, should provide work for scores of researchers for many years to come. The fact that the search for answers is ongoing indicates that it is incomplete. That means that the facts we will be reviewing probably do not constitute a definitive answer. This does not mean, however, that we cannot consider the policy implications of what is known now. We will do that because the policies being advanced currently by those in a position to promote and enact them may have profound effects, possibly positive and possibly negative, on the health and life expectancy of the entire population.

Analytical Framework

Now that the course of this venture has been laid out, we need to do one more thing in preparation. We need to develop a clearer, shared understanding of the kind of things we are searching for. Committing oneself to using a scientific approach means that one cannot settle for something like the definition of pornography employed by some members of Congress, namely, "I know it when I see it." Accordingly, chapter 2 is devoted to outlining the tools we will be using throughout the book, giving special emphasis to definitions. Chapter 3 focuses on the extent of the variation in health status that is revealed in data for the population as a whole. Each of the remaining chapters focuses on one or more factors or variables that we identified above and its role in determining health and life expectancy.

So far I have suggested that we will deal in facts, data, and research findings. As you know, saying that something is a fact will not necessarily convince all listeners of the truth of that assertion. We regularly see and hear experts in many fields arguing about interpretations of facts, even the validity of the facts. In some cases, experts come at the same issue from different perspectives, use complicated measures, and emphasize distinctive aspects of the issue. In many cases, it is not so much that they disagree, but that they are trying to answer somewhat different questions even as they address similar topics. This happens because the experts in one field do not read what the experts in other fields have to say about the topic. Experts in related fields end up creating separate bodies of knowledge which, under ideal circumstances, should come together to create a more fully developed set of answers. In many fields, this scenario persists without anyone becoming overly concerned.

What is happening in the area that we are about to launch into is special because experts from different fields of study are very much aware of one another's work. Anyone associated with this body of research will tell you that this is a very exciting time to be focusing on the questions we will be addressing. Researchers with very different kinds of expertise are not only aware of the findings on related topics produced by researchers in other fields, they are incorporating those findings into their own work. The knowledge base is becoming broader and complex explanations are becoming more widely accepted by researchers who come to this area of work bringing with them very different analytical perspectives.

My training is in sociology, and it is the perspective from which I see the world, so what I say will certainly proceed from this worldview. However, the material you will be encountering here will include research produced by epidemiologists, practicing physicians, basic science researchers, public health researchers, statisticians, political scientists, economists, and social-psychologists, to name a few of the disciplines that contribute to the body of knowledge that is becoming known as the study of *population health*. Others label it *social epidemiology*, which describes the primary focus of what we will be looking at very well. What you will not find in the body of the text is much effort to interpret findings from any particular theoretical perspective. This is especially true of later chapters, which is where the health status of large groups of people, rather than the health of individuals, becomes the central focus of discussion. At that point, we will be comparing the differences in the health status of large populations of people by neighborhood, city, state, and country.

The explanation for why researchers from so many different disciplines have been able to come together to address questions in this field unlike so many other fields is interesting. It seems that researchers from each of the disciplines I just mentioned kept coming up with partial answers to the questions they were asking. Reports kept ending with statements indicating that the researchers were frustrated by the lack of more complete and satisfying explanations. Their reports repeatedly concluded with statements advocating further research on questions that they readily admitted fell outside of their own areas of expertise.

The biggest hurdle that stood in the way was the contrast between the focus on the individual patient's problems that medicine has traditionally employed and the focus on patterns exhibited by entire groups of people employed by researchers in many of the other fields that are now involved. This is not to say that doctors did not understand that all those other aspects of a person's life were important. It is just that they were convinced that the physical indicators exhibited by individuals were the crucial determinants of a person's health status. Many doctors continue to think that even as the research published in medical journals indicates that an increasing number of medical scientists are now very interested in the range of factors other than physical indicators being addressed in the population health literature. Medical researchers who are considering a broader range of factors affecting patients' lives are finding that such an approach helps explain why the same disease proceeds faster and is more devastating in the case of some patients than others. Findings reported by researchers in other countries, who were concluding exactly the same thing, further advanced this research agenda.

It is not that researchers had been ignoring data coming from other countries in the past. It is just that a heightened interest in sharing knowledge began to evolve over the last few decades, possibly because of the increasing ease with which it can be accessed, thanks to the Internet. Growing international interest in achieving answers to similar questions accelerated the process of generating common indicators and scales to measure health. That has made cross-national research findings, which we will examine in the final chapters of the book, more comparable in recent years. The amount of data revealing comparable results that is accumulating makes the similarity in the conclusions being reported by researchers from different countries impossible to ignore.

Because this area of research is moving at a very fast pace, there are very few comprehensive texts. Accordingly, I will be referring to articles and reports presented in a wide range of publications. As you will see, the vast majority of articles were published over the past decade. This is not to suggest that earlier research is unimportant. It is just that most of it has been incorporated into more recent work. If you decide to search for additional information, be prepared to find a great deal more and to find it in scattered places.

As I have said, it is an exciting time to be considering the topics we will be discussing here. With that—let us begin this adventure.

CHAPTER TWO

~

The Tools: Definitions, Measures, and Data Sources

The primary objective of this chapter is to discuss the analytical tools we will be using throughout the book. The first item on this agenda is the matter of defining what we mean by such terms as health and illness. This is an important step because the verbal definition is meant to pinpoint exactly what is being measured and how it is measured. That turns out to be far more complicated than one might think. We will also discuss data sources. Only then will we actually examine some tables that report on such things as life expectancy and mortality. We see in this chapter a table that compares the health status of Americans to that of people in other countries, plus a couple of other tables that provide some comparative information on the health of people in this country.

Epidemiology

The tools we discuss in this chapter are basic to the work done by epidemiologists. As long as we are going to be defining concepts, we might as well begin by defining epidemiology. The root word, "epidemic," pretty much explains it all. It is the study of the spread of disease. It stems from the Greek for "about or upon" (epi), "people" (demos), and "study" (logos). Hippocrates, a physician-philosopher writing during the fifth century BC, is credited with the earliest exposition of the factors implicated in the distribution of illness. Modern epidemiology is generally traced back to John Snow. He identified the Broad Street water pump as the source of contaminated drinking water responsible for the spread of the outbreak of cholera in London during the middle of the nineteenth century. He did it by using a map to locate the addresses of the people who died. It became clear that the greatest concentration of deaths was in a community where people relied on the Broad Street pump to obtain their drinking water. Attributing cholera to contaminated water was a revolutionary idea. It was certainly not immediately accepted as the most likely explanation. Unfortunately, we cannot stop to explore the process of discovery or the nature of discussions that eventually convinced skeptics that it was an accurate assessment. Besides, there are a number of more recent, very well publicized cases to consider.

Jumping to the latter half of the twentieth century, let us consider an epidemiological episode that received a great deal of media attention in 1976. The Legionnaires' Disease story unfolds much like a gripping "whodunit" mystery. The site is Philadelphia, where a number of conventions were taking place. The biggest was the one organized by the American Legion. Toward the end of the convention period, an unusually large number of people began getting sick with what appeared to be the flu. But it was midsummer and it is unusual to see so many people getting the flu in the middle of summer. It was clearly some kind of epidemic. When people began dying from whatever this was, the Centers for Disease Control and Prevention (CDC) became involved and the investigation kicked into high gear.

Where would you start to investigate? The epidemic was obviously due to something that the people attending conventions in Philadelphia all had in common. Something they ate or drank? Extensive tests revealed that there was nothing in what they all consumed that could have produced the symptoms. By now the investigators knew that the epidemic was due to something that could be spread like a virus or bacterial infection, but it was not like anything they had seen before. How else could whatever this was be spread? Through the air? The investigators searched the air ducts and air-conditioning units, and looked for deposits of toxic materials that could be inhaled. Nothing! The fact that there was no clear answer began to inspire fear and paranoia. Maybe this was some secret material developed by a foreign power, by what was still the Soviet Union, for example, to poison Americans. We were in the Cold War period, but everyone knew that things could escalate very rapidly.

Eventually the contaminant was traced to standing water in the hotel water-delivery system and the conclusion was that the infectious agent was waterborne. The disease was named Legionnaires' Disease. Since then, it has been identified in the water sitting in shower heads that are not used very regularly in a variety of institutional settings. Shortly after the CDC announced that it had identified the infectious agent, Americans began to relax and tell each other that we were all becoming unnecessarily paranoid. It seems nostalgic to recall a time when the threat of a potential epidemic could be so effectively resolved and we could all go back to feeling safe.

There have also been cases where an epidemic was initially suspected but turned out to be a criminal case instead, with a human culprit playing the central role. The Tylenol case, which took place in Chicago in 1982, may be one of the most notable examples. Seven people died from ingesting Tylenol laced with cyanide, all purchased at the same drugstore. The perpetrator was never caught. One person tried to extort money from the company that makes Tylenol. He was caught and sentenced. He claimed that he did not do the poisoning and there was never enough evidence to prove otherwise. What followed in the wake of this case was passage of regulations governing the packaging of pills and other edibles. That is why bottles of pills and jars of foods now have seals on them that show if they have been tampered with.

Moving on to epidemiological developments taking place during the first decade of the twenty-first century brings us to the anthrax threat that followed in the wake of the September 11, 2001, terrorist attack. A number of letters that contained anthrax spores were sent to media figures and politicians. Everyone in the country was paying attention to who was getting those letters and how they fared after they opened them. By the time the scare ended, five people had died. Both the 9/11 attack and the anthrax scare contributed to the urgency with which city officials all over the country were working to protect people from terrorist attacks.

The newly established Homeland Security office raised the stakes by issuing alerts, including warning mayors and local health departments about the potential of poisonous substances being distributed through water systems and airways in public buildings of all sorts over the next five years or so following 9/11. Statements made by representatives of the CDC as well as local health departments on how we should all deal with a wide range of risks were suddenly getting a lot of attention. We learned that the heads of these agencies had been fighting with little success for more funding to improve their facilities and enhance their capabilities. Suddenly, Americans were all in favor of increasing their funding. Indeed, there is good reason to think that twenty-first-century epidemics will require even more money and attention than we have allocated thus far. Clearly, our collective level of anxiety regarding risk to our health and safety has changed a lot, undoubtedly because we now live in an era of heightened fear of attack by fanatics willing to die for their cause.

The CDC lists at least fifteen devastating syndromes that most of us generally do not hear about. When whatever is causing the outbreak is identified somewhere else in the world and we think that there is a low chance of it affecting Americans, we go on with our lives and do not spend time thinking about it.

You may remember a high degree of concern being registered by the media in 2003 telling us about the speed with which the severe acute respiratory syndrome (SARS) virus was spreading. According to the World Health Organization (WHO), SARS first appeared in Asia but went on to infect 8,098 people worldwide; 774 of them died. Shortly after SARS dropped out of the headlines, we began to hear about bird flu or avian influenza, which was causing people handling diseased poultry to become ill. Domestic birds had been infected through contact with migrating birds. Between 2003 and 2004, about one hundred million domestic birds in eight Asian countries either died from the disease or were killed. Epidemiologists began to think that such drastic measures had eradicated the problem. However, new outbreaks occurred toward the end of 2004. The fear that bird flu might evolve into a form that could be spread from person to person, which had been very rare thus far, meant that epidemiologists had good reason to keep very close watch on who was becoming infected.

In the spring of 2009, the CDC issued warnings about the risk of contracting swine flu. The number of cases increased so fast at first that both the CDC and WHO began warning of the potential of a "pandemic." The media focused a great deal of attention on the topic, which led to pig farmers complaining that the label was causing people to avoid pork products. They wanted it referred to by its scientific identifier—H1N1 flu strain. Over the span of a few weeks, the CDC and WHO determined that H1N1 flu was in fact acting in a way that put it much closer to a mild version of ordinary flu, which was nevertheless reaching pandemic proportions. It is curious that there was relatively little interest in comparing the course of this outbreak to the one that occurred in 1976 during the Gerald Ford administration, when there was an all-out effort to obtain enough vaccine to vaccinate everyone (Markel and Potts 2009). In the end, the 1976 H1N1 outbreak was determined to be far less significant than initial talk of an epidemic had suggested. There were fewer than two hundred cases and one confirmed death. In that case, the head of the CDC ended up losing his job because he and other experts who were expressing concern were charged with fearmongering for political purposes.

Then there are the bacteria, as opposed to viruses, that have been evolving into strains that are far more difficult to control. The medical community has been aware of the risk of the spread of MRSA (methicillin-resistant Staphylococcus aureus) among hospitalized patients for some years. The fact that the number of such cases has been rising is worrisome—the number of people dying from the infection has tripled over four years from 2001 to 2005. According to the CDC, there were 94,360 cases of infection and 18,650 deaths in 2005. Infectious disease specialists say that there is no excuse for the increase because prevention is so simple—greater attention to hygiene, especially hand washing. What is becoming even more troubling is that people with no connection to health-care settings are becoming infected. In fact, according to the CDC, about 14 percent of infections reported in 2006 were community based rather than hospital based. The spread of community-based MRSA is not well understood, so the spread of the infection is proving more difficult to control.

Two other drug-resistant bacteria are being closely watched: C. diff (Clostridium difficile) and XDR TB (extensive resistant tuberculosis). Both occur in response to overuse of antibiotics. C. diff occurs when previous use of antibiotics suppresses normal bacteria in the colon. The Agency for Health-care Research and Quality found that there were over two million cases of C. diff in U.S. hospitals between 1993 and 2005. According to the WHO, there were about 9.2 million new cases of TB in 2006 throughout the world, about 5 percent of which were multidrug-resistant (WHO Report 2008). Americans heard a great deal about drug-resistant TB in 2007, when a passenger who knew he was infected flew halfway across the world. Everyone he had come into contact with during the trip was identified, contacted, and tested. You can imagine how broadly the infection could spread as a result of an international trip. He was quarantined as soon as he arrived in the United States, and to the best of the CDC's knowledge, no one became infected. The fact that no one was infected came as somewhat of a surprise, certainly a welcome surprise.

While the number of people currently affected by these bacteria is still relatively small, the fact that the bacteria do not respond to antibiotics is obviously alarming. Pharmaceutical companies have been working on new antibiotic formulations and have actually produced a small number of potentially effective new drugs. However, the drugs that have come into existence are not only extremely expensive, but they have not been used long enough to have an experience record. Nor has anyone been running studies to see if some combination of older, less expensive drugs would work. Scary? Yes, but not unforeseen. Physicians have known for some time that many people in this country were overusing antibiotics and that this was fostering the emergence of bigger and more resistant "superbugs." Others who track the shifts in causes of death have also been aware of this development. We will return to the issue of how the profile of what we die from has changed over time in the following chapter.

The most familiar application of epidemiological tracking occurs in cases of food poisoning. The most common agents include the E. coli and salmonella bacteria (*bacteria* is plural; *bacterium* is singular). Both are generally traced to food workers who have violated the most basic rules of cleanliness like washing their hands after using the bathroom. There have been several cases of contamination linked to peanut butter and to chicken over the last few years. There have also been instances in which people got sick from eating fruit contaminated with a strain of salmonella. Washing the fruit would prevent that.

Admittedly, these illustrations of epidemiological data collection activity are somewhat atypical in that they recount specific episodes. The focus of our attention in the discussion to follow will be on information that is collected on a regular basis. We will be looking at shifts in trends over time and at variations in those trends exhibited by different groups within the population. Our ultimate purpose is to try to identify what accounts for better health and longevity and what produces worse health and shortens people's lives.

Before we leave the topic of epidemiology, let us stop to define two relevant terms used in epidemiological research that will come up later in our discussion—*prevalence* and *incidence*. *Prevalence* refers to the number of cases that exist in the population. *Incidence* is the number of new cases. Bubonic plague provides a good illustration. Because the prevalence of bubonic plague in this country is typically zero, when a case of bubonic plague is reported from time to time, it stands as a prevalence of one. When the second case appears, there is prevalence of one and an incidence of one. The addition of one new case means that there has been a 100 percent increase in the number of cases. The appearance of the third new case comes on top of a prevailing rate of two; so the increase by one more case constitutes a 50 percent increase in the incidence rate. By the way, we do see reports of cases of bubonic plague in the Southwest. That happens when children go into weeds surrounding golf courses to search for golf balls and get bitten by rats that are infected by fleas that carry the plague. The bites can be treated and the children do get well.

What Is Health?

So now that we have begun to consider some terms used in counting the persons who have a disease, we must confront the central problem, namely—

how will we distinguish the people who are healthy from those who are sick? You can see why a clearly stated definition is important. "Knowing" who is healthy and who is not is not good enough. We must agree on what we have in mind when we make that determination. Here are some of the attempts to come up with a definition that I have heard, plus the criticisms that followed:

- Someone who exercises and eats right. Actually that says something about a person's behavior and nothing about his or her health status. After all, a person who has a terminal disease can look fine, eat right, and exercise during the initial stages of the disease. Would you say that person is healthy? As a matter of fact, some people say yes and others say no. The point is we need to agree.
- Someone whom a doctor examines and finds healthy. That, too, is not enough. Doctors don't make such assessments just by looking at someone. They use various kinds of tests but there is no single test designed for this purpose. What kinds of tests/measures do you want doctors to base their judgments on? Even if you don't feel qualified to comment, don't you want to be sure they are using exactly the same tests to make this determination? There is also no battery of tests that fulfills the definition of a "complete physical." As a matter of fact, a full range of tests would be very expensive and still might not be able to predict a sudden death from a heart attack. Got any ideas on how you might want to resolve that?
- Someone who is well enough to go to work or school. Yes, but that focuses on behavior again. What about people who have a chronic illness, asthma or diabetes, for example, but work steadily? Or how about people who have physical disabilities and cannot get around without braces, crutches, or wheelchairs but do go to work or school?

Not easy, right? The more you think about it, the more complicated it seems to get. Keep these three possible sets of answers in mind. This initial attempt to define health turns out to be relevant to the measures of health that statisticians responsible for coming up with this information actually use.

Many interested parties have considered the question of what it means to be healthy and they did come up with clear verbal definitions. We could simply adopt the most popular one. The definition that is most widely quoted comes from the WHO. Unfortunately, the fact that it is widely quoted does not mean that all those who cite it do so because they think it is ideal. Indeed, in the view of many, the WHO terminology exacerbates the problem of finding a definition we can all agree on. According to the WHO, health is: "the state of complete physical, mental, and social well-being and not merely the absence of disease and illness." What's the problem with this definition? My answer is: how many mornings over the last year have you gotten up and been able to assert that you were in the state of complete physical, mental, and social well-being? You have to admit, attaining that level of health on a regular basis is a lot to expect. It might be too idealistic a standard to aim for.

Maybe we can't come up with a single definition. Maybe we should try to separate the components of the definition that the WHO uses. Since physical health, mental health, and social health are very different dimensions of health, maybe we should try to define and measure each separately first.

Looking at the meaning of health from a theoretical perspective, we can identify the assumptions from which each of the three dimensions of health identified by the WHO proceeds. The most well-developed approach to health is generally referred to as the "medical model," so we will treat the other two perspectives as models as well, namely, the sociocultural model and the stress model (Wolinsky 1980).

I. The Medical Model focuses on the absence of disease. It assumes that:

- There must be observable, objective signs of disease
- Only physicians can diagnose disease
- It is solely a physiological phenomenon
- It is appropriate to focus on nonhealth as opposed to health

As you might expect, the medical model has been criticized from both a theoretical and practical, or patient, perspective. The model says that objective, physical indicators of disease must exist for a person to be diagnosed as ill. Critics say that the medical model is mechanistic. It encourages doctors to treat the body like a machine composed of parts that can be examined, treated, repaired, and even replaced. The whole person is ignored in this perspective.

The model asserts that there can be no medical diagnosis of disease if doctors cannot find an objective indicator or if the symptoms patients present do not fit a recognizable syndrome. Whether or not the doctor thinks that any particular patient is a hypochondriac and whining unnecessarily or whether the doctor believes the symptoms are real but still cannot do anything about it may influence how sympathetic the doctor is. That does not alter the fact that the patient will leave the doctor's office without a diagnosis of disease. From the medical perspective, doctors cannot and should not try to treat something they cannot identify. From the patient's point of view, the fact that doctors cannot identify it does not mean that it does not exist or that it is not a legitimate complaint requiring some kind of treatment. The second approach provided by the sociocultural model corrects for this by putting the patient's perspective at the center.

Critics go on to say that this model shows how much power doctors have over us as individuals and in the broader society. They are in a position to legitimate one set of problems by calling it a disease but not another set. The problem is that if they do not legitimate a particular set of problems, then the people experiencing those symptoms are not considered to be really sick and that has all kinds of social consequences. In fact, those who claim to be sick but are not diagnosed with an identifiable illness are likely to meet with social disapproval and social sanctioning. That brings us to the question of social functioning; that is, carrying on with one's work.

II. The Sociocultural Model focuses on the capacity to function socially. It assumes that:

- Social performance and functioning are of primary importance
- Health is relative depending on one's role and its requirements
- Nonperformance of one's role is deviant; therefore, being unhealthy is deviant (and socially sanctionable or punishable)

In this model, persons who are chronically ill, disabled, or diagnosed with a fatal illness but go to work, school, and fulfill their responsibilities on a regular basis are considered healthy. It is also true that since the kinds of efforts and abilities required by people's jobs vary so much, whether one can be considered healthy depends on one's role, job, or position in life. That is, people who load trucks with heavy boxes need a great deal of physical strength and cannot risk back strain, which would prevent them from lifting those boxes. By contrast, accountants need good eyesight and cannot risk headaches that would interfere with their ability to concentrate on a long list of figures. Then there are persons who seem to be perfectly healthy, but do not fulfill their responsibilities and claim to have an illness. From the perspective of this model, the latter are persons are taking unfair advantage, which must be discouraged.

So far, one model emphasizes physical health to the exclusion of the way a patient feels and the other emphasizes how a person acts regardless of the presence of disease, disagreeable symptoms, or the patient's feelings about any of that. Obviously neither of these models captures the complete picture of what health is. Let us move on to the third model.

III. The Stress Model focuses on a general feeling of well-being. It assumes that:

- Well-being depends on the situational context, which can only be determined by an individual's own view of the situation; that is what ultimately establishes whether the person experiences stress and whether that experience will have detrimental health effects.

Finally, in this model we have an approach that acknowledges the importance of feelings, specifically the feeling of well-being, as indicated by how much stress a person experiences quite apart from any physical symptoms or readiness to fulfill responsibilities. The problem with the model is that efforts to measure stress levels are not well enough developed to produce an objective measure of stress that would permit comparison of one person's stress level to another person's. Yes, there are various "instruments" that measure stress levels by asking people about their stress. However, there is no single instrument that everyone who studies stress has agreed is the best one to use. There is nothing like a blood test for which there are norms or standards indicating what is normal and what is not normal plus a reasonable level of consensus regarding the levels that predict certain health outcomes.

While this model does focus on the whole person, which society generally regards as a good thing, the model does not pinpoint who is sick and what kind of treatment will take care of the problem.

So there you have it. The three prevailing perspectives focus on very different approaches to health. I have outlined them to show how they differ. While some people continue to critique one or more of these perspectives, we will not be doing that. We will continue to concentrate on the facts without attempting to interpret them from any theoretical perspective. My objective in reviewing the three models we have just considered is to make the point that they are so different that it is difficult to see how they could be combined to create a single measure. That brings us back to the central question. If we can't agree on a model or perspective leading to a verbal definition, how can we differentiate those who are healthy from those who are not? If we were to assess the health of a single individual, even a group of people, we might be able to agree on a number of tests and measures, combine them, and come up with a score. However, if we want to say something about the health of large numbers of people, those in one city versus another or in one country versus another, then we really do have to find a single indicator, something that can be represented in numerical terms.

To illustrate, education and income come with their own numerical values or quantifiable indicators, as in number of years of education and annual earnings, respectively. This is in contrast to religion, which has a *nominal* value with no numerical dimension or *operational measure* attached. This becomes a problem if your objective is to determine if being more or less religious makes a difference to whatever you are studying. As a matter of fact, there is a small body of research that tells us that people who are more religious are healthier. (We will review the literature on this topic in chapter 6.) How do you establish who is more religious? It is certainly not as easy as saying who is more educated. Nevertheless, researchers who wish to determine whether people who are more religious are indeed healthier must come up with a way to measure "religiosity." Furthermore, they must tell the rest of us what that measure is so that we can decide whether we think that it really measures what the researchers say it measures. Interesting intellectual puzzler, isn't it? However, this is just one of many hurdles that we will encounter.

The basic problem we are addressing here is the challenge of developing an operational measure for health. Perhaps we will have to settle for measuring what we can actually measure with a greater degree of confidence, which is not exactly the same thing as a measure of health. Like it or not—it is easier to measure nonhealth than health. As a result, from this point on we will focus on nonhealth even though our ultimate objective is to come up with something that will ultimately advance health.

Morbidity and Mortality

That brings us to such portentous topics as *mortality* and *morbidity*, which we must first define and operationalize (move from a nominal value to a quantifiable indicator). Coming up with verbal definitions of the two terms is the easy part—mortality is death and morbidity is illness and disease.

Mortality is pretty straightforward—one is either alive or dead. This is not to deny the fact that it would be easy to get distracted by getting into a discussion on exactly when death occurs. Historically, a person was considered dead when he or she stopped breathing and/or the heart stopped beating. However, now that a respirator can keep a person's heart beating and lungs functioning artificially, we no longer use the presence of a heartbeat as evidence of viability. The measure is now brainwave function. As you know, that is not without its own set of controversies. Does a flat brainwave mean the person has no chance of recovery? The answer is—that depends on whether the brain stem is fatally damaged. To determine that, a clinical neurological examination must be carried out. This involves a series of neurological tests, confirmatory laboratory tests, and determination of the cause of coma (Wijdicks 2001). For purposes of this discussion, the existence of a death certificate will serve as the indicator of death.

Morbidity is not nearly so easy to define or measure. It is basically the nonhealth side of the coin that raises all the same issues that we encountered in trying to define health. Persons who have been diagnosed with particular diseases can, of course, be counted. However, what do you do about those who don't know they have a disease or who have a disease that they have reason to deny? The former is illustrated by hypertension or high blood pressure, which is implicated in death from heart disease, yet even people who are at high risk are asymptomatic. The latter is illustrated by HIV infection (human immunodeficiency virus) which leads to death from AIDS (acquired immunodeficiency virus infection). The measure that an increasing number of researchers are using as the best measure of health is *self-assessed health*. We will get back to weighing the pros and cons of this measure of morbidity later in this chapter.

Life Expectancy

Life expectancy is the measure that is most often used to describe the health of large groups of people; for example, in comparing the health status of the people from one country to another. Life expectancy figures are generally reported separately for males and females. Let's consider how life expectancy is calculated. Since there is no way of knowing what will happen in the future to increase or decrease our life expectancy, we must rely on the facts that are available to us right now. Life expectancy figures represent how long people are living currently. We say that an infant born this year will live to the age that adults in the society are living right now. This is the way life expectancy is calculated by actuaries, who set life-insurance tables, as well as by epidemiologists.

A related measure, Years of Potential Life Lost (YPLL), has been appearing with greater frequency in recent years. It is calculated as the sum of the number of years "lost" between age of death and age sixty-five (or some other specific age; eighty-five, for example). The number of years lost by whole categories of people is summed to capture the impact of premature death on specific populations. The result is generally referred to as "excess" death.

Data Sources and Health Statistics

The federal government collects and reports mortality and morbidity statistics for the entire U.S. population. It also calculates life expectancy tables. The National Center for Health Statistics (NCHS) has primary responsibility for compiling this information. It operates under the auspices of the CDC, which is, in turn, a branch of the U.S. Department of Health and Human Services. In other words, this branch of the federal government assembles "health" information on all Americans. We will be relying on these statistics throughout the book.

We will examine the latest tables available at the time this manuscript is being written. In fact, I will be treating the NCHS publication as a supplementary text. I will summarize some of the tables, but I encourage you to update this information by looking up the numbers released for the current year, after this book is in print. Access to the information is free and downloadable from the Internet site operated by the NCHS. The address of this site is www.cdc.gov/hchs/hus.htm. It is easiest to go to *Health, United States 2008* (or whatever the latest year listed is). Next, go to the heading Trend Tables. Before considering the information presented in these tables, we need to consider the measures the NCHS employs and discuss the process through which it obtains that information.

The National Vital Statistics System is charged with the responsibility for compiling the vital statistics collected by the states. Vital statistics refers to births, deaths, marriages, and divorces. The information is reported on a monthly basis plus additional supplements and special reports in a publication entitled *National Vital Statistics Reports*. The NCHS compiles the vital statistics information collected by each state to produce a comprehensive profile of the vital statistics of the whole country.

Mortality data (*data* is plural; *datum* is singular) are based on death certificates. State laws require that a death certificate be completed for every death and be signed by a doctor, medical examiner, or coroner indicating cause of death. The death certificate asks for a fair amount of information. In addition to the cause of death and any underlying causes, it asks for the time, date, and place of death (e.g., home, hospital, or nursing home) plus sociodemographic information including age, marital status, occupation, and education. Obviously, the accuracy of this information depends on how well the person signing the certificate knows the deceased, whether the patient's health record is readily available, or if a family member is present and can answer the questions.

The government collects morbidity data using three different approaches. This is where our earlier discussion on what we mean by "health" becomes relevant. First, the most straightforward data collection method is the one used in the Health Records Survey. Initially, only records of hospital visits were gathered. Doctors' records were included a little later. Hospitals report treatments or procedures and how long the patient stayed. Doctors report the number of patient visits and reasons for the visits. Both sets of reports indicate charges and information on patient demographics; for instance, age and sex of patients. The Health Records Survey was initiated in 1962.

For obvious reasons the data reported in the Health Records Survey cannot be treated as though this provides an accurate picture of the health of Americans. For one, some people do not seek treatment because they cannot afford to do so. Two, others don't seek treatment for other reasons, such as fear, denial, or because they are not experiencing any symptoms. Three, there are always some people who seek treatment even when they don't really need to do so. What would give us a more complete picture? Records based on a standardized physical examination?

As a matter of fact, the government does exactly that through the second measurement approach—the Health Examination Survey, which was established in 1961. It operated on a periodic rather than an annual basis until recently. This is a very expensive proposition even if only a small number of people, a sample of the population, undergo a comprehensive physical exam. The objective, however, is an important one, namely, to obtain information about the level of undetected disease. The survey, renamed the National Health and Nutrition Examination Survey (NHANES), produced a series of three reports, NHANES I, II, and III, covering the following periods: 1971–1974, 1976–1980, and 1988–1994. As of 1999, the government began using a semi-trailer completely outfitted to perform thorough physical examinations. It is now a continuous survey with no breaks. The semi-trailer travels across the country to obtain a cross-national population sample of people who are selected to participate on a voluntary basis. This method of collecting data was instituted to reduce costs and produce more regular reports.

That still leaves the matter of how people feel about their health out of the picture. The third measurement approach to collecting health information is designed to address that issue. The National Health Interview Survey (NHIS) came into existence in 1957.

The survey was redesigned in 1997. It collects information on all household members in the population for the Family Core portion. In another section, the Child Core portion, an adult reports information on a randomly selected child under age eighteen; and a randomly selected adult answers question about him/herself in the Adult Core section. The NHIS gathers data on health conditions, health-related behaviors, and health-seeking experiences. Additionally, it asks about the family's health-care coverage, for instance, insurance, and whether respondents have had difficulty getting care. These two questions address the family's level of *access* to care. Respondents are asked where they usually go for their health care, and about *utilization* of health-care services; for instance, how much care they sought over the last year. The survey asks about health conditions and injuries, and more specific questions about AIDS, from attitudes and knowledge about it to getting tested for it. Questions about behaviors related to health include the following topics: use of tobacco, alcohol, and other substances; level of physical activity and exercise; and receiving immunizations.

There is one question on the general health status, for which interviewees are given four options: excellent, very good, fair, or poor. This is where the survey addresses the question of how a person feels. The answers to this question have been attracting increased attention over the years. Some researchers have concluded that self-assessed health is a highly sensitive indicator of morbidity, which turns out to be predictive of health-seeking behavior, disability, even death (Ferraro and Su 2000; Bierman, et al. 1999; Kawachi, Kennedy, and Glass 1999; Ware and Sherbourne 1992). It is also true that some researchers have been finding that blacks who rate their health as poor have a much lower chance of dying than whites who rate their health as poor (Lee et al. 2007). The explanation offered by the researchers is that blacks may value aspects of health that are less closely associated with mortality, which, in turn, may be related to educational level and interpretation of assessments presented by health providers. Nevertheless, self-assessed health continues to be the most commonly used indicator of health status, as will become obvious in other chapters of the book.

Calculations

Mortality and morbidity data can be expressed using different kinds of calculations. Actual or whole numbers are of course reported. But whole numbers are not good when you want to compare one group of people to another. It is better to use *rates* of death or disease. This measure is superior to using either whole numbers or percentages because it allows for comparisons of populations of different sizes. In calculating a rate, the base number is the same for all the populations being compared, for example, the number of deaths for every one thousand or one hundred thousand persons of a specific age group, sex, or race. Rates also allow for comparisons across time and place. The calculation overcomes the fact that the total number of people in the population has changed over time and that the speed at which different sectors of the population are increasing varies.

Death rate is calculated as the number of deaths, divided by the population at midyear, multiplied by one thousand.

$$\frac{\text{\# deaths}}{\text{\# persons in the population at midyear}} \times 1{,}000 = \text{death rate}$$

This is the calculation for the *crude death rate*. A more accurate version of this measure is the *age-adjusted death rate*. It is calculated the same way for each age category that is reported. The rates for each age category are then summed up to arrive at the more accurate number. The age-adjusted death rate is considered more accurate than the crude death rate because the risk of death is higher at some ages than at others. If the population has a particularly high number of young people, for example, who are at low risk of dying, the total death rate will be lower than it is in a population that is older and includes more people at greater risk of dying. The age-adjusted rate overcomes that variation.

To illustrate—infants can be treated as a separate, clearly identifiable population. The infant mortality rate is calculated as deaths of persons under one year of age per every one thousand births. You should know that infant mortality is a very commonly used measure because it is considered to be an even more sensitive indicator of the health of an entire society than the mortality rate or life expectancy. Why is it considered to be a more sensitive measure? Because human beings are particularly vulnerable during infancy. They are totally dependent on adults. How well a society cares for its most vulnerable members is generally regarded as the best indicator of a society's ability to care for all of its members.

Life Expectancy Tables

A good place to begin looking at the wealth of information that is available to us is the life expectancy data—ours compared to that of people in other countries. The table reports figures for 2004, the latest year for which these data are available.

Interpretation

What do you consider to be the most significant facts found in this table? Does the rank in which you find the United States surprise you? Consider-

Table 2.1. Life Expectancy at Birth by Sex for Selected Countries in 2004

Males			Females		
Country	1980	2004	Country	1980	2004
Hong Kong	71.6	79.0	Japan	78.8	85.6
Japan	73.4	78.6	Hong Kong	77.9	84.7
Switzerland	72.8	78.6	France	78.4	83.8
Sweden	72.8	78.4	Spain	78.6	83.7
Australia	71.0	78.1	Switzerland	79.6	83.7
Israel	72.2	77.9	Australia	78.1	83.0
Canada	71.7	77.8	Sweden	78.8	82.7
New Zealand	70.0	77.5	Canada	78.9	82.6
Norway	72.3	77.5	Finland	77.6	82.3
Spain	72.5	77.2	Norway	79.2	82.3
Singapore	72.6	77.1	Puerto Rico	76.9	82.3
Netherlands	72.5	76.9	Israel	75.8	82.2
England and Wales	70.8	76.8	Austria	76.1	81.5
France	70.2	76.7	Singapore	74.7	82.0
Greece	72.2	76.6	New Zealand	76.3	81.7
Austria	69.0	76.4	Belgium	76.8	81.5
Costa Rica	71.9	76.4	Germany	76.8	81.5
Northern Ireland	68.3	76.0	France	76.1	81.4
Germany	69.6	75.7	Netherlands	79.2	81.4
Belgium	70.0	75.6	England and Wales	76.8	81.1
Cuba	72.2	75.4	Portugal	75.2	81.0
Finland	69.2	75.4	Northern Ireland	75.0	80.8
Denmark	71.2	75.2	Costa Rica	77.0	80.7
United States	70.0	75.2	Chile**	76.9	80.6
Portugal	67.7	74.5	United States	77.4	80.4
Scotland	69.0	74.2	Denmark	77.3	79.9
Puerto Rico	70.8	74.1	Cuba**	76.9	79.8
Chile**	71.1	74.0	Scotland	75.2	79.3
Czech Republic	66.8	72.6	Poland	74.4	79.2
Poland	66.0	70.7	Czech Republic	73.9	79.0
Slovakia	66.8	70.3	Slovakia	74.3	77.8
Bulgaria	68.5	69.1	Hungary	72.7	76.9
Hungary	65.5	68.6	Bulgaria	73.9	76.3
Romania	66.6	68.3	Romania	71.9	75.6
Russian Federation*	61.4	59.1	Russian Federation*	73.0	72.4
Italy***	70.6	76.8	Italy***	77.4	82.9
Ireland***	70.1	75.2	Ireland***	75.6	80.3

Source: Health, United States, 2008, Table 25: Life Expectancy at Birth and at 65 Years of Age, by Sex: Selected Countries and Territories, Selected Years 1980–2004.
*The Russian Federation is the only country in which life expectancy is lower in 2004 than it was in 1980.
** Life expectancy data are available for 1990 but not 1980.
***Life expectancy data are available for 2002 but not 2004.

ing that we are the richest and most technologically advanced nation in the world, shouldn't we expect to have the longest life expectancy of anyone in the world? What accounts for the fact that people in so many other countries live longer than we do? If life expectancy is in fact an important indicator of health, what does this say about the health of Americans? These are precisely the kinds of questions we will be addressing in the chapters that follow.

Another observation that is hard to miss in this table is that females live longer than males in all the countries on the list. No, the explanation is not perfectly obvious. No, it is not because men have more stress. This is one of those cases where what "everybody knows" to be true turns out to be a lot more complicated. The conventional wisdom explanation, which we will be considering shortly, has oversimplified the issue. Because the topic of sex differences inspires a good deal of controversy, you might be surprised to hear what some of the alternative explanations are. We will explore that topic in chapter 4, where we focus directly on age and sex.

Finally, there is the fact that life expectancy decreased in one country. The fact that the long-standing trend toward increasing life expectancy reversed in Russia has inspired a great deal of scholarly attention. In actuality the same thing happened in the other countries formerly associated with the Soviet Union, including Romania and Bulgaria during the late 1980s and early 1990s; however, the downward trend had already shifted toward longer life expectancy by the end of the 1990s. We will return to this issue in chapter 11, when we focus on international trends more directly.

Earlier I said that the infant mortality rate is considered to be the most sensitive measure of health used in making international comparisons. It turns out that those rates are even more troubling than the adult mortality rates. We will discuss infant mortality rates in greater detail in chapter 4, when we focus on age as a *variable*.

Although the definition of *variable* is self-evident, it might still be useful to state what we mean by it so that we are all operating on the basis of shared understandings. Clearly, a variable is something that varies. That is, of course, tautological, meaning that it is redundant and uses the word we wish to define in the definition. Nevertheless, that definition captures the essence of what we are interested in. We will be exploring what explains variation in mortality, morbidity, and life expectancy by identifying the factors or variables that could help explain it. If we find some clear differences, then we can go on to investigate what it is about those variables that is responsible for differences in the health of the population we are looking at or as we agreed, differences in nonhealth; that is, mortality and morbidity. We will discuss one or more of the variables we identify as possible explanations for health variations starting with chapter 4.

At this point we are ready to examine a table that provides us with information on life expectancy among Americans. Let's begin with data on how long we are living these days and how much that has changed over time. Clearly, we have achieved an impressive increase in life expectancy over the twentieth century. However, further examination reveals that there is considerable variation in life expectancy when we start separating the population into differentiated categories. You already know that life expectancy differs for men and women. Let's add another variable—race.

What observations can we make about the data we see in this table? The first thing that you might point to is that this is a very limited picture of the racial composition of the U.S. population represented in this table. That is certainly true. However, that is the record that is available to us if we want to go that far back in time. There is a lot more to say about using race as a variable and/or about the need to report figures for other racial/ethnic groups. We will get to that in chapter 5, where we focus on race and ethnicity. For now, let's limit our observations to what we see here. The fact is—all four categories of people made significant gains in life expectancy. Females of both races have had, and continue to have, an advantage over males. Whites had an enormous advantage over blacks to begin with. Blacks made bigger gains, but the differential remains large. It is the differential that we will be paying attention to as we proceed with this discussion. (I am using and will

Table 2.2. Life Expectancy in the United States from 1900 to 2005 According to Sex and Race

Year	All	White Male	White Female	Black Male	Black Female
1900	47.3	46.6	48.7	32.5	33.5
1950	68.2	66.5	72.2	59.1	62.9
1960	69.7	67.4	74.1	61.1	66.3
1970	70.8	68.0	75.6	60.0	68.3
1980	73.7	70.7	78.1	63.8	72.5
1990	75.4	72.7	79.4	64.5	73.6
2000	77.0	74.9	80.1	68.3	75.2
2005	77.8	75.7	80.8	69.5	76.5

Source: Health, United States, 2008, Table 26: Life Expectancy at Birth, at 65 Years of Age, and at 75 Years of Age, by Race and Sex: United States, Selected Years 1900–2005.

continue to use the labels used by the government to designate race/ethnicity. Black and white were the primary designations used until quite recently; African American is used in some but not all tables.)

That brings us to the next table, which provides us with considerably more information on variation in mortality rates because it employs a larger number of racial/ethnic categories. New ethnic/racial categories were introduced during the 1980s. However, that means that the information does not go back far enough to allow us to reach any conclusions about trends over time. In fact, the rates that are reported are sometimes summed over three-year periods to even out random "blips" (i.e., erratic increases or drops in rates) that occur from year to year but are inconsequential over the long term. In other words, you can't conclude that something is a trend if you only have information for a few consecutive years. Tables that provide information over five decades serve as far more reliable sources of information for interpreting trends, but that kind of data was not being collected on the basis of ethnicity. With that let us consider the latest mortality statistics which are reported by sex and race or ethnicity.

This table makes clear how much differentiation in death rates you are likely to find as you proceed to subdivide the population. It becomes clear that some categories of people are dying at significantly higher rates than others. This raises the same basic question that keeps coming up in this chapter and the question that we will be dealing with throughout the book—what accounts for the variation? The way the statistics are presented cannot help but suggest that there is something inherent in people's genetic makeup that

Table 2.3. Death Rates by Sex and Race per 100,000 Persons for 2005

All Persons	798.8		
Males	951.1	Females	677.6
White	933.2	White	666.5
Black	1,252.9	Black	845.7
American Indian/Alaska Native	775.3	American Indian/Alaska Native	567.7
Asian/Pacific Islander	534.4	Asian/Pacific Islander	369.3
Hispanic	717.0	Hispanic	485.3
White, non-Hispanic*	945.4	White, non-Hispanic*	677.7

Source: Health, United States, 2008, Table 34: Death Rates for All Causes, by Sex, Race, Hispanic Origin, and Age: United States, Selected Years 1950–2005.

*White, non-Hispanic is self-explanatory. It includes whites of European descent. People identify themselves as belonging to particular categories. We will discuss why the data are reported using these categorizations in chapter 5.

explains the differential. However, that is misleading. While researchers are beginning to find that there is a greater degree of genetic difference by race and/or ethnicity than we were ready to acknowledge even a few years ago, no one is prepared to say that differences in genetic makeup can account for much of the differential in death rates. (We will return to genetics in chapter 8.)

Let's assume that you are willing to accept my statement that differences in genetic makeup are not primarily responsible for the high level of variation in death rates. Does that suggest to you that it must be something that people are doing that causes some to end up with either better or poorer health? Actually it is even more complicated than that. That brings us to three additional variables, namely, *health behavior*, *medical care*, and *stress* that need to be considered in explaining the variation in mortality rates we see in this table.

There is one more variable that we have not discussed so far but it is one that most people would agree is a significant factor in explaining variation in mortality rates, namely, *poverty*. That covers all the variables we will be addressing in the following chapters except one, i.e., *inequality*, but we have to explore each of the other factors first before we get to that one because it is the most controversial. That completes the list of all nine variables we will be discussing: *age*, *sex*, *race*, *poverty*, *health behavior*, *medical care*, *genetics*, *stress*, and *inequality*. Before we begin focusing on the impact of any one of these variables, we need to discuss what kinds of things people are dying from to see whether that helps explain the variation in mortality rates. We will do that in the following chapter.

Summary and Conclusions

The chapter started out by discussing health and illness. Having considered the matter of defining health and attempting to measure it, we discovered that the problems related to measuring health status were difficult to overcome. Accordingly, we found that we would be paying a lot more attention to death than health. To be precise, it became clear that we would be focusing on mortality rates throughout the rest of the book because they can be counted with a greater degree of confidence than other indicators of health and illness. To the extent that we do discuss health and illness, we will generally be relying on people's self-reported assessments of their own health status.

Our initial examination of death rates over time revealed a considerable amount of variation by sex and further variation by race and sex. The rate of death for different causes is the subject of the following chapter.

CHAPTER THREE

~

The Causes of Death

The tables we looked at in the last chapter made clear that there has been an impressive increase in life expectancy since 1900 in this country. In this chapter we will examine more closely what Americans were dying from then and what they are dying from now. As you will see, there is a direct link between the shift in what we are now dying from and the fact that we are living so much longer.

The Shift in Causes of Death over the Twentieth Century

Let's begin by looking at the change in causes of death from 1900 to 2005.

Even without knowing very much about disease, you can probably see a significant difference between the leading causes of death in 1900 and 2005. In 1900, five out of the top ten causes of death were due to infection. In 2005, only two of the top eleven causes we are infectious diseases; six were chronic illnesses. It is important to realize that doctors could not do much for people who contracted an infectious disease before antibiotics became available, which happened around the middle of the twentieth century. Before then, the basic treatment was bed rest and, in some cases like tuberculosis, quarantine to protect others from the infection. That is very different from what doctors are able to do now. They may not be able to "cure" heart disease, cancer, or stroke, but they certainly have many more tools at their disposal to diagnose these illnesses at earlier stages, stop the progress of the diseases, and prolong life.

Table 3.1. Top Ten Causes of Death in the United States per 100,000 Persons

1900		2005	
Cause	*Rate*	*Cause*	*Rate*
Heart disease*	345	Heart disease	211
Influenza/pneumonia	202	Cancer	184
Tuberculosis	194	Stroke	47
Gastritis	143	Lung disease	43
Accidents	72	Accidents	39
Cancer	64	Diabetes	25
Diphtheria	40	Pneumonia/influenza	20
Typhoid	31	Suicide	11
Measles	13	Liver disease/cirrhosis	9
Cirrhosis of liver	13	Assault	6
Whooping cough	12	HIV	4

*This category was originally labeled: Major cardiovascular renal diseases and stroke.
Source for 1900: Death Rate, for Selected Causes: 1900 to 1970. Series B 149-166. *Historical Statistics of the United States from Colonial Times to 1970,* vol. 1 (Washington, DC: U.S. Bureau of the Census, 1975).
Source for 2005: Health, United States, 2008, Table 28: Age-Adjusted Death Rates for Selected Causes of Death, by Sex, Race, and Hispanic Origin: United States, Selected Years 1950–2005.

Looking at the table one more time—would you say that there has been a dramatic decline in the rate of death from heart disease? It looks that way until you realize that the 1900 rate combines the heart disease and stroke rates. There is no question that the rate of death from heart disease has declined during the twentieth century. How much it declined is more controversial because that is difficult to establish with absolute certainty. Causes of death were not as reliably identified and recorded then as they are now, so we cannot always be absolutely sure whether the decline in a particular cause reflects more accurate diagnosis and recordkeeping or an actual change in the rate at which we are dying from any particular cause. It is worth keeping this observation in mind when we begin considering factors linked to current death rates.

The Transition from Infectious to Chronic Illness

The change in the list of leading causes of death over the twentieth century in the United States is pretty dramatic. Going back further in time and looking at causes of death throughout human history is even more revealing. An overview of the types of illnesses people have been dying of throughout the world can be organized into four epidemiological phases:

- Phase One: the pestilence and famine phase
- Phase Two: the receding pandemics phase
- Phase Three: the degenerative man-made diseases phase
- Phase Four: the delayed degenerative diseases and emerging infections phase

During Phase One, the pestilence and famine phase, people had virtually no control over their fate. If there was a famine, they had less to eat, became weak, succumbed to disease, and died. If the famine was prolonged, more people died. Phase Two marks both the declining threat of "pestilence," that is, decline in the spread of infection, and greater stability in the food supply, which helped more people to avoid illness. On the negative side, the resulting growth and concentration of population fostered a rising rate of infectious disease among larger numbers of people (McKeown 1976). Phase Three brings a shift away from infectious illness to chronic illness. Phase Four is marked by the increase in degenerative diseases, like lung or kidney disease, and all the newly emergent infectious diseases that we discussed in the last chapter, including C. diff., SARS, avian flu, MRSA, and AIDS.

These four phases map out the process of *epidemiological transition* (Omran 1971). Given that the same phases can be observed throughout the industrialized world, it is not surprising to find that countries at an earlier stage of development and industrialization are at an earlier stage of this process. How fast they go through the phases is not easy to predict. The fact that they must go through each of the phases is inevitable.

The epidemiological transition process has consequences for the *demographic transition* process. *Demography* is the study of population change. Later in the discussion we will be referring to *demographic* characteristics of the populations we focus on. That means we will be looking at factors that describe a population of people—their age, sex, and race. To produce an even more complete picture, we will be looking at *sociodemographic* characteristics, which brings in education, income, occupation, and any related factors on which we can find data. For now, let's get back to what we mean by demographic transition and how it is related to epidemiological transition.

The Relationship between Epidemiological and Demographic Transition

Demographic transition captures the rate at which the size of a country's population changes. There are only four ways that can happen: through birth, death, immigration, and emigration. The demographic transition process considers shifts in birth and death rates. The First Phase in the demographic transition process is the "pre-transition" stage, which roughly corresponds to Phase One of the epidemiological transition process—the pestilence and famine phase. At this stage, people are motivated to have many babies in an effort to guarantee that at least some children, primarily boys, will survive to support their parents when the parents become aged and can no longer provide for themselves. Infant mortality is high because infectious diseases are prevalent and infants are the most vulnerable and susceptible to infection. When there is plenty of food, people marry young and proceed to have as many children as nature will provide. There are now more people who need to be fed. If the crop fails, it does not take long before people experience famine. That makes them weaker and less able to fight off infection. Therefore, any infectious disease that comes on the scene is all the more devastating. Historically, there were continuing waves of plenty followed by waves of famine and pestilence before the onset of demographic transition.

In Europe, but not in other parts of the world, things began to stabilize during the second half of the eighteenth century. That is when the Second Phase, or "early phase," in the demographic transition process took hold. This parallels Phase Two of the epidemiological transition process when the food supply becomes more stable and the risk of death less threatening. What happens in terms of population growth during this phase is interesting. The death rate starts to decline, as fewer people are faced with either famine or pestilence. However, it takes awhile for people to be convinced that the drop in mortality will last. People continue to have many children, just in case. The drop in birth rates signals the beginning of the Third, or "late" Phase in the demographic transition sequence. This is when population growth stabilizes, because the population exhibits a drop in both the birth rate and the death rate. This also marks the epidemiological shift from infectious disease to chronic disease. That brings us to the Fourth, or "post-demographic" transition Phase, which is characterized by a stabilized, even declining, rate of population growth. During Phase Four people are living longer but experiencing a higher rate of both degenerative disease and the newly emergent and devastating infectious diseases, which we noted in discussing epidemiological transition.

In some of the most highly industrialized European countries, the current population growth rate is lower than the rate of replacement. In other words, people in those countries are having fewer than one baby per person in the population. The rate in the United States is slightly higher than the rate of replacement. There are also many countries that are just beginning to industrialize, meaning that the demographic transition process they are experiencing is producing extremely rapid population growth. In fact, a number of countries are *doubling* the size of their populations at what some observers think is an alarming rate, every twenty-five years in the most extreme cases. The problem is that they are not able to feed themselves during years when they are not able to produce enough food. When they succumb to famine, disease is quick to follow. When there is enough food, the population increases at an extremely rapid rate. This is exactly the same cycle that advanced, industrialized countries went through much earlier. The difference is that now rich countries can and do offer aid to poor countries to prevent famine and disease. That is not the same as help that would result in the stabilization of population growth.

The countries that have gone through the demographic transition process in the distant past are not only stable but also rich, which means that they must decide how much aid, in the form of food and medicine, they will provide to poor countries. The rich countries must choose between watching the developing countries' populations grow at a very high rate because death rates drop dramatically when there is plenty. This reduces adult mortality as well as infant mortality while birth rates continue to be high. The alternative is watching people suffer the ravages produced by pestilence and famine and die at exceptionally high rates until both birth and death rates stabilize. As we know, this takes more than one or even two generations (Farmer 2001). The pace at which the demographic transition process is proceeding in poor countries is not likely to move much faster because rich countries do send aid. Yet, the poor countries themselves are not yet at a stage of development that would permit them to institute policies that would reduce the reliance on the next generation of sons. Thus, their birth rates continue to be high even as their death rates decline, with all the social problems this produces.

Whatever your reaction to this wrenching dilemma, there is another even more pressing, related problem. Those involved in matters of world health say that there is an urgent need to intervene to prevent the spread of the newly emergent infectious diseases that could grow to epidemic proportions. The reason for this concern is that viruses change. There is no way to know whether the viruses will become more virulent or less virulent or how they might change. For example, a virus could suddenly transform itself so that it can be spread far more easily, through droplets that are airborne; that is, through sneezes. The risk is that this could pose a new threat to parts of the world where infectious diseases have been under control for more than two centuries. This is obviously an agonizing topic, which deserves serious attention. We cannot do justice to it here. We must return to the central topic that we said we would address in this chapter, namely what accounts for the variation in mortality rates in this country. Okay, we are now ready to begin looking at tables that make the degree of variation explicit.

How Much Do Death Rates Vary?

Let us begin by considering how much the death rate has fallen over time.

To discuss the information that this table offers, we should agree on some basic table reading principles and talk a little about the causes themselves. The numbers going across are *rows*; the numbers going down are *columns*.

The National Center for Health Statistics tracks the eleven leading causes of death. Let's consider what they are more closely. A few of the classifications may be somewhat unfamiliar. Cerebrovascular disease is death from a stroke. The difference between a stroke and diseases of the heart, and more specifically ischemic heart disease, is that a stroke occurs when a blood vessel breaks in the brain. Death from ischemic heart disease occurs when the blood vessels involved are in the heart. This is what is commonly known as a heart attack. Doctors call it a myocardial infarction (MI). As we noted earlier, stroke and heart attack were grouped together as death from diseases of the heart. This continued until well into the twentieth century. Neoplasm is the scientific word meaning cancer. In the case of chronic lower respiratory disease, which is lung disease, the dashes in table 3.2 mean that the death rates were not recorded until 1980. There are a number of diseases that fall under this label; emphysema may be the most familiar one. Statistics on HIV were also not available before 1980 because it was not identified until the middle of that decade. Most other categories are self-explanatory, except for the assault category. This category was labeled homicide and legal intervention until 1998, labeled assault for ten years, and then homicide as of 2008. The mention of legal intervention adds

Table 3.2. Leading Causes of Death for All Persons in the United States in 2005 and Selected Prior Years, Rates per 100,000 Persons

	1950	1970	1990	2000	2005
All causes	1,446	1,223	939	869	799
Heart	587	493	322	258	211
Cerebrovascular disease	181	148	66	61	47
Malignant neoplasms	194	199	216	200	184
Chronic lower respiratory disease	—	—	37	44	43
Influenza and pneumonia	48	54	37	24	20
Chronic liver disease and cirrhosis	11	18	11	10	9
Diabetes mellitus	23	24	21	25	25
HIV	—	—	10	5	4
Unintentional injuries	78	62	38	35	39
Suicide	13	13	13	10	11
Assault (homicide)	5	9	9	6	6

Source: Health, United States, 2008, Table 28: Age-adjusted Death Rates for Selected Causes of Death, by Sex, Race, and Hispanic Origin: United States, Selected Years 1950–2005.

a dimension that you might not automatically think of. It refers to death as a result of a confrontation with law-enforcement officers.

The information presented in table 3.2 should equip us to discuss the shift in causes from 1950 to 2005. The only other point to keep in mind concerns interpreting trend data. Be careful to distinguish between changes in rates from year to year and changes that show a pattern of change from decade to decade. The longer the time period involved, the more convincing the inter-pretation that there has been a more permanent, rather than a fleeting, shift in causes. Given that the first two intervals, 1950 to 1970 and 1970 to 1990, span twenty years and the last interval, 2000 to 2005, spans only five years, the three periods cannot be treated as comparable. We will simply have to watch trends evolve for a longer period of time before we can be sure that the changes in death rates that we see occurring now will continue.

The only other advice I have is to start reading the tables from the left-hand corner; begin by looking at the first row and after you see the main idea there, go on to look at the first column. Starting with the first row, table 3.2 tells us that most causes of death have declined significantly over the last half century. It is worth keeping in mind that reducing the rate of death is a highly laudable objective, but that we must all die of something. The problem is that people die at very different rates and from differing causes depending on sex and race or ethnicity.

If we rank the top eleven causes of death for all persons, then rank the causes separately by sex for the latest year that we have available, the list looks like this:

Table 3.3. Leading Causes of Death in Rank Order per 100,000 Persons for 2005

Cause	All Persons	Males	Females
Heart disease	211	261	172
Cancer	184	225	156
Stroke	47	47	46
Lung disease	43	51	38
Accidents	39	54	25
Diabetes	25	28	22
Influenza	20	24	18
Suicide	11	18	4
Liver disease	9	12	6
Assault	6	10	3
HIV	4	6	2

Note: I have substituted conventional labels for some causes of death.
Source: Health, United States, 2008, Table 28: Age-adjusted Death Rates for Selected Causes of Death, by Sex, Race, and Hispanic Origin: United States, Selected Years 1950–2005.

You already knew that women live longer than men. Now we see that men die from *all* the leading causes of death at a higher rate than women. That definitely requires an explanation. Wait until you see how large the differences in rates are when we break down the rates further by race/ethnicity as well as sex in the next table. I have created the following table by combining data reported in a series of tables. Because the NCHS reports this information for eight of the eleven leading causes of death, the following table is limited to those causes.

Table 3.4. Leading Causes of Death by Race/Ethnicity and Sex per 100,000 Persons* for 2005**

Males	White	Black	American Indian/ Alaska Native	Asian/ Pacific Islander	Hispanic	White, not Hispanic
Causes						
Heart disease	258	330	173	141	192	262
Cancer	222	294	148	133	153	227
Stroke	45	71	31	42	38	45
Lung disease	53	44	35	23	25	55
Accidents*	22	23	34	10	21	22
Suicide	20	9	19	7	9	21
Assault	5	37	11	4	12	4
HIV	4	28	4	1	8	3
All causes	933	1,253	775	534	717	945

Females	White	Black	American Indian/ Alaska Native	Asian/ Pacific Islander	Hispanic	White, not Hispanic
Causes						
Heart disease	168	228	116	92	129	170
Cancer	155	180	106	95	102	160
Stroke	44	61	37	36	34	44
Lung disease	41	23	26	10	15	42
Accidents*	9	8	15	6	8	9
Suicide	5	2	6	4	2	5
Assault	2	6	4	2	2	2
HIV	<1	12	2	**	2	<1
All causes	667	846	568	369	485	678

* The accident rate refers to deaths due to motor vehicle accidents only.
** Too few cases to obtain an accurate count.
*** The table applies to persons who live in the United States and identify themselves as belonging to these ethnic/racial categories.
Source: Health, United States, 2008, Tables 34, 35, 36, 37, 40, 41, 43, 44, and 45: Age-adjusted Death Rates for (Each of the Eight Causes of Death), According to Sex, Detailed Race, and Hispanic Origin: United States, Selected Years 1950–2005.

As you can see, the variation in rates is pretty amazing. The most startling difference is obviously the one between the total rate at which Asian/Pacific Islander females die (369) and black males die (1,253). We know that the difference between male and female rates means that we probably are better off avoiding making comparisons across sex lines. Restricting comparisons to racial/ethnic categories within the same sex still reveals enormous differences. There are a couple of ways to think about the differences. In looking at the male rate, for example, we can compare the death rate of the five racial/ethnic categories to one another or we can compare each to the *all person male* death rate. In either case, the concept that applies is *excess mortality*. To illustrate, if 261 (see table 3.2) is the all person rate for mortality from heart disease for males, then anything above that for a particular racial/ethnic group of males can be considered excess mortality because it exceeds the standard for all males. The reasoning behind the concept goes something like this: The difference between the exceptionally high rate for black males in comparison to the rate for all males is due to factors that it is reasonable to assume can be controlled. If some people within a certain population, men in this case, can achieve a lower rate, then other men within that population should be able to attain it as well. Human beings are not that different from one another. So it is humanly possible to attain death rates that are not so different. We will talk at length about a variety of factors that contribute to the differences in death rates across different racial/ethnic groups—genetic differences, lifestyle or behavior differences, as well as income differences that allow some people to buy more of the things that make for a better, possibly longer, life to see how much each contributes.

Returning to the issue of differences by sex, the fact that the rate of death from the leading cause of death for everyone, heart disease, is so much lower for women than it is for men is a topic that continues to interest researchers. The steady decline in the rate of death from heart disease and cerebrovascular disease for both sexes is intriguing. Why was there such a major drop in heart disease mortality? No one knows for sure. Some analysts argue that the high cardiovascular death that we experienced during the twentieth century was really an epidemic and it is now declining of its own accord (Nieto 1999). Others suggest that the drop is due to increased awareness of the factors that are responsible and a change in people's behavior.

According to Dr. Dan Jones, the president of the American Heart Association (AHA), the AHA is celebrating the fact that the goal it set in 1999 to reduce the death rate from heart disease from heart disease and stroke by 25 percent by 2010 was achieved five years ahead of time (American Heart Association 2008). The reduction equates to approximately 160,000 lives saved in 2005, the latest year for which data were available when the state-ment was released. According to Jones, multiple factors led to the reduction in deaths. He pointed to the following: improved emergency treatment for heart attacks, stroke, and blocked arteries; widespread use of cholesterol-lowering statin drugs; aggressive management of high blood pressure; tobacco excise taxes; and antismoking and clear-air legislation. He also identified factors that have prevented the rates from falling further, including the fact that "39 percent of Americans are physically inactive couch potatoes," that rates of obesity and type 2 diabetes are going up, and that there are disparities "across economic, education, gender, race, and geographic lines" (DeNoon 2008). Nevertheless, the AHA remains optimistic, saying that it projects continuing decline in heart disease and stroke in the future.

The cancer death rate has also been declining at the rate of 1.1 percent per year since 1993, and at twice that rate since 2002, according to the Ameri-can Cancer Society (ACS). ACS reports that death rates have decreased by 18.4 percent among men and 10.5 percent among women since the early 1990s (ACS 2008). Why there hasn't been an even more significant drop in cancer rates is related to the fact that cancer is really not just one disease, so the cancer rates are calculated separately for different sites or organs. It seems that cancer (this is true of most other diseases, as you will find as we proceed) is linked to demographic factors. For example, cancer of the skin was more prevalent among the poor until the second half of the twentieth century. Things changed as poor people began spending more time working indoors rather than working out in the field. By contrast, rich people began sunning themselves to excess and developing skin cancer (Rimpala and Pukkala 1987). In other words, the mortality rate does not necessarily drop for a particular cause of death at a steady pace largely because when some people stop doing something that increases risk, others begin doing it. Smok-ing presents another good illustration. As the male rate of smoking began to level off, the female rate started to rise and was reflected in the rising female lung cancer rate.

There is almost as much controversy and debate regarding causes of death that seem perfectly clear on the surface, homicide, for example. The homi-cide rate doubled between 1950 and 1980 (from 5.1 to 10.4 per one hundred thousand) and declined steadily since then to nearly the same rate as we saw in 1950 (6.1 per one hundred thousand in 2005). Before we ask why, let us look more closely at the demographic profile that reveals who was involved. The rate peaked in 1990 for men ages twenty to twenty-four (at 36.9 versus 7 for females of the same age). Looking at the differences between white and black men (data on other groups don't go back far enough), we find that the black male homicide rate was highest for men twenty-five to thirty-four years old, at 154.5 per one hundred thousand in 1970, when the white rate for the same age group was 12.5 per one hundred thousand. The comparative female figures during that year were 25.3 for black females and 3.3 for white females. What explains such a significant drop in homicide since 1970 in light of the added information on race and sex?

According to politicians and police chiefs across the country, they should receive the credit for success because of all the increased attention to crime control training, technology, et cetera. Economists and other social scientists say that it is because our economy improved. Epidemiologists and demographers point out that it may have more to do with the rise and decline in the number of people in the population who are most likely to engage in criminal behavior. You don't have to be a demographer to see the logic here. Who is most likely to become involved in violent criminal activities? It is not grandmothers and grandfathers. It is younger people, in fact younger men, who are most likely to be involved in crime. Accordingly, as the number of young men in the population dropped (in line with the declining birth rate), the homicide rate dropped as well.

We will be returning to the question of why there is so much variation in homicide death rates at several points in the book. We consider two relevant variables—age and sex in the following chapter, and then we will turn to race in chapter 5. We return to the topic of race and violence once more in the final chapters of the book to reconsider what might explain the sharp decline in the homicide rate, including deaths due to legal intervention, over the last couple of decades.

As an aside, you might be interested in the proportion of homicide deaths that are specifically due to legal intervention. The rate is probably much smaller than you might have guessed. The rate from 1979 to 1997 averaged out at about 0.14 of all deaths per year (Sikora and Mulvihill 2002).

Summary and Conclusions

This chapter illustrates the process of epidemiological transition that we discussed in the last chapter. The primary causes of death in this country at the beginning of the twentieth century were infectious diseases. By the end of the twentieth century, Americans were less likely to die of an infectious disease, and more likely to die of a chronic disease. Separating Americans into categories differentiated by sex and race/ethnicity, we find tremendous variation in death rates. We learned that epidemiologists refer to rates that are much greater than the average for any particular category of persons as excess mortality. Focusing on excess mortality is the first step in the search for an explanation. Indeed, that is the basic question to which we will be devoting our attention from here on in, namely, what explains why some people die at a younger age and at a higher rate than other people?

Talking about such issues in a thoughtful way introduces dimensions based on solid research that go well beyond what everyone already knows based on that good old source—the conventional wisdom. Not only are recent research findings intriguing, they are consistent in their conclusions regarding a whole lot of things that are otherwise hard to explain—like why people do things that they know are detrimental to their health. Finding a convincing answer to that question would be satisfying, wouldn't it? We will get there, but it will require persistence and patience on your part. We must first examine the separate effect of each of the variables we set out to investigate before we can bring all of them together to produce a more complete explanation.

I realize that we are identifying more questions than we can answer at this point. And I recognize that this is frustrating. My prognosis is that you will get over that feeling by the end of the book. Expect your patience, persistence, and effort to consolidate an overwhelming amount of material to be rewarded in the end. As you will discover, developing a sense of control, in this case, control over a body of knowledge, is a powerful asset that will equip you to discuss the topics we consider with just about anybody you encounter.

CHAPTER FOUR

~

Age and Sex

This chapter aims to outline what we know about variations in morbidity and mortality in relationship to age and sex. The chapter begins with some observations on age and health. We turn next to the differences in the health of males and females. However, age and sex are so intertwined that it is not always easy to keep them separate. Accordingly, we will soon be tying in findings that focus on both.

On the surface, age and sex are not complicated variables. They are relatively easy to use in carrying out research since age comes with its own measure, and we are basically given only two alternatives in identifying our sex. By the way, sex is the correct term to use in this context even though many people use sex and gender as if these two words were synonymous. As a point of clarification, sex is biology; gender is how one acts out one's sex role or what society says is the appropriate way to act out the role. To illustrate, in our culture colors carry gender connotations. Although not nearly as bad as it was in past generations, it is still bad to dress a little boy in anything that is pink, which is the color most closely associated with femininity. Females are raised to be expressive, males are raised to be stoic. These traits are not inherent. In other words, we are still likely to hear that it "natural" for women to be emotional and that explains why they cry. We internalize the idea that men who cry, especially in public, are exhibiting signs of weakness and lack of control, which is generally treated as highly inappropriate by some and "unnatural" by others. Accordingly, it makes us uncomfortable to see that happen.

Curiously, we have been exposed to a fair number of emotional retirement statements being made on TV by successful athletes who are usually thought to epitomize masculinity. Given how much attention Americans pay to what celebrities are doing—will it suddenly be OK for men to become tearful in public when they experience something similar? We'll see.

The Relationship Between Age and Health

Let's begin the discussion on age with some basic questions. What do you think is the single most dangerous time in life and what is the safest, using death rate as the basic indicator? You might be surprised to hear that the most dangerous year of life does not occur sometime in one's declining years. Yes, many more people die then. But they don't all reach year X and die during that one year. (Or as one of my students put it: people don't come in batches with a set expiration date.) Death is more spread out than that. By contrast there is one age during which people are at most risk of dying, and that is during infancy—the first year of life. Because of this, infant mortality receives special attention.

Similarly, the safest years of life are not what you might expect either. People are not least likely to die during their late teens or early twenties. This period is often nominated as the safest period because it precedes what are presumably more stressful years that begin once people begin taking on increasing levels of responsibility through work, marriage, child rearing, and so on. In actuality, the safest years are between five and fifteen. Think about it, what might people of that age die from? Accidents, right, but little else. If a child gets past the first four years with no signs of serious illness leading to death, then the chances are good that he or she will live to the age of fifteen. After that, the chances of dying start to increase. You probably did not expect to hear that the chances of dying start to increase after age fifteen, did you?

As we have all observed, people do not age at the same rate. Some people look and feel better at older ages than others do at younger ages. Research on the physiology of aging indicates that the level of stress a person experiences is implicated. It seems that stress has cumulative negative effects. The more stress a person experiences in life, the faster a person ages (Sapolsky 2004, 239–51). Is it only stress? Maybe it is genetic. Maybe it is lifestyle. We will deal with each of these possibilities in later chapters.

It is interesting to note that those who live to be sixty-five increase their chances of living quite a bit longer (*Health, United States, 2008*, table 26). American males who live to sixty-five can expect to live another 17.2 years, to a little over eighty-two. American females who live to sixty-five can expect to live another twenty years, to eighty-five. The average life expectancy in this country in 2005 for females was 80.4. For males it was 75.2. Clearly, men gain a bigger advantage if they make it to sixty-five. That does not affect the fact that a larger proportion of men than women are likely to die before sixty-five. Before we focus on sex differences, let's go back to life expectancy in general for a moment.

How many more years do you think it is humanly possible to add to current life expectancy? In other words, what do you think is the outer limit of a normal human life span? The current projection made by those who study these kinds of things is 120 years. The Census Bureau estimates that as of 2003 there were more than seventy thousand people over one hundred years of age, that is, "centenarians." Of those, 56,091 were females and 14,013 were males. Indeed, there has been a good deal of attention being paid to the fact that the fastest-growing cohort of Americans are those eighty-five years and older.

Not particularly surprising is finding that regular exercise is associated with significantly better health, and smoking and being overweight are associated with significantly worse physical functioning. One other piece of good news is that autopsies performed on centenarians reveal that they generally do not have any sign of Alzheimer's disease. Those who live longest may have a range of chronic health problems, but they seem to be at less risk of the one disease that many older people are particularly concerned about because of its effects on a person's mental faculties. Another point of good news is that of the men who reach a very old age, 68 percent report that their health is excellent or very good (Yates et al. 2008).

Whether you think a very long life is a blessing or a curse, people who live to a ripe old age have to support themselves for all those years after they stop working, probably while needing increasing levels of care. This is a problem that goes beyond the individual level. Policy makers in all highly developed countries are struggling to come up with good solutions, since populations in all such countries are aging at an unprecedented rate. In case it is not immediately obvious, the worry is that at some point people retire and go on to live many more years after they stop earning a steady income, so their savings decline while the cost of living continues to rise, particularly the cost of health care. The fact that the baby boom generation is now reaching retirement age makes the issue more salient and the need to develop constructive public policy more pressing. We have known for some time that older persons are likely to become sicker, poorer, and increasingly more isolated (Neugarten and Reed 1996). Something to think about, isn't it? While aging is a topic that raises a host of significant social concerns, we cannot stop to give them the attention that they deserve here if we are to continue addressing the topics that we outlined at the beginning of the book.

Another complication connected to old-age survival brings us back to the age/sex link. The sex ratio at age sixty-five is 122 females for every 100 males. By eighty-five, it is 259 females for every 100 males. What do you think explains that? Women just have it easier—that's why they live longer, right? The nature-nurture argument always produces some "lively" conversation. With that caveat—let the arguments begin!

The Relationship Between Sex and Health

As we have already observed in the table on international life expectancy in the previous chapter, women in all those countries live longer than men in the same countries. This has been true of women in economically developed countries for a long time (Lorber 1997). Their life expectancy increased for a number of reasons, but one of the most important reasons is that they were no longer dying in childbirth. Women in some underdeveloped countries do not live as long as men even now for the same reasons. The fact that women live longer in most industrialized countries is an important observation and deserves to be carefully examined. The basic question is this—does biology or gender role provide a more powerful explanation for the difference in life expectancy between males and females? That is the essence of the *nature versus nurture* debate.

Nature versus Nurture

Which side of the argument do you favor? The nature side of the argument says that females live longer because of a biological advantage. The nurture side of the argument says that women live longer because of the advantages offered by their gender role. If it is biology that explains why women live longer, then that must be true across all human populations. Consider this bit of information—the age at which females begin to outnumber males in the United States, that is, the "crossover" point, is thirty-nine among whites and fifteen among African Americans (Lane and Cibula 2000). Employing a biological framework would mean that African American females have that much greater a *biological* advantage over African American males in comparison to the advantage that white females have over white males. Such a statement makes it obvious that there must be more to the explanation.

If it is not biology, maybe it is due to the social roles that women and men are expected to play. That means that there has to be something that is characteristic of women's and men's roles across all cultures. You don't have to be an anthropologist with field experience to know that isn't true.

Would you be surprised to hear that such sociobiological issues inspired considerably more argument a couple decades ago than they do now? That's what facts do. They throw a wet blanket on some pretty good arguments grounded in what people believe or "feel" to be true, as opposed to incontrovertible facts coming out of scientific inquiry.

That does not mean there is far less to argue about, only that new and different concerns have captured people's attention. To begin with, there is the question of whether we have enough research that deals with sex differences to make generalizations. Until relatively recently, females were excluded from samples of the populations health researchers were studying. That began to change during the 1960s with the rise of the feminist movement. Members of this movement identified the problem as a matter of dominance on the part of male doctors who were dismissive of women's health concerns. The Boston Women's Collective, born out of the women's movement, responded with a groundbreaking book entitled "Our Bodies, Our Selves," first published in 1971 and revised a number of times, with the latest revision coming in 1994 (Ruzek, Clarke, and Olesen 1997). The book used mainstream medical literature to explain body functions, symptoms, and treatments to enable women to do more for themselves to stay healthy. That has continued to be a central focus of the women's health movement.

The lack of medical research on women's health began to receive greater attention in the United States during the 1980s (Harrigan et al. 1997; Collins and Sharpe 1994; Clarke and Olesen 1998). However, it took an act of Congress to cause women's health issues to be addressed in earnest. The Congressional Caucus for Women's Issues, chaired by Patricia Schroeder, began looking into women's health issues in 1989 in response to the publication of a widely publicized report indicating that men would reduce their risk of cardiovascular disease by taking aspirin, but said nothing about whether it would help women. That resulted in the passage of the Women's Health Equity Act of 1990, which established the Office of Research on Women's Health (ORWH) within the National Institutes of Health. The ORWH received $9.4 million of funding to carry out ten years of research focusing on women's health issues, which was increased to $20 million in 2000 (U.S. General Accounting Office 2000). ORWH continues to receive funding and has been releasing a steady stream of research findings over the last few years.

The rationale for excluding women from clinical research prior to the 1990s was grounded in the following reasons: (1) the general belief among researchers that men and women do not differ significantly in response to treatment in most situations; (2) the inclusion of women introduces additional variables (e.g., from hormonal cycles) and decreases the homogeneity of the study population; and (3) women might become pregnant; protecting the fetus from unanticipated negative side effects outweighs other possible research objectives. However, once the Public Health Service Task Force on Women's Health Issues took up the topic and published its findings in 1985, the National Institutes of Health (NIH) responded by announcing a policy urging the inclusion of women and requiring justification for exclusion. What was public policy since 1986 became public law in 1993 when Congress passed the NIH Revitalization Act, requiring inclusion of women and minorities in clinical research.

The ORWH makes the following statement to explain why attention to research on women's health is so important.

Many conditions and diseases disproportionately affect women in terms of incidence, diagnosis, course, and response to treatment. Further, factors such as biology, genes, culture, education, income, access to and quality of care, and access to opportunities for inclusion in clinical trials and studies can contribute to adverse health outcomes for many populations of women. In order to better document, describe, prevent and treat disease in women and girls, research should take into account this diversity of experience and population-specific topics.

The ORWH goes on to say that the study of women's health is shifting to an interdisciplinary approach as the interrelatedness and complexity of human health and disease is better understood. The topic was addressed in some detail by the Institute of Medicine in a 2001 report entitled: "Exploring the Biological Contributions to Human Health: Does Sex Matter?" The authors of the report make a number of interesting observations to support the recommendation that much more research is needed. For example, functional magnetic resonance imaging (MRI) reveals that females rely on both sides of the brain for certain aspects of language, while men primarily rely on the left hemisphere. That may explain why women who suffer a left-sided stroke do not experience as much decline in their language performance. On the other hand, we also learned that they have far greater risk of developing life-threatening ventricular arrhythmias in response to a variety of potassium channel-blocking drugs.

A number of government agencies have recently cooperated in creating an online course covering the latest findings on sex-based differences in biology in an effort to highlight the need for more research. It carries continuing medical education credit but is available to anyone who is interested. The course is entitled: The Science of Sex and Gender in Human Health.

Given all the attention that women's health has been receiving, it should not be surprising to hear people beginning to argue that men's health is being ignored (Riska 2004). The question that some people believe deserves greater attention is—what explains the continuing disparity between women's and men's health status and life expectancy?

The Nature Side of the Argument

Turning to the nature side of the argument, we find that there are some other provocative sex-linked findings to consider, such as the sex ratio at birth. There are more male babies born than female babies. That is because more male babies are conceived. The historic ratio was about 115 males to every 100 females conceived, which allows for more male fetuses to be lost before birth, at birth, and in infancy. The explanation is simple and, like it or not, substantiated by reality. The biological weakness of males is compensated for by the higher rate of male fetuses conceived compared to female fetuses, which allows for the greater loss of male fetuses. To the extent that this argument is convincing, it does make you wonder how the idea that women are the "weaker sex" became so firmly entrenched.

Sociobiologists also argue that *nature* allows males to die at a steadily increasing rate once they pass the age at which they are expected to fulfill their primary biological function, namely, to father children and stick around to support the mother and child while they are most vulnerable. A corollary of this observation is that nature gives women an advantage over men while they are in their childbearing years. Once women move past that age, they lose their advantage and are at just as much risk of dying from the major killer diseases as men.

It is also true that this assessment deserves greater scrutiny. Is it possible that this conclusion has less to do with nature or nurture than long-standing conventional wisdom that members of the medical community share? It may be that institutional policies grounded in the conventional wisdom have translated that belief into statistical reality. The fact that women are not expected to die of heart disease during their childbearing years may explain why doctors do not look for it and do not find it. The higher heart-disease death rate recorded for males may be due to the fact that a higher proportion of deaths among younger women are ill-defined, meaning that deaths from heart disease among women are not being recorded accurately (McKinlay 1996, 17).

Many scholars have noted that women do have a biological advantage, but one that can be canceled out by social disadvantage. To illustrate, the sex ratio in India fell from 972 women per 1,000 men in 1901 to 935 women per 1,000 men by 1981, but steadily increased in the industrialized world (Doyal 1995). The explanation is not very complicated: female children are not as highly valued as male children in some parts of the world, so they get less food and medical care, which makes them more susceptible to illness and death (Lorber 1997).

However, the social policies adopted by some regions within underdeveloped countries like India show that the ratio can be altered. Amartya Sen, the 1998 Noble Prize winner for economics, refers to the lower ratio of women to men as the phenomenon of "missing women" (Sen 1998). He points out that in Kerala, India, the ratio of women to men in 1993 was about 104 to 100 males, which is almost equal to that of European countries, where the ratio at the end of the twentieth century was about 105 to 100. India as a whole had a female/male ratio of 93 to 100 during this time. According to Sen, a number of factors contribute to this phenomenon, including much higher female literacy, matrilineal property inheritance, and political activism.

Far harder to explain is the declining ratio of males to females at birth in industrialized countries. It has dropped from what was generally thought to be the standard ratio of 115 males to 100 females to about 106 to 100 over the last few decades (Davis, Gottlieb, and Stampnitzky 1998). What accounts for that? Something males are doing? Something that is happening to our environment? There is no shortage of contaminants that might be blamed. A recent report on chemicals and pharmaceutical products, including hormones, found in the tap water we drink makes this clear. Drinking bottled water is no better, not only because it is, after all, tap water from somewhere, but it seems that chemicals used in the production of the plastic containers may be leaching out into the bottled water. (As those who say this point out, to be bottled, the water comes through some kind of pipes and taps.) In short, something is happening to our environment and we are not all sure how it is affecting our health right now, and we certainly have no way of predicting the long-term impact.

Statistical analysis of sex ratio by age of mother and birth order indicates that the sex ratio decreases with the age of the mother (Matthews and Hamilton 2005). In other words, the number of boys born to mothers over the age of forty is lower than it is among younger mothers. The same is true as the number of babies a woman gives birth to increases.

One of the newest findings is that the sex ratio varies with latitude (Bakalar 2009). It seems that there are large differences between tropical and temperate regions of the world—the warmer the climate, the lower the ratio. Researchers note that the same is true in the case of mice, voles, and hamsters. Why this is the case is not at all clear.

In the meantime, the sex gap of the population as a whole has been getting smaller over the past couple of decades. According to the Census Bureau, the ratio of males to females in 2005 was 97.0 to 100. However, the difference is not spread evenly throughout the age groups. Boys outnumber girls up to the age of eighteen. Women are in the majority after age forty. Among people in their nineties, the ratio of men to women is 38 to 100. One must look at the age pyramid to see how the ratio changes from one age group to another and to see the bulge that the baby boom generation makes in the pyramid. That bulge explains how it is that age group between fifty-five and fifty-nine grew by 29 percent between 2000 and 2005. Those over eighty-five are not far behind, at a 20 percent rate of growth.

Conventional Wisdom Explanations for Why Women Live Longer

We have not yet focused on what the conventional wisdom tells us is the most obvious explanation for the difference between male and female life expectancy. There are several parts to this explanation. Let's start with the firmly held belief that women are more willing to seek medical care for their problems, while men are more likely to deny that they have a problem and delay seeing a doctor until things get so bad that they are forced to do so. Sound familiar? The conventional wisdom goes on to say that women are generally more willing to talk about their problems, ailments, and frustration. That is closely connected to the second firmly held belief—that women are better at managing stress. Men, it is said, keep everything inside, building up a really high level of stress, and that is what contributes to the higher male mortality rate, particularly from heart disease. The question is how much is just that, a firmly held belief, as opposed to fact based on hard evidence.

The third part of the explanation revolves around the idea that men experience more stress because they have more demanding jobs. They have a greater burden of responsibility at work plus carrying the major responsibility for supporting the family. Having raised these issues, I am going to frustrate you by suggesting that we will have to leave the discussion about the impact of work stress on male life expectancy, the third firmly held belief, to a later chapter. The reason is that there has been so much new and significant research on stress that it will take a full chapter to examine it in any detail. For now, let's focus on the first part of the explanation that women live longer because they are more likely to go to the doctor.

As a matter of fact, women do go to the doctor more often than men. According to the Chartbook on Women's Health compiled by the National Center for Health Statistics, women between the ages of fifteen and sixty-four made four times more visits to physicians' offices than men in 1992 (National Center for Health Statistics 1996). However, there is more to this story that most people never hear. Women's higher rate of visits to doctors may have less to do with gender role socialization and more to do with the kinds of health problems women experience in contrast to the kinds of problems men experience. For one, women see doctors for some things that men do not have any experience with, namely, childbirth and gynecological problems. However, even apart from sex organ–related health care, women see doctors more. What the conventional wisdom does not tell us is that women go to the doctor more because they actually experience more illness. The shorthand explanation is that "women get sicker, but men die quicker" (Lorber 1997).

Recent findings indicate that the gender gap is smallest for *life-threatening conditions* throughout adulthood, but that men do increasingly worse with age (Gorman and Read 2006). The evidence shows up as a statistic in the *self-reported health status* measure. Men are more likely to report excellent health at younger ages, but with increasing age the gap closes. Not only do women report experiencing a significantly higher level of functional limitation, the disadvantage increases with age. Women experience a higher rate of nonfatal chronic illness including musculoskeletal problems, most digestive disorders, thyroid diseases, anemias, migraine headache, urinary conditions, and varicose veins. Women are 50 percent more likely to have arthritis than men. These conditions "bother but do not kill." By contrast, men have higher rates of fatal chronic illnesses. Men are at greater risk than women of dying from heart disease, infectious and parasitic diseases, accidents, and cancer (Waldron 2001).

Getting back to the fact that women go to the doctor more than men, it seems that when morbidity levels are considered, the difference between the male and female rates of doctors' visits decreases (Verbrugge 1990). Moreover, men and women ultimately die of similar diseases. It is what happens to them before they die that differs. Men suffer less discomfort during their lives but experience fatal conditions, which shorten their lives. Women experience considerably more morbidity in the form of nonfatal conditions that cause discomfort and disability for many more years than is true for males. In the end, the trade-off is between higher female morbidity versus higher male mortality. Neither alternative looks like a good bargain, but then, we really don't have all that much choice about it anyway.

As an aside, you might be interested in hearing that research specifically devoted to the question of whether women "over-report" symptoms indicates that there is no difference in reporting between men and women (Macintyre, Ford, and Hunt 1999). However, given that we know that women actually experience more ill health, some investigators have begun to rethink this long-standing bit of conventional wisdom. Is it possible that the level of morbidity among women is being underestimated because women are in fact under-reporting (Macintyre 1993)? This is an intriguing question that researchers have not tackled directly to date because the research would be difficult to carry out.

Research designed to answer a different question does sometimes unexpectedly provide new insights, in this case, on how under-reporting morbidity and the higher level of disability among women might be connected. Researchers attempting to understand why women do not do as well after hip-replacement surgery as men found that women delay undergoing surgery. They found that women are generally in worse shape by the time they do undergo the procedure (Holtzman, Saleh, and Kane 2002). Thus, women end up enduring more disability and pain both before and after hip-replacement surgery. Of course, it is possible that the women involved were accurately reporting the level of pain and disability they were experiencing but simply not moving toward the next step. That does, however, mean that women may not be as quick to seek treatment as men, which is what constitutes the challenge to the conventional wisdom on this topic.

It is also possible that women delay going to the doctor for economic reasons. Since women have more doctors' visits in part because they are dealing with conditions exclusive to women, it follows that more visits translate into higher costs (Kjerulff et al. 2007). The fact that they live longer and generally earn less during their working years contributes to the possibility that they put off going to the doctor due to the costs involved.

Nature and Nurture in Combination

The more we look at sex differences the more we see that the combination of biology and social roles offers the best explanation for the differences in mortality rates between males and females. The total rate of death from unintentional injuries for males is 54.2 per 100,000 and for females it is 25.0 per 100,000. Let's consider the variation in mortality rates for motor-vehicle accidents by sex and age because there is more detailed information for this.

The following chart indicates that the male mortality rate is 21.7 and the female mortality rate is 8.9. However, the age distribution makes clear that there is more to it.

That certainly looks like evidence for the nurture side of the argument. In other words, young men are far more likely to die of motor vehicle–related injuries than young women. While the difference is even more extreme at the other end of the age spectrum, considerably more effort has gone into trying to explain the difference in rates at an earlier age. The generally accepted explanation goes like this. Boys in this society grow up learning that engaging in risky behavior is a sign of masculinity. Furthermore, whether you and I like it or not, cars have, perhaps more so in the past than now, been treated as extensions of our identity. A great deal of money and talent has gone into convincing us that the kinds of cars we drive say something about who we are. Driving a fast, expensive sports car tells people that the owner, even if he is a pretty ordinary-looking, middle-aged man, must be rich, successful, and willing to spend money on the good things in life. If a person could not drive an expensive, fast car, then driving any kind of car fast was the next best thing. It established a person's, mainly a male person's, identity as daring. Women have not needed to be daring. The ceaseless message to women, at least according to the public media, is that they need to be sexy and otherwise attractive to men, which does, of course, sometimes result in women ending up at risk of death in a car driven by a male out to prove his

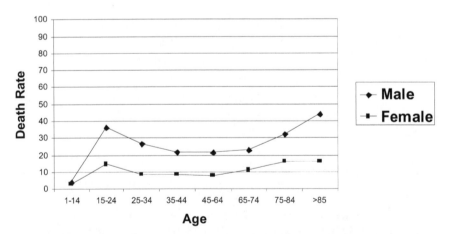

Figure 4.1. Death rates from motor vehicle–related injuries in 2005. *Source: Health, United States, 2008,* Table 43: Death rates for motor vehicle–related injuries, by sex, race, Hispanic origin, and age: United States, selected years 1950–2005.

masculinity. In the end, how much of the variation between young males and females in death due to motor-vehicle accidents can be explained by gender-role socialization is not clear, but their higher rate of alcohol consumption is considered to be a major factor.

The belief that male sex hormones predispose males to more aggressive behavior persists even though the evidence is inconsistent (Waldron 2001). For a while there was some excitement about the idea that men who have an extra Y chromosome might be especially prone to violent behavior. That hypothesis has not received much support. Yet there is no question that men are far more likely to engage in violent behavior. One of the top ten causes of death that gets a considerable amount of attention in this country—homicide—confirms the point.

The male rate of homicide in 2005 was 9.6 per 100,000 versus the female rate of 2.5. To what extent is that due to sex-role socialization as opposed to an inherent predisposition to violence in males? Let's look at the age and sex distribution.

That certainly looks like biology must be playing a significant role. However, if that explanation is to hold up, then it must be true of all males regardless of race or ethnicity, right?

Let's go back to the male homicide rate and look at the difference in death rates by race for the same year. The *total* white male death rate was 5.3

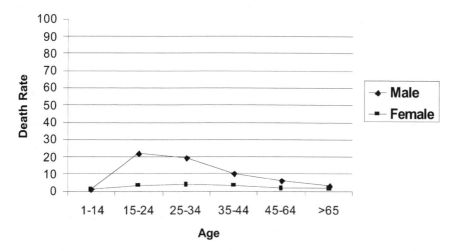

Figure 4.2. Death rates due to homicide by sex per one hundred thousand persons in 2005. *Source: Health, United States, 2008,* **Table 44: Death rates for homicide, by sex, race, Hispanic origin, and age: United States, selected years 1950–2005.**

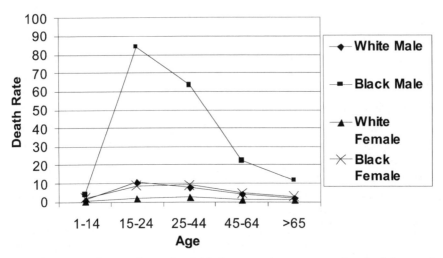

Figure 4.3. Death rates due to homicide by sex and race per one hundred thousand persons in 2005. *Source: Health, United States, 2008,* Table 44: Death rates for homicide, by sex, race, Hispanic origin, and age: United States, selected years 1950–2005.

compared to the *total* black male death rate, which was 37.3. That suggests that race is a critical factor. However, if race is so important, then the black female rate should look more like the male rate, or we will be forced to conclude that there is something more complicated happening here. The chart above makes this point very graphically.

Clearly age, sex, and race must all be considered in coming up with a convincing explanation for the variation in homicide rates across the four demographic categories represented in this chart. Why black males, especially young black males, are at greater risk of homicide than white males and females of either race is a question that deserves a serious answer, an answer grounded in facts. Additional facts that contribute to the answer will accumulate with each chapter and we will return to examine this question more directly in chapter 11. By then we will have a great deal more information to consider, which should lead to a much better-reasoned and informed set of understandings about the questions we have raised thus far.

Getting back to the two variables that are the central focus of this chapter, age and sex, for now would you agree that the variation in motor-vehicle mortality rates by sex and age is best explained by the interaction between nature and nurture? We know that there are some basic differences between male and female *morbidity*, which leads to differing *mortality* rates.

The nurture side of the explanation exacerbates that outcome. What males are taught about what it means to be manly in this society leads to behavior that increases the level of risk of death for males. Boys learn from an early age that risk taking is associated with masculinity. Smoking, drinking, engaging in sports that cause injuries, and playing through pain are all behaviors that symbolize masculinity. Drinking in combination with any other risky behavior explains a large share of the difference in mortality rates between males and females.

Summary and Conclusions

The impact of age and sex on health status comes down to this. Men experience fatal chronic conditions earlier than women, which explains their higher rate of mortality at an earlier age. Women experience nonfatal chronic conditions earlier than men, which explains their higher rate of morbidity. The fact that women's earlier morbidity is chronic rather than fatal explains the difference in life expectancy.

There are five hypotheses being pursued to explain sex differences in life expectancy: (1) biological risks, that is, genetic and hormonal differences; (2) acquired risks connected to work and leisure activities; (3) psychosocial aspects connected to symptoms and health-seeking behavior; (4) health-reporting behavior, which may be learned; and (5) prior health care or how previous care affects future health (Waldron 2001).

Does the preceding discussion leave you with the feeling that we have identified more questions than we could answer? I warned you that this would happen but that the feeling will dissipate as you move forward through the chapters in the book. We will return to the questions that have come up thus far, after we consider a number of other relevant variables.

You might find some comfort in discovering that virtually all the researchers who focus on the issues we have considered here end by saying that we need more research. Where they diverge is in their recommendations regarding the kinds of research they believe are likely to produce the greatest benefit. Do we need more basic medical research? Do we need research that is more inclusive, focusing on a broader range of variables encompassing dimensions associated with social roles? In my view, we need it all.

Helping people to manage their own health better has received a great deal of attention from mainstream researchers as well as the most vocal critics of mainstream medicine. Those engaged in biomedical research see more funding of mainstream research as the best solution. Their critics have been aggressively promoting alternative medicine (Budrys 2005, 84–95).

Almost everybody agrees that improving media coverage of health issues is sorely needed. Few people would disagree with the assessment that what we hear and read can be described as "hype" more likely to inspire hysteria than a better understanding of health risks.

There have also been some more specific policy recommendations directed to improving women's health. Women's health centers have been promoted by some. The idea behind the emergence of such centers is that women's health care is fragmented, which leads to the duplication of some routine tests, while others are missed. To what extent these centers are actually improving upon existing health care for women is not clear. Another recommendation aimed at improving women's health is creating a medical specialty to address women's health issues. This has not received much support from the medical community.

We will now leave the age and sex variables to focus on race and poverty in the following chapter. We will first examine how well race functions as an explanatory variable, going on to consider why it is so often linked to another variable, poverty.

CHAPTER FIVE

~

Race and Poverty

This chapter focuses on race, poverty, and the connection between the two. The concepts have become closely linked because poverty is the one variable that is consistently found to be significant in research attempting to explain racial/ethnic variations in health. Before we get to that, we will focus on race more specifically. The initial question we will be considering in discussing race as a variable is: what do people mean when they invoke the concept of race? We will then go on to discuss poverty in greater detail, outline how it is measured, and briefly reflect on what we, as a society, are doing, if anything, to alleviate poverty. The chapter ends by considering a number of other factors that might account for the exceptionally high mortality experienced by blacks in this country.

The Concept of Race and What We Mean by It

What is meant in discussions on race varies depending on time and place. References to the topic can be traced to the ancient historical writings of both the Greeks and Romans (Williams 2007). The concept reflects social understandings, values, and beliefs, which change over time. When we hear that someone belongs to a particular race, the first thing that comes to mind is the way the person looks. Is there anything else beyond physical characteristics involved? That depends on time and place. Race as a concept has been associated with a range of meanings, including: (1) race as biology, (2) race as culture, (3) race as ethnicity, (4) race as nation, and (5) race as social class (Herman 1996; the following is based on Herman).

Race as biology was abandoned long ago by social scientists and health-care researchers alike who are unanimous in saying that such distinguishing characteristics as skin pigmentation, facial characteristics, and hair texture used to delineate race have little biological significance. Such characteristics matter because they are so outwardly conspicuous, but they are arbitrary as indicators of anything beyond looks. Historically, race was defined as "blood," but this meaning was rejected a century ago when medical science could find no evidence of biological differences between races based on blood type. In fact, scientists concluded that there is as much biological variation within races as there is between races. Second, race as culture is grounded in the recognition of differences in language, religion, and customs. While such differences could be treated as relative rather than hierarchical, that is not what happens. Differences are generally further interpreted in such a way as to imply superiority or inferiority, which turns into the basis for discrimination. Third, race as ethnicity has been gaining increased popularity because it sounds more pleasing. But the increasing use of race/ethnicity as a construct means that the two terms are being conflated and being used for the same boundary-setting functions that operate when race as a concept is being invoked. Both conceptualizations reflect attributions of biological and/or cultural superiority and inferiority. Fourth, race as nation has less salience for Americans than it does for people in some other countries. We can see it operating in such settings as South Africa before the official end of apartheid and more recently in the former Yugoslavia. It functions to establish an "us versus them" mentality and justifies characterizing the other as inferior. Racial and ethnic slurs and other negative labels may even provide support for seeing the other as less than human. Finally, race as social class is the meaning that has become established in this country. It serves as an index of social standing allowing for assumptions regarding level of education, distinctive linguistic qualities, and residential location.

Those who are members of the racial *majority* in this country—whites—have little reason to concern themselves about what meanings are attached to the concept of race on a day-to-day basis. Those who belong to racial and ethnic minorities are far more sensitive to the social attitudes and stereotypical images they confront on a daily basis. In other words, it is not one's race per se that matters. It is what people say about it that matters. And what people say is based on what they have heard other people say. You get the idea—what people say becomes part of the larger cultural belief system that we all share regardless of personal experience. Or, as sociologists put it—the meaning of race is *socially constructed*.

The Institute of Medicine (IOM) agrees that race is a social construct and recommends abandoning it and replacing it with "ethnicity" as the differentiating variable. While this recommendation is addressed to the NIH, it is ultimately aimed at the U.S. Office of Management and Budget (OMB), which sets the standards for classifications to be used in data collection by all government offices (Oppenheimer 2001). Whether this will ever happen and whether such a change would alter social attitudes remains to be seen.

Similar arguments and proposals have appeared sporadically in the past. However, they have appeared far more frequently in recent years (Navarro 1991). Paradoxically, at the same time that the call for shifting the focus from race to some other form of identification attracts increasing support, research on a wide range of topics, morbidity and mortality included, continues to search for and discover differences, indeed large differences, by race. Accordingly, expect to find race coming up as a point of discussion in virtually every chapter to follow.

Race and Data Collection

Given that race is an abstract, socially constructed concept, which is not grounded in biological differences, we know that there are problems associated with using it as a distinguishing variable. It does not take long for the problems associated with using race in data collection to become apparent.

One of the most recent attempts to address the problem came in the form of changes introduced in the 2000 census. Prior to the 2000 census, people of mixed race had little choice but to opt for "other" as their racial category. They objected. The obvious solution—to allow people to indicate more than one category—is not so self-evident when you consider what the purpose of the census is, namely, to count all of us. The 2000 census revealed that nearly seven million people identified themselves as members of more than one race (Schwartz 2001).

So how do you count someone who checks off more than one racial/ethnic category? As one-quarter of an Asian person, for example? We count the person separately for every category checked, but that would result in an inaccurate total count. As you can see, racial classification is fraught with problems. As of the 2000 census, the Census Bureau allowed us to select from up to six racial categories (white, black, American Indian or Alaska Native, Asian, Native Hawaiian, or other Pacific Islander) and one ethnic classification, Hispanic. Beginning with the 1990 census, people were asked whether they were Hispanic or non-Hispanic first and then which of five racial categories they belonged to (in previous census counts Asian and Pacific Islander were combined into a single category). In the 1990 census, the Census Bureau had ten categories to deal with. With the changes in the 2000 census, the possibilities increased geometrically. The Census Bureau now has 126 possible racial/ethnic combinations to sort out.

The fact that Hispanic or non-Hispanic is the first option means that some people report themselves as Hispanic and white while others report that they are non-Hispanic and white. The differences between the two categories as far as health status is concerned are minor. That may be changing because the Hispanic white category has been registering slightly better mortality and morbidity statistics than the non-Hispanic white category. That is interesting, isn't it? We will be exploring possible explanations.

Government agencies responsible for collecting health information struggled with and resolved one dimension of this issue, race of child at birth, a couple of decades ago. How would you assign racial identity to an infant? To be specific, in filling out a birth certificate, what racial category would you assign a child born of a white father and a black mother (LaVeist 1994)? Black, right? How about a black father and white mother? Black again? Not necessarily, at least not anymore. Before we untangle that, what about a white father and a Japanese mother? Japanese, right? What about a Japanese father and a black mother? Japanese or black?

The way classification of the race of a child worked in this country historically was that the race was generally determined by the race of the father, unless the father was white and the mother was black. In that particular case, the child was classified as black. As of 1989, however, the policy changed. Children are now classified according to the race of the *mother* regardless of the race of the father.

The way birth certificates have been filled out reveals a major problem for anyone who is interested in analyzing trend data. Because the data on the race of children at birth are not based on a consistent measure over time, the data on birth rates by race are not as accurate as they might be. Accuracy of such data matters, for good reason. Both policy and social attitudes are built on data about birth rates, for example, particularly teenage and unmarried birth rates. In an effort to overcome such difficulties, the government reported both the pre-1989 and post-1989 counts for some years before dropping the pre-1989 definition (Williams 1996).

Then there is the death certificate. How is race determined in the case of a person who dies in a strange place, as a result of an accident, for example (Williams 1996)? The answer is that the emergency-room doctor fills out the death certificate, without having known the person when he or she was alive. The doctor simply classifies the person's race based on what the person looks like. Could the doctor make the wrong designation? Does it matter? To the person who died, it does not matter at all. It matters quite a bit for recordkeeping purposes.

How confident can we be that the data on race regardless of when they are gathered are accurate? And turning the question around, should we be paying so much attention to a classification that has no biological basis? Some people argue that it cannot be disregarded because there are major social consequences associated with race, namely, racial stereotyping and racial discrimination, that is, racism. Those who argue that we should abandon race agree that racism is a major factor. They say, however, that if that is what we are interested in then we should be focusing on racism directly and not struggling to come up with improvements for conducting racial counts. (Bhopal and Donaldson 1998; Fullilove 1998; Williams 1994). That is, of course, a "catch-22" situation. How do you know when racism occurs unless you collect data on how many people of particular groups are involved to determine if the racial minority is being treated unfairly?

Why do we continue to use this variable even though there are so many problems associated with it? There are at least two practical reasons. One is that we have been collecting information based on race all along. Discontinuing it would mean all the trend data we have collected in the past could not be compared to data being collected now. Another reason for not dropping race as a variable is that it is not easy to come up with alternatives. Health statistics collected by other highly developed countries are reported using classifications other than race. Use of race as a distinguishing category in this country stems from our history of slavery and the need to count free people in contrast to enslaved people, and then go on to count the free people eligible to vote and so on. Most other countries classify people by social class.

Social Class as a Variable

Using social class in this country is not a viable option. Why? What do you think most Americans say when asked what their social class is? It has long been observed by social scientists that nearly 90 percent of us say that we are middle class. If we are pressed into classifying ourselves further as working class or middle class, that near 90 percent figure splits in half, which does not allow for enough differentiation to be useful. How is it that other countries can use this variable and we cannot? The answer is that people in other countries identify with the social class they belong to. We obviously do not.

Not only are people in other countries—England, for example—ready to embrace their social-class designation, they are prepared to argue for more benefits and rights for their class. When they fill out forms, they simply indicate which of the five social-class categories they belong to as defined by English custom. Just as those in the lower classes make every effort to have more social benefits come their way, those in the upper class make every effort to protect traditional privileges and pastimes—fox hunting, for example—which has come under fire from animal-rights activists.

People in other countries believe that the class one is born into matters a lot and that rising above "one's station" is rare. Americans are convinced that just the opposite is true. There is no question that some people do move into a higher social class than that of their parents. But it does not happen as often as many people would like to think and it is not more likely to happen here than elsewhere. However, our belief system is adamant about asserting that this is the land of opportunity and we can all "get ahead" with a little luck, if we really want to.

Americans like to think there are no real class differences in this society. Yes, some people have more money than others, but because everybody has a good chance of getting rich, class does not matter. That is certainly what the cultural belief system says even if there is an enormous amount of evidence to indicate that people who are born rich are much more likely to stay rich and those who are born poor are much more likely to stay poor. What varies over time is how much richer the rich are at any time and how much poorer the poor are. By the end of this book you will see that poverty status or near-poverty status may not matter nearly as much as the broader concept of socioeconomic inequality and the extent to which inequality explains differences in mortality.

Social class, which is sometimes used synonymously with socioeconomic status, like race, is an abstract concept, but one that does have very clearly identifiable components according to social scientists. Maybe we could use those and get rid of race as a major differentiating classificatory category. Let's consider that possibility. Social scientists consider social class to consist of three basic components—income, education, and occupation. It is important to understand that social class is a combination of all three. Therefore, a person who wins the lottery isn't automatically catapulted into the upper class. If you think about it, you should not be surprised to hear that. What makes someone a member of the upper class? The most certain indicator is how long the family has had its wealth, which is not the same as a high income. In fact, it can take several generations of wealth to gain membership in the upper class. During that time the children will have had the opportunity to attend excellent schools, possibly enter into prestigious careers, join the right organizations, develop the right friendships—fit into the role. By that time, the source of the original wealth, which could have come from dirty, even dishonest, work, is not so important, even if some people can still remember what the original source of the family's wealth actually was.

Occupation is the hardest of the three components to use because it is a "nominal" concept without a clear-cut operational measure attached. It is not easy to "operationalize" this concept, that is, to attach a numerical value to occupational status that can then be ranked along with other occupations. There really is no single reliable and stable scale that everyone can agree on. When someone delves into this topic, they generally list occupations in order of prestige without going further. So we still don't have a fixed indicator of *how much higher* the prestige of one occupation is versus another.

How about income? Income is good because it comes with its own quantitative measure, but it is not problem-free. If you use income in reporting death rates, income at what stage of life would you want to know about? Would you use income at time of death? That is probably not the same as income at the time the person was at the peak of his or her earnings. If the person is retired and has been out of the workforce for a long time, then peak earnings will be low by current standards, even if that level of income was considered high at the time. Getting accurate income information at any time of life after a person dies might not be possible in any case. As a result, we collect income data in connection with morbidity but not mortality. In other words, you can ask living people directly about their current income and their current health status. We don't have income data linked to mortality for individuals. It is possible, however, to compare the average income of large groups of people, a whole state, for example, in conjunction with the mortality rates for the entire population of the state. We will look at those findings in a later chapter.

That leaves education as the only other indicator of social status that is left to us. Because it, like income, comes with its own measure and is stable in the sense that it cannot drop, it is gaining in popularity as an important indicator. A growing body of research confirms that it is, in fact, a powerful indicator of health status. As a result, it has been appearing with increasing regularity in conjunction with mortality statistics collected by the government. Now all we have to do is identify what it is about education that causes this effect. We will do that in one of the final chapters of the book.

At the same time, knowing that education is a very powerful indicator of social status, which predicts to a range of social advantages including health, does not mean that it is likely to replace race as the basic differentiating variable we use to collect data in this country, if only because we have collected data based on race for so long. If we decided to stop using race, for whatever reason, that would mean all the data we have collected in the past would have only historical value and could not be used to track ongoing shifts in health status. Since we keep seeing significant differentials by race, neither can we ignore those differences, nor can we stop collecting data based on race.

The Evidence on Racial/Ethnic Variations in Health

As you might suspect when we discuss health and race/ethnicity, we will be most concerned with the categories of people who have high mortality rates rather than those who have low mortality rates. In other words, we will not be discussing the health of Asian Americans in any detail because their health status is not considered to be problematic and is therefore not the focus of much research. Furthermore, while it is clear that Asians do live longer, why they live longer is not so clear. Rather than sift through a lot of speculative explanations and inconclusive evidence, we will concentrate on topics that have received a great deal of attention and have been extensively researched. We will be directing a great deal of attention to the question of why African Americans have such high mortality rates. Most comparisons are made between the health of blacks and whites because more complete statistics are available on these two categories of people. When possible we will consider the health of other ethnic groups as well.

Poverty and Its Relationship to Health

The main reason that race and poverty are linked is that a higher proportion of blacks than whites are poor. How do we know that? Table 3 in *Health, United States* reports poverty levels by race. The percentage (notice that this is not a rate) figures, as I have abstracted them, look like this for 1995 and 2005, the last year for which we have information at the time of this writing. I am comparing the data for these two years because the poverty rate rose steeply during the decade of the 1980s and declined during the late 1990s. The poverty rate began to rise again during the first decade of the twenty-first century; however, we will have to follow this trend for a few more years to see if it continues in the same direction.

Table 5.1. Percentage of Persons Below the Poverty Level in 1995 and 2005

Race/Ethnicity	All Persons		Children <18		Children < 18 in Female-Headed Household	
	1995	2005	1995	2005	1995	2005
All races	13.8	12.6	20.2	17.1	50.3	42.8
White	11.2	10.6	15.5	13.9	42.5	38.8
Black	29.3	24.9	41.5	34.2	61.6	50.2
Asian	12.2	11.1	18.6	11.0	42.4	25.6
Hispanic Origin						
Mexican*	31.2	22.9	39.3	29.5	65.9	51.4
Puerto Rican*	38.1	25.6	53.2	32.1	79.6	55.3

* The Mexican and Puerto Rican statistics are for 2000.
Source: Health, United States, 2008, Table 3: Persons and Families Below Poverty Level, by Selected Characteristics, Race, and Hispanic Origin: United States, Selected Years 1973–2005.

Race as a Proxy Measure

As you can see, this table presents us with some pretty shocking information. One of the most troubling facts it forces us to confront is that such a large percentage of American children are poor. Being poor as an adult is bad enough, but children who are poor have even less chance of overcoming the disadvantages associated with poverty, because, as a growing body of evidence indicates, poverty during childhood has a range of lasting detrimental effects. We will get back to this topic in later chapters. For now, let's focus on the relationship between poverty and race in general. Although the 2005 rate of poverty for blacks at nearly 25 percent is higher than it is for any other racial/ethnic group, it is now lower than it has ever been. It was over 50 percent during the 1960s and roughly 30 percent until the last years of the twentieth century. The fact that such a high percentage of blacks are poor has long been used as a marker of something other than race. It has been used as a *proxy measure* for the effect of poverty.

What do you think of interpreting the data on variations in health using race as a proxy measure for poverty? No one would argue that it is ideal. The rationale for doing so in the past was as follows: since we do not have data on income, this is the closest thing to it. It is also true that once we started collecting data on Hispanics we found that some Hispanics are often just as poor or even poorer than blacks. However, poverty is generally not used to nearly the same extent in assessing the health status of Hispanics as it is used to explain the health status of blacks. In short, while no one is eager to defend the use of race as a proxy for poverty anymore, that application has not been completely eliminated either. Considering that we put so much thought into developing precise operational measures for the other variables we were using, and that there were teams of specialists working to improve data collection methods, it is curious that we have been willing to settle for this really inadequate proxy measure for poverty for so long.

Discussions that focus on the relationship between race and poverty sometimes mention historical context. The idea is that slavery is a major factor in explaining the economic disadvantage that African Americans continue to experience in this country. When researchers looked into living conditions and life expectancy of slaves, however, they discovered that slaves had a higher level of consumption of goods and lived longer than industrial workers in both Europe and the United States during that time period (Sen 1999, 28–29). Slaves nevertheless made every effort to escape from bondage. That tells us that availability of goods alone does not explain the essence of social deprivation. The lack of freedom is far more important.

Determining Who Is Poor

By now, the question of how we determine who is poor and who is not may have started to bother you. The answer goes back to the early 1960s. There is some interesting history here that is deeply grounded in what is basically a socially constructed explanation for poverty. It goes like this. Historically, here and elsewhere, poverty was considered to be a misfortune confronting individuals who were thought to have brought much of their misfortune upon themselves. That explains why poor people who fell into debt were thrown into debtors' prisons in England during earlier centuries. Americans saw things exactly the same way. In other words, there was no need to bother about such people. No one was particularly interested in determining who they were or how many of them there were.

It was not until the Great Depression of 1929 that people in this country recognized that good, upstanding, hard-working people could become poor through no fault of their own. That is what brought Social Security into existence in 1935. Social Security was designed to provide a safety net for people who retired after a lifetime of work with little in savings and no other source of income to sustain them during their remaining years. Two facts are worth noting with regard to this momentous turning point in American social thought. Life expectancy at the time was fifty-seven, and people could be forcibly retired at age sixty-five. As you know, life expectancy is now, on average, seventy-eight, and companies are not permitted to retire people at sixty-five. That is age discrimination and it is illegal.

These statistics should tell you why politicians keep warning us that the Social Security Fund will go broke and why there is unending debate about how to fix it. There was no problem with funding when life expectancy was shorter so that there were more people paying into the fund than the number of people eligible to receive it. Nor were they receiving Social Security payments for as long as they are now.

Getting back to the topic of poverty, it turns out that with the passage of Social Security legislation, we, as a society, moved on to other concerns, namely World War II. Once the war was over, this country entered a period of unprecedented prosperity. Everyone seemed to be better off financially. The topic of poverty moved off the sociopolitical radar screen. People were buying new houses, buying things to put into those houses, buying cars. That happened because wages were frozen during the war and factories were producing war goods. People had not been buying consumer goods because they weren't being produced. After the war ended, peacetime production went into high gear. The economy surged ahead. Personal income increased by about 37 percent between 1950 and 1956 (Bureau of Labor Statistics 1978, 5). Right in the middle of this period of great prosperity, a small number of critics appeared on the scene to say that things were really not as rosy as we were being led to believe. They said that there were people being left out and falling further behind even as the rest of society was enjoying the benefits of economic growth.

However, there was not enough factual data to support or refute the critics' assertions. The government was pressed into providing information that would do so. The only way that could be done was to count the number of people who were poor. How would you do that? Yes, you need to count the number of people falling below the poverty line. The crucial question is—how do you determine where the poverty line stands? Simply picking a percentage of the population and saying that they are the ones who are poor was not acceptable. There was no agreement on what percentage would be appropriate—5 percent, 20 percent, 50 percent, more, less? Besides, some politicians were arguing that there was no problem. In spite of the lesson learned during the Great Depression, Americans still really believed that only a small number of people were poor and that those who were brought it on themselves—they drank, gambled, had too many children, were lazy, and so on. Yes, there may have been some people, widows for example, who were not to blame for their impoverished circumstances, but churches and charities were assisting them. Some might note that this sounds very much like what some Americans, especially some politicians, say now.

So, back to the problem of counting who is poor. The agreed-upon solution identified during the early 1960s was to use the existing "cost-of-living" index, which the Bureau of Labor Statistics first created around 1918 for purposes of determining a fair-wage scale to be used for setting wages in shipbuilding yards (Bureau of Labor Statistics 1978). The National Consumer Price Index (CPI), published periodically since 1921, measured the cost of a "market basket" of essential goods and services being purchased by families. The categories have been fairly stable after they were initially identified. They include: food, housing, apparel, transportation, medical care, recreation, education and communication, a catchall category called "other goods and services," plus some special indexes, most notably energy (that encompasses gas, oil, and electricity). The measurement mechanisms have undergone several revisions. The 1959 revision improved on earlier versions by extending the survey to cover the entire country rather than selected cities. The CPI is now widely used for a broad range of purposes. Companies use it to determine wages, salary, and pension increases from year to year. It serves to evaluate economic growth in general. The differences in the speed at which different components of the CPI are increasing provide fodder for policy arguments. If you are interested in the CPI, you can find that information in tables published in the NCHS publication we refer to throughout the book (*Health, United States*). The tables report trend data on selected CPI items to compare the rate at which medical-care costs have been rising in comparison to other costs. However, you might be interested in the difference between how much the cost of clothing, for example, has risen compared to medical costs. It will also be worth noting how much the cost of energy, oil and gas more specifically, has risen over the past few years compared to other components.

The poverty level calculated on the basis of the CPI market basket of essential goods and services was announced for the first time in 1961. It turned out to be $2,973 for a family of four. Since then the poverty line for families of different sizes has been calculated. The Census Bureau website makes that information readily available. (It also tells us that the Department of Health and Human Services uses a "poverty guideline" measure for the current year for administrative purposes while the Census Bureau reports the "poverty threshold" for the previous year based on actual changes in costs. The two are similar but not identical.)

So how many people do you think fell below the poverty line the first time the count was taken? It was 22 percent. That is over one-fifth of the entire population! That was an enormous political embarrassment. When Census Bureau statisticians took a closer look, the situation became even more difficult to justify. It became clear that poverty was not evenly distributed. While 22 percent of the total population was poor, 29 percent of those over the age of sixty-five were poor; 50 percent of people in female-headed households were poor; and 56 percent of African Americans were poor. What followed in the wake of these revelations came in the form of the Great Society initiatives of the Lyndon Johnson administration. New programs were introduced to deal with some of the inequities. Civil rights legislation, Medicare and Medicaid programs, and financial aid for education were some of the most groundbreaking initiatives.

As we saw in the table above, as of 2005 only 12.6 percent of the population fell below the poverty line. Does that mean that we have been successful in our efforts to overcome poverty? The answer to that question is far from settled. Some observers argue that the proportion of people who fall below the poverty line constitutes an overcount. They say that even fewer people would be counted as poor if we included all the benefits that people receive such as food stamps, housing assistance, Medicaid, and so on. Others dismiss that argument by asking how many of us could make it on $10,210 a year—the 2008 poverty line for a person under sixty-five. Or how about $20,650, the 2008 rate for a family of four—two adults and two children? They say that it is hard to imagine how one could survive on that income, regardless of what the CPI market basket of goods indicates, so they conclude that there are really many more people who are poor than we are actually counting. In case it is not perfectly obvious, this debate is steeped in a system of social and political beliefs about how much the country should be doing for people who are not making it on their own. (In saying this, critics use "the country" to mean "the government" rather than private philanthropy, which almost everyone now agrees is doing a great deal of good but is not equipped to provide assistance equally and equitably across the country to all those who need assistance.)

Health statistics are increasingly being reported by poverty status. Three categories are typically used to present health-status statistics by poverty status: (1) 100 percent of poverty or under, (2) 100 to 200 percent of poverty, and (3) 200 percent of poverty or over. Using actual 2008 income figures for a family of four, this means we are talking about families at 100 percent of poverty or under earning $20,650 or less; families at 200 percent of poverty or over earn $41,200 or more. That really doesn't tell us whether those families who are far better off have better health. Would families with incomes at 300 percent of poverty, or $61,950, have better health than those at lower income levels? Or 400 percent of poverty, which is $82,600? Or even 500 percent of poverty, which is $103,250? As we will see in later chapters, using a 200 percent of poverty cutoff does not seem to provide a wide enough range to reveal significant differences in health status.

Poverty and Welfare

Without getting too distracted by yet another highly controversial topic, let us consider for a moment what our government does to help those who cannot make it on their own. How much does this society dole out in welfare? Like everything else we have taken up thus far, we must first specify what we have in mind before we discuss welfare. Where do you draw the line between welfare and social programs that are not welfare? For example, do you consider financial aid to college students to be welfare? No? Why not? What makes welfare, welfare? How about tax write-offs for corporate executives who go out for fancy lunches? Even convention expenses for academics like me? Not welfare? How about government bailouts of banks that have issued too many risky loans? Then there are all the economic "incentives," from outright monetary gifts to help establish new offices to release from property taxes that corporations are offered for bringing their businesses to a city or state. Some people consider that to be corporate welfare—what do you think? Isn't welfare essentially a matter of the government giving money to someone? There is no question of what people have usually meant when they talked about welfare, namely, giving money to poor, unmarried women with children. Why is giving them money different from giving it to college students or corporations? The answer is that the value system in this country says that poor people brought their situation on themselves and they should not be rewarded for it. That attitude may change depending on how stories about those who have lost their homes because they could not pay the mortgage turn out—are we to understand that the majority are hard-working people, who did most things right except for taking out a questionable low-interest loan, or are these greedy people who knew that they should not be taking out such a loan and don't deserve much sympathy?

The welfare program that so many Americans thought was so objectionable, the Aid to Families with Dependent Children (AFDC), ended in 1997. That is when the Temporary Assistance to Needy Families (TANF) program was legislated. It was designed to give financial assistance under strict conditions, primarily requiring recipients to look for a job. If the recipients cannot find a job, then they are required to enter a job-training program so that they will be able to find work. In all cases, financial aid is limited to sixty months over a person's lifetime. What happens after that, in those cases where someone still cannot cope, is something that states have been trying to figure out how to handle, since federal welfare funds are not available.

There are a few other programs, such as supplemental social security insurance (SSI), for which disabled persons may qualify; supplemental food assistance for women, infants, and children (WIC); and the food-stamp program. (Again, not to get too distracted, but it is worth considering that the food the poor are receiving is not a matter of charity. The poor are actually purchasing the food but the government is subsidizing those purchases, so that stores, major food-producing companies, agribusinesses, and so on, all make money on the transactions. Doesn't that mean that the food-stamp program is also providing welfare to food producers?)

In case you have not noticed—healthy adults without dependent children are not eligible for any of the government aid programs. All adults, healthy or not, over the age of sixty-five are eligible for Medicare. Medicare is, however, generally considered to be an "entitlement" program, which is not the same as welfare. People over sixty-five are entitled to the benefits this program offers because they have earned it. We will discuss it and other forms of health insurance in much more detail in chapter 7.

Explanations for Racial Variation in Health

Although there is complete agreement among researchers about the existence of significant racial health disparities, the reasons responsible for the disparities are far from clear. That there is a long history of systematic racial inequality in health care going back to the seventeenth century is documented by Byrd and Clayton in a book of two volumes (2000, 2002). Interest in identifying the causal factors gained momentum in the 1980s with the publication of the *Report of the Secretary's Task Force on Black and Minority Health* issued by the Department of Health and Human Services in 1985. The report pointed out that the health status of blacks had improved dramatically since 1900; when average life expectancy at birth for all Americans was 47.3 years, it was 33 years for blacks. However, the report went on to say that there were sixty thousand excess annual deaths attributable to health disparities. A widening gap between black and white mortality during the decade of the 1980s heightened the sense of concern (Ng-Mak et al. 1999).

An article published in the *New England Journal of Medicine* in 1990 probably did the most to capture the attention of policy makers and researchers alike. The authors reported that the mortality rate in Harlem was more than double that of U.S. whites and 50 percent higher than that of U.S. blacks, which might not have attracted nearly as much attention if they had not also noted that this meant that black men in Harlem were less likely to reach age sixty-five than were men in Bangladesh (McCord and Freeman 1990).

David Satcher, the former surgeon general under President Bill Clinton, and his colleagues drew attention to the topic again by reporting how much progress in reducing racial disparities there has been over the last four decades of the twentieth century across a range of social determinants (Satcher et al. 2005). They found that income rose from 65 percent to 84 percent for blacks compared to the median income of whites. The ratio of African American to white high-school dropouts declined; racial segregation declined. Only the difference in wealth between African Americans and whites remained the same, with African Americans continuing to have about 7 percent of the wealth of whites. However, the main point the researchers wanted to make was that by comparison, the black/white health ratio had not exhibited any improvement over this time period. Using 2002 statistics, they reported that 83,570 excess deaths could have been prevented if the black–white gap were eliminated. Moreover, they stated that the infant mortality rate and the mortality rate for African American men over the age of thirty-five actually worsened over the same period.

The fact that health disparities have not diminished and have even been increasing for some age groups led Congress to direct the Agency for Health-care Research and Quality (AHRQ) to begin tracking disparities in health-care delivery to determine the extent to which the health-care delivery system was responsible. That led to the first National Healthcare Disparities Report, released in 2003. The National Health Disparities Report, 2007, states that three key themes characterize the report: (1) overall, disparities in health-care quality and access are not getting smaller; (2) progress is be-ing made, but many of the biggest gaps in quality and access have not been reduced; and (3) the problem of persistent lack of insurance is a major barrier to reducing disparities.

The fact that health disparities remain has still not been fully explained has motivated the NIH to launch a new effort "to help move research related to the complex factors underlying health disparities into the 21st century." The NIH announced the creation of the Center to Study Genomics and Health Disparities in March 2008.

One of the basic questions that health researchers have been struggling to answer in recent years is: What is it about the consequences of the poverty that minorities experience that results in health disparities? Is the main prob-lem that poor people don't get medical care when they need it because they can't afford it? Or is it that they get inferior medical care? Some researchers say that inferior care is a major factor (Freeman and Payne 2000). Others have argued that they can't afford the fresh fruit and vegetables that are better for their health than cheaper and more filling fast food. Then there are the disadvantages of living in a neighborhood that is dangerous and possibly more polluted. Are they forced to take jobs that are dangerous? It is probably all these things. Doesn't that explain everything? Well, no, it doesn't.

When researchers began tracking black mortality rates, they discovered that the rates were not the same from place to place. Researchers knew that people who live in poverty-stricken areas have higher death rates, but they could not explain why the effect was more extreme for blacks. To illustrate, boys in Harlem who live to age fifteen have a 37 percent chance of surviving to age sixty-five, while girls have a 65 percent chance (Geronimus et al. 1996). This is in contrast to the mortality rate of blacks in the Queens/Bronx area, who have mortality rates similar to the national average for whites.

If poverty offers the main explanation for higher mortality rates among blacks, then why is it that Hispanics with similar incomes have much lower mortality rates? As you recall from chapter 3, Hispanics have lower rates of mortality from heart disease and stroke. What researchers want to understand is how it is that Hispanics at the same income level as blacks experience far lower mortality for the two causes (Karter et al. 1998). One group of researchers came up with a potential explanation that they went on to test. They called it the Salmon Hypotheses (Abraido-Lanza et al. 1999). You know that salmon (yes, the fish) return to the place where they were born when they are ready to spawn. They die shortly thereafter. Get it? Maybe the lower rate of mortality among Mexican Americans can be explained by the observation that many go back to Mexico in their declining years. The researchers did not indicate surprise when they found that they had to reject this hypothesis. It seems that the number of Mexicans who leave the United States and die in Mexico is just not that high. It does not explain the difference in mortality rates between Hispanics and African Americans.

There is also evidence to indicate that African Americans have more chronic health problems than other racial/ethnic groups. In effect, they have a higher rate of morbidity in addition to a shorter live span (Hayward et al. 2000; Hayward and Heron 1999; Ferraro and Farmer 1996). They are far more likely to qualify for Medicare disability coverage before age sixty-five than whites, about one-third of African Americans versus 12.9 percent of whites (Short and Weaver 2008). The factors that might explain these disparities, and the extent to which poverty is involved, have been examined repeatedly, including lifestyle choices, like smoking; health insurance; education; and net worth (Sudano and Baker 2006). We will consider the role played by lifestyle in greater detail in the following chapter and the role played by health insurance in the chapter after that. That a range of factors is involved continues to stand as the conclusion reached by the majority of researchers.

Biomedical Research Focusing on Racial/Ethnic Variation

Let's look at a few examples of medical research focusing on the relationship between race and particular diseases. I want to emphasize that the following in no way represents a review of the existing literature, which is voluminous. The following discussion is meant to serve as a sample of the kinds of questions researchers have asked and the answers they have come up with. It is worth noting that one of the complaints that some researchers have is that there is an absence of clinical test data on the health of minorities for the same reasons that there were insufficient data on women until relatively recently—they simply were excluded from clinical trials, which results in an information gap (Maxey and Williams 2007).

Starting with coronary heart disease, a review of the research indicates that factors related to the higher rate of mortality among blacks include the following: higher prevalence of smoking, hypertension, diabetes, and obesity. At the same time, blacks are less likely to undergo appropriate diagnostic testing (coronary angiography) and treatment (coronary revascularization) (Francis 1997; Geiger 1996). Researchers invariably conclude that more research is needed to determine the extent to which personal behavior, such as smoking, increases risk in contrast to other factors, including the health system's failure to deliver appropriate care.

In examining the factors that are responsible for the high rate of mortality from stroke, the data indicate that blacks have higher rates of hypertension (high blood pressure) and diabetes, which are the two main risk factors associated with stroke. However, when researchers control for those two factors, blacks are still more likely to die from stroke. (Controlling for the two factors means that the death rates from stroke for whites with similar rates of hypertension and diabetes are being compared to the rate for blacks with the same health problems [Kittner et al. 1990].)

Recognition of the high rate of cancer mortality among minorities captured the attention of the IOM. The IOM organized a panel to examine the progress in research on cancer in 1999. The panel concluded that the National Cancer Institute is doing an excellent job in advancing cancer research, which has resulted in a sustained decline in cancer mortality rates. However, it also pointed out that not everyone is sharing in the progress. While stating that it is basically opposed to using race in collecting data, it advised the National Cancer Institute to devote more attention and a greater share of resources to studying racial/ethnic disparities.

The findings related to breast cancer, which are particularly perplexing, provide a powerful illustration of the IOM's critical observation regarding cancer care. Black women experience a slightly lower incidence of breast cancer than white women. Therefore, the question that researchers have been struggling to answer is why their mortality rate turns out to be consistently higher than that of white women (Lannin et al. 1998). The single most important reason that seems to explain this is that black women seek medical care at a more advanced stage of disease than white women. By now, you probably won't be surprised to hear that researchers cannot explain why this occurs.

Unraveling these issues is not a simple assignment. Consider the complexity associated with the following pieces of information. Blacks have a higher mortality rate for lung cancer than whites. At the same time, there is clear evidence that blacks are less likely to undergo lung cancer surgery, which plays a major role in reducing their survival rates (King and Brunetta 1999). When the rate of surgery is the same, the survival rate is similar for blacks and whites (Bach et al. 1999). Which still leaves us with the question of why aren't blacks undergoing as much surgery? Is it that doctors are not diagnosing black patients early enough? Not offering comparable treatment? Not discussing the risks associated with smoking? One possibility is that smoking affects blacks differently than it affects whites. Cotinine, which is what becomes of nicotine when it is metabolized and absorbed into the blood, can be found at a higher level in the blood of blacks than of white or Mexican American smokers with similar levels of smoking (Caraballo et al. 1998). It is not clear why this occurs, but it is clearly linked to the increased carcinogenic risk experienced by blacks.

Of course, you also have to ask why more blacks began smoking and fewer quit smoking even as the majority of Americans were quitting (Kiefe et al. 2001). The researchers who report this say that the variables that are most closely associated with the rise in smoking among blacks are education and other socioeconomic variables. On the surface the relationship may seem obvious, but it is actually quite complex. It is certainly unlikely that they do not know that smoking is linked to cancer. We will get back to the effects of education and socioeconomic differences later in the book.

Just in case any of this suggests to you that researchers are ignoring the possibility of genetic differences, be assured that they are not. Consider the high rate of kidney failure among blacks. In 1997 the *incidence* of end-stage renal disease, which requires dialysis or transplantation, was four times higher in blacks than in whites, and *prevalence* was almost five times greater (Young and Gaston 2000). Hypertension, or high blood pressure, is primarily responsible for kidney failure. It is tempting to assume that this exceptionally high rate of hypertension and ultimate kidney failure among blacks in comparison to whites must be genetic. The problem with that conclusion is that the majority of African Americans come from the sub-Saharan region of Africa where the population typically has low blood pressure, which translates into low levels of hypertension. It would be unreasonable to argue that only those with a flaw in this genetic trait somehow landed in the United States. This is not to say that there is no genetic component involved. It is to say that the whole issue is far more complicated than that.

Given the high rate of renal failure among blacks in addition to the fact that end-stage renal disease treatment (dialysis and kidney transplantation) is covered by Medicare, one might expect that a comparable number of blacks would be undergoing transplantation. That does not turn out to be the case (Young and Gaston 2000). Why this is so given that inability to pay for the procedure is not an obstacle is a matter that has received a great deal of attention from researchers. The list of possible explanations is extensive, starting with lack of donors providing a good match to the rules for allocating organs used by the United Network for Organ Sharing, which is the central organ bank in the country. Then there is the fact that cost of transplantation is covered, but the high cost of immunosuppressive drugs after the first three-year postsurgical period is not.

According to the IOM, racial and ethnic minorities receive lower quality of care (Smedley, Stith, and Nelson 2003). The explanation behind this assertion is not entirely clear. Maybe doctors do not provide the same level of care for African Americans. Maybe the way the health-care system is set up results in discrimination and that is what explains the higher level of morbidity and mortality African Americans suffer. We will consider these possibilities in greater detail in chapter 7, when we consider the importance of medical care in explaining differences in overall mortality.

Summary and Conclusions

To sum up this discussion, we have been confronted with a number of well-grounded facts and a much larger number of inconclusive findings. We find that poverty and race are consistently linked in the literature, making it difficult to identify their respective effects on health status. The question that continues to require a more complete explanation is: how does the fact that a higher proportion of blacks are poor than are persons belonging to other racial/ethnic categories translate into health disparity? Poverty does of course have some obvious consequences that help to explain why blacks have such high mortality and morbidity rates, but it is also clear that not all the pathways between poverty and health disparity have yet been fully explored.

We reviewed the debate on the use of race as a major differentiating variable in the collection of national health statistics, which needs to be explained given that researchers agree that biological differences are not sufficient to explain racial health disparities. That is when we found that race has been serving as a proxy measure for poverty. We also found that no one argued that it is a good proxy measure in the past when a greater proportion of blacks were in fact poor than is the case now. The fact that the poverty rate for blacks has been declining and the research on what is responsible for variation in health is now more extensive and complex makes it clear that poverty alone is far from an adequate explanation for the existence of the wide health disparity between blacks and whites.

We also find some observers arguing that, with all its flaws as a differentiating variable, we cannot simply abandon race in collecting health data because we need continuity in the data collection process to understand changes in mortality and morbidity over time. More importantly, the fact that large differences in mortality and morbidity rates by race are consistently reported has led to the conclusion that there is a pressing need to identify the factors that are responsible for those differences. Thus, rather than abandoning race as a variable, we have begun to collect statistics that differentiate by ethnic background as well as race not so much because anyone is arguing that these designations are meaningful, but because such data have important policy implications.

A number of researchers have made the point that race and ethnicity, like sex, must be understood as a matter of social experience (Smaje 2000). Social experience has powerful structural and psychological effects that translate into significant health consequences. While race in and of itself has relatively little effect on health, the social consequences of being identified as belonging to a particular race, or sex or age group for that matter, may have important effects on a person's health. In short, race as biology cannot explain why blacks experience excess mortality and morbidity. Racial discrimination or racism, which has practical as well as psychosocial ramifications, provides a far more powerful explanation.

Let's explore that idea a little further. The conventional wisdom says that racism, like poverty, has been largely overcome. It holds that members of minorities do not experience nearly as much racism now as they did prior to all the legislation that struck down segregation and other forms of discrimination. There is evidence to suggest that the reality is just the opposite. Let's consider the evidence.

As we have already seen, a smaller percentage of blacks are poor now than was true in the past. That clearly supports the idea that increasing numbers of blacks are better off across a range of indicators—income, college enrollment, occupational advancement, and so on. Does this mean that we are seeing a decline in racial discrimination? A review of attitudes surveys conducted in this country between 1963 and 1995 may surprise you.

Trend analysis of the attitudes expressed by white Americans with regard to racial inequality as recorded by the Gallup Organization and other surveys from 1963 through 1995 indicates that there has been a significant change in social attitudes (Schuman and Krysan 1999). In 1963, 43 percent of whites said that whites were to blame for the disadvantages blacks were facing; 19 percent said blacks themselves were to blame. By 1995, the percentage of whites who said that whites were to blame dropped to 14 percent; the percentage who said that it was blacks themselves who were to blame rose to 56 percent.

This clearly constitutes a dramatic shift. No one argues that it can fully account for the health disadvantages blacks face. However, it obviously has social consequences. Indeed, the trend in social attitudes has recently shifted in the opposite direction from what the conventional wisdom tells us about racial tolerance in this country. The Barack Obama presidential campaign had the effect of bringing the topic much closer to the center of public discourse. That produced a number of media surveys. The results of a survey conducted on March 19, 2008, by CBS found that 42 percent of those polled said that racism is a serious problem, compared to 10 percent who felt that way about sexism (United Press International 2008).

In the end, the literature we have reviewed here has the effect of raising more questions than providing clear answers. That simply means we will have to keep looking for a more complete answer by considering these questions from the perspective provided by other variables. Maybe it is neither poverty nor race. Maybe it's people's behavior or lifestyle that offers a better explanation for variations in mortality. In that case, race and poverty may be implicated as factors underlying certain learned habits and practices. Behavior related to health is the subject of the following chapter.

CHAPTER SIX

~

Lifestyle and Health Behavior

We have long known that our lifestyle is a major factor determining how healthy we are. What has changed is that we are now able to determine exactly how the specific behaviors we engage in are affecting our health because a number of easily accessible tools have come into existence to tell us that. Dr. Michael Roizen was certainly not the first to argue that some of the things we are doing are damaging our health, but he was undoubtedly the first to receive so much attention for attaching numbers, as in months of life lost, to those activities. It all started with his 1999 book entitled *Real Age: Are You As Young As You Can Be?* Since then he established a corporation, RealAge Inc., which offers sixty-five health tests and tools on his Internet site so that one can not only personalize one's understanding of one's real age, but figure out what to do to become healthier. The basic instrument he created tells people how to calculate the number of months of life they are losing due to their behavior both because of the things they do (e.g., eat fatty foods) and things they don't do (e.g., exercise). There are now many competitors with books of their own. Also, some health insurance companies and associations dedicated to increasing awareness of specific diseases are introducing their own versions of such an instrument. A more direct, main-stream application of this idea has been adopted by British doctors who use a lung function test that calculates the patient's "lung age" to show how much damage smoking is doing, in an effort to convince patients to quit smoking (Parkes et al. 2008). This is obviously a growing phenomenon.

The question such developments raise is—why is it that so many people visit all these websites but not nearly as many follow all the advice the sites offer for achieving a longer and healthier life? The answer is not that complicated. Let's face it—it is difficult to resist the temptation to indulge in all that delicious-looking, rich, and comforting food that we are enticed with by slick and sophisticated advertising campaigns. Exercise is hard work and time consuming. Flossing is boring. And so on. Besides, aren't we all basically convinced that those love handles and thunder thighs are due to our genes and impossible to alter anyway? Indeed, there is some evidence that it is our genes after all. We will get to that bit of evidence later in the chapter.

That brings us to the basic question we will be discussing here. How much of what we hear about healthy behavior is based on evidence and how much of it is based on conventional wisdom? This chapter reviews recent research findings on the impact of lifestyle and behavior choices on health. It focuses more specifically on the following topics: smoking, exercise, and diet. We will also examine briefly the relationship between religion and health, which may not strike you as "behavior," but seems to fit into this chapter better than into other chapters. We will relate this information to the three basic demographic variables we have examined thus far, namely, age, sex, and race. Our ultimate aim, remember, is to identify factors that will explain variation in mortality and morbidity. The chapter begins by discussing why health behavior receives so much attention these days.

One explanation for why we are hearing so much more about what we should be doing to improve our health is attributable to the shift in disease patterns, that is, the shift from infectious illness to chronic illness. In contrast to infectious illness, the negative effects associated with chronic illness are either reduced or aggravated by certain behaviors. There is often not that much that can be done to slow down the progress of chronic illness except lifestyle change.

Advice on Health Behavior

While there have been many expositions on the effect of behavior on health over the years, there are two that stand out. One is the 1974 book by Victor Fuchs, *Who Shall Live?* Fuchs, a health economist, compared the lifestyles and health indicators of the population of Nevada and Utah. There is no question that people in Utah came across looking a lot healthier than people in Nevada. According to Fuchs, this was because the residents of Utah were living orderly lives, did not smoke, drink, gamble, get divorced, leave family and friends to move to a place where they would not know anyone, and so on.

The other person who had a major impact was John Knowles, an MD who was then the head of the Rockefeller Foundation. In his 1977 book entitled *Doing Better, Feeling Worse*, he stated that health is largely a matter of individual responsibility. He did say that society has some responsibility too, but that part of his argument was overshadowed by his assertion that 99 percent of us are born healthy (Knowles 1977). He argued that those who followed the seven basic health habits he identified would enjoy better health. He developed a list of recommended health habits based on some early conclusions reached by researchers who were analyzing data gathered in Alameda County, which encompasses Oakland, California (1977). By the end of the chapter we will consider more recent interpretations of the research findings that come from this database. For now, let's focus on the health habits Knowles recommended more than three decades ago: (1) three meals a day at regular times and no snacking, (2) breakfast every day, (3) moderate exercise two or three times a week, (4) adequate sleep (seven or eight hours a night), (5) no smoking, (6) moderate weight, and (7) no alcohol, or only in moderation.

How could anyone object to this list? Those who were critical of it at the time pointed out that such advice reflects a middle-class bias regarding how one should live. They pointed out that people who did not have steady nine-to-five jobs would have trouble following this advice. As increasing numbers of people have jobs that do not fit that description, we are finding that eating, sleeping, and exercising on a regular schedule may be difficult for an even greater number of people. The only thing on the list that has changed since the time it was announced is the advice on snacking, which is no longer considered objectionable. The idea that 99 percent of us are born healthy drew considerably more criticism.

Advice on improving one's health has always been around. The topic is undoubtedly receiving more attention of late because entrepreneurs are continually introducing us to new products that they claim will assist us in our efforts to improve our health behavior. There are products to help us lose weight by following somebody's special diet book or buying the recommended foods; quit smoking with the assistance of various gums, patches, and so on; shape up by joining a health club, et cetera. In the past, we were more likely to simply be told to rely on the strength of our character to shape up. Much of the behavior that Knowles and Fuchs recommended was already familiar to most people. Even before they wrote, people from childhood on were advised not to overindulge, not to go out in cold without buttoning up, and to get enough rest. On the other hand, people growing up during the 1950s were also told to finish everything on their plates because there were starving children in Europe or China or wherever. (Don't try to figure out the logic—people couldn't explain it then either.) Mothers were advised to serve meat three times a day to insure that everyone in the family was getting enough protein. Soldiers were given cigarettes as part of their army rations during the war because smoking was said to have a calming effect. They got into the habit of smoking at an early age and found it hard to quit later, even as everyone joked about cigarettes being "coffin nails." It was not until the surgeon general issued his report in 1964, definitively stating that cigarettes cause cancer, that people started taking the joke seriously. In other words, people were as likely to be exposed to bad advice as good.

Personally, I am not so sure things have gotten that much better. It is just that we are now getting our advice from sources other than family members, most notably, from various so-called experts willing to be interviewed by the media and from individuals whose expertise is not always made explicit over the Internet. There is also the problem of persons with respected scientific credentials telling us about risks, then turning around and changing their minds. Not long ago, we were told to stop eating eggs because eggs increased cholesterol; then we heard that it wasn't the eggs at all but all the fatty meats we were eating alongside them. We were told that aluminum foil causes Alzheimer's disease; later we were told that was a mistake. We were advised to take zinc to reduce symptoms when we have a cold, even though others were telling us that there is no clear evidence that zinc does any good. We continue to be advised to take megadoses of various vitamins and minerals, while hearing warnings that this could be damaging.

Coffee provides an excellent current example of the problem with advice on health behavior—it may lower the risk of developing type 2 diabetes, the risk of Parkinson's disease, and gout; it is a source of healthful anti-inflammatory and antioxidant compounds; but, it may increase the risk of rheumatoid arthritis, produce headaches, aggravate various gastrointestinal problems, and so on. It seems that even when there are good data, we still have to deal with very mixed messages.

There is a similar argument going on with reference to the value of vitamin D. Recent research indicates that vitamin D deficiency is related to heart disease and possibly breast cancer, but other studies have not come up with the same results (Wang et al. 2008). Careful monitoring of blood sugar, which has been the primary piece of advice doctors could give to patients at risk of diabetes, turns out to be of questionable value. In short, every day brings new information that seems produce more questions than answers.

Given how confusing all this information is, it is not surprising when we hear people say they suspect that medical researchers and pharmaceutical companies are denying the benefits of alternative medicines to keep us from making ourselves healthy because that would put a dent in their incomes.

Let's consider the most recent evidence on the most commonly discussed risk-producing health behaviors with the understanding that researchers will very likely continue to come up with newer, more refined measures and findings, with the potential of turning around what we now think is fact.

Smoking

According to a 2006 statement issued by the CDC, tobacco remains the leading preventable cause of death. The numbers are staggering. Smoking causes an estimated 438,000 deaths per year, or about one out of every five deaths; if current trends continue, twenty-five million Americans will die prematurely from smoking-related illnesses; on average smokers die fourteen years earlier than nonsmokers; for every death, there are twenty more people living with smoking-related illnesses. (Unless otherwise indicated, all references to CDC data on smoking come from CDC fact sheets, which provide citations.)

The good news is that there has been a huge decline in the number of people who smoke in this country over the last four decades. The bad news is that the decline may have stalled. The most recent estimate based on the 2006 National Health Interview Survey indicates that 20.8 percent of Americans smoke—that is, about forty-five million. Statistics on smoking are generally tracked back to 1965, the year that the surgeon general issued the first major warning on the health risks associated with smoking. As you will recall, we did not begin collecting statistics on other racial and ethnic groups until the 1980s. So we only have data for blacks and whites going as far back as 1965.

Table 6.1 tells us that the percentage of people who were smoking in 2006 is about half of the percentage who smoked in 1965. The percentage of males who smoked in 1965 was considerably higher than the percentage of females. The percentage of females who smoke currently is only slightly smaller than the percentage of males who smoke. As of 2006, black males between the ages of forty-five and sixty-four were the most likely to smoke (at 33 percent) and black females between the ages of eighteen and twenty-four were the least likely to smoke (at 15 percent). (There has been a very sharp increase over the last five years in the percentage of black men ages eighteen to twenty-four smoking, from around 20 percent to 31 percent. This may be a temporary aberration that does not require much attention or it may be an indicator of a significant change that does demand further investigation.)

Table 6.1. Smoking by Percentage of Persons 18 Years of Age and Over in 1965 and 2006

	1965	2006		1965	2006
All persons	42	21			
All males	51	23	All females	34	18
White	50	24	White	34	19
18–24 years	53	29	18–24 years	38	21
35–44 years	57	26	35–44 years	44	22
Black	59	26	Black	32	19
18–24 years	63	31	18–24 years	37	15
35–44 years	67	22	35–44 years	43	21

Source: *Health, United States, 2008,* Table 63: Current Cigarette Smoking Among Adults 18 Years of Age and Over, by Sex, Race, and Age: United States, Selected Years 1965–2006.

The rate of smoking among other racial/ethnic groups has not been tracked in the past. Table 65 in *Health, United States, 2008,* reports the average rate of cigarette smoking for the 2004–2006 period by race, ethnicity, and education. We find that the rate of smoking among those who identify themselves as belonging to two or more races is far higher than it is for other categories, at 35.5 percent for males and 33.1 percent for females. This is in contrast to the lowest reported rate among Asian females, which is 5.2 percent; 18.1 percent of Asian males smoke. Everyone else comes closer to the average rate, which is 18.4 percent over the 2004–2006 period. By education, we find the highest rate of smoking among whites with no high school diploma—40.8 percent; and blacks at 30.3 percent. By contrast, only 15 percent of whites and 13.3 percent of blacks who have some college or more smoke. This is in contrast to the 9.5 percent rate among Hispanics who have no high school diploma and the 10.6 percent rate among those who have some college. I have seen no discussion of these clearly odd patterns.

Obviously, what explains the variation in smoking behavior is not clearly understood. There is some evidence that negative external factors, such as an unsafe neighborhood or personal physical trauma, increase the likelihood of smoking (Ganz 2000). The health consequences of smoking and of quitting are, however, unmistakable.

Based on an examination of nearly nine hundred thousand respondents to the Cancer Prevention Study II, there is a significant increase in life expectancy attributable to smoking cessation (Taylor et al. 2002). Male smokers who quit at age thirty-five gained 6.9 to 8.5 years; women gained 6.1 to 7.7 years. Those who quit at younger ages gained more. Those who quit at age sixty-five gained, but gained less. A review of 665 publications showed a 36 percent reduction of risk of death from heart disease from quitting (Critchley and Capewell 2003). The benefits of quitting appear quickly. Researchers find that quitting at least a month before certain forms of cardiac surgery results in considerably less angina (crushing chest pain) after surgery (Haddock et al. 2003). What is particularly troubling is finding that people with tobacco-related chronic illness are more likely to continue smoking than those who are not sick (Stapleton 2007).

The CDC estimates that smoking increases the risk of death from twenty-three causes (GAO 2003). The most common smoking-related deaths in 2005 were: lung cancer (124,000), heart disease (108,000), and chronic lung diseases of emphysema, bronchitis, and chronic airway obstruction (90,000). Smoking is also implicated in cancers of the bladder, oral cavity, pharynx, larynx, esophagus, cervix, kidney, lung, pancreas, and stomach, and causes acute myeloid leukemia.

According to a 2009 CDC report, the risk of dying from lung cancer is more than twenty-three times higher for men who smoke than it is for those who do not smoke. More striking is finding that the risk of lung cancer for women who smoke is thirteen times higher than it is for men. Because a steadily increasing number of women began to smoke during the second half of the twentieth century, female deaths from lung cancer increased as well—by more than 600 percent between 1950 and 2005. By 1987, lung cancer had surpassed breast cancer as the leading cause of cancer-related death. It is worth noting that smoking has effects for women that men do not experience; it increases their risk of infertility and preterm delivery, as well as stillbirth, low birth weight, and sudden infant death syndrome (SIDS) for their children. Menopausal women who smoked earlier in life have lower bone density and are therefore at increased risk for hip fractures.

There are a number of other intriguing findings related to childbearing that have attracted attention. It seems that prenatal smoking increases the risk of antisocial behavior in the offspring and it is even possible that it is a risk factor for serious mental illness (Wakschlag et al. 2002). Then there is this finding: "A child whose grandmother smoked during pregnancy may have almost twice the risk of developing asthma as one whose grandmother did not smoke—even if the child's mother was a nonsmoker." (Bakalar 2005). The researchers explained that a mother's smoking may alter the mitochondrial DNA, which is the genetic inheritance that is transferred only through the mother.

There are also racial differences. Based on a study of differences in the risk of lung cancer among 183,813 people, researchers found that African Americans and Native Hawaiians are more susceptible to lung cancer than whites, Japanese Americans, and Latinos (Haiman et al. 2006). Part of the explanation for the differential effects comes from the National Institute on Drug Abuse (NIDA). NIDA researchers have found that, while black teens smoke fewer cigarettes per day, 15.1 versus 19.6 for white teenagers, they exhibit similar levels of cotinine (the product formed by the body from nicotine) concentrate and similar levels of nicotine dependence (NIDA 2006). It is possible that this is due to the preference that African Americans have for menthol cigarettes, which may be more addictive (Harvard School of Public Health 2005).

The health costs to individuals are obvious. There are also broader social costs of cigarette smoking. The most comprehensive initial attempt to calculate the costs, presented in 1993 by the Congressional Office of Technology Assessment (COT), a governmental agency created to advise Congress on matters that require accurate technical information, estimated that the cost was $2.59 per pack of cigarettes (MacKenzie, Bartecchi, and Schrier 1994). The COT used three sets of calculations to come up with this figure. First, costs to employer: work absence at 6.5 days per year more than nonsmokers—decreased productivity, plus the increased cost due to health-care claims. Second, costs to society as a whole were calculated on the basis of lost productivity due to premature death ($47 billion per year in 1990) and loss of productivity due to passive smoking ($8.6 billion in 1990). The cost of fires caused by smoking materials was estimated at $552 million in direct property damage. The report went on to say that none of this takes into consideration the social-psychological as well as financial costs sustained by family members of the person who develops a smoking-related disease and dies from it. Finally, as the cost of cigarettes increases, "opportunity costs" (the lost opportunity to use the money for something else) become more significant. Maybe that money could be used to buy healthier foods and make other consumer products that enhance one's standard of living, from air conditioners to running shoes.

The CDC released an updated assessment of the social costs associated with smoking in 2002 (Landers 2002). By its calculations, each pack of cigarettes sold resulted in $7.18 in medical care costs and lost productivity. That is more than $150 billion per year between 1995 and 1998, a figure that is not only higher than previously thought but more than the estimates used in the landmark tobacco settlement, which we will get to shortly.

Secondhand Smoke
The National Institutes of Health's National Toxicology Program's Report on Carcinogens lists "environmental tobacco smoke" (ETS), or second-

hand smoke, as a Group A carcinogen, which means that it is known to cause cancer in humans. According to the National Cancer Institute (a unit within the National Institutes of Health), about half of secondhand smoke comes from the end of a cigarette, cigar, or pipe. This is called side-stream smoke. The smoke that is exhaled by a smoker is called mainstream smoke. The consensus is that ETS causes about thirty-five thousand deaths from heart disease and about three thousand lung cancer deaths among adult nonsmokers.

A full analysis of the chemicals that are in tobacco and those that are added to tobacco has not been completed. According to the National Cancer Institute, about four thousand chemicals have been identified in tobacco smoke, but there may be more than one hundred thousand. Of the chemicals that have been identified, sixty are known carcinogens. How do we know that these chemicals are affecting us? Exposure is measurable as the level of cotinine present in the body.

The fact that secondhand smoke constitutes a serious health risk is something the tobacco industry was fully aware of for decades. The documents uncovered by the lawsuit launched against the tobacco industry by forty-six state attorney generals, which resulted in the Master Settlement Agreement of 1997, revealed not only what the tobacco industry knew about the health risks associated with smoking, but what it did to make sure that the public did not learn about those risks both in this country and in other countries. The settlement had the effect of making thirty-two million pages of material open to public scrutiny:

> In 1978, a confidential study for the US Tobacco Institute concluded that public concern about second-hand smoke (ETS) and "passive smoking" was "the most dangerous threat to the viability of the tobacco industry that has yet occurred." (Ong and Glantz 2000, 1254)

The tobacco companies had not been concerned about the potential decline in smoking in Europe until the European coalition of researchers associated with the International Agency for Research on Cancer (IARC), a branch of the World Health Organization, reported that they found a 16 percent increase in lung cancer among nonsmokers in 1998 (Ong and Glantz 2000). Philip Morris wasted no time, taking on the task of spearheading a strategy to counter the agency's findings by devoting $2 million to the effort to shape public opinion and up to $4 million on research.

We know that the rate of smoking has been declining. One fascinating piece of research on smoking cessation tells us that people tend not to quit smoking on an individual basis. They tend to quit in clusters (Christakis and Fowler 2008). It seems that people who are more educated quit earlier, which is not particularly surprising. Those who continue to smoke, whether they are well educated or not, are increasingly being marginalized. Recognizing that they are being pushed farther from the center of the group to which they belonged in the past may give them added motivation to quit on an individual basis.

How much of the litigation that produced the 1997 legal settlement contributed to the decline is less clear. The settlement required the states to drop pending legislation in return for $200 billion to be divided among the forty-six states that were party to the suit. The public health benefits were not as great as expected because most states failed to devote most of the money to efforts designed to reduce smoking. Estimates by the CDC indicate that the 10 percent increase in the price of a pack of cigarettes that took place as a result of the settlement led to a 9 to 15 percent decrease in smoking among adolescents, but only a 3 to 5 percent decrease among adults. It also produced less than the predicted effect on prenatal smoking, which declined by half of what was expected (Levy and Meara 2006).

There is good reason to think that the smoking saga has not ended. The decline in smoking very likely still has a way to go considering that the price of cigarettes continues to increase, states continue to pass laws expanding tobacco-free space, and insurance companies entice nonsmokers to give it up by offering lower insurance premiums to nonsmokers. Also, the effects of a lawsuit filed by six individuals in Florida who were awarded $145 billion in 2007 have not been fully realized (Vernick, Rutkow, and Teret 2007). States attorneys may have agreed not to sue; individuals made no such commitment. Thus, the tobacco industry may still have to deal with innumerable suits, filed by individuals, with unpredictable outcomes but with the certainty of high costs to the industry.

If you are still not convinced that smoking will kill you and that the tobacco companies know it, consider a widely reported story regarding the argument presented by one tobacco company in support of smoking (USA Today 2001). The Philip Morris Tobacco Company came up with the following argument in trying to discourage the Czech government from instituting an antismoking policy. Philip Morris calculated that the Czech government saved $30 million in 1999 thanks to the "indirect positive effect" of smoking. In other words, the government benefited from the premature deaths of people who smoked, saving the government money that it would have otherwise had to spend on health care, pensions, and other social payments.

When the story was leaked to the press, the president of Philip Morris confirmed that the story was true.

Diet and Weight

Obesity is now considered to be "epidemic" in the United States. According to a Rand Corporation analysis of the Behavioral Risk Factor Surveillance Survey conducted by the CDC, which includes 1.5 million people, the proportion of Americans who are one hundred pounds or more overweight has increased by 50 percent from 2000 to 2005 (RAND 2007). The method for estimating this is based on evaluating the relationship between weight and height using the Body Mass Index (BMI) calculation to assess body fat. The BMI is calculated as weight in kilograms divided by height in meters squared. According to the National Heart, Lung, and Blood Institute (NHLBI), a BMI of between 25 and 29.9 is overweight, 30 to 34.9 is mildly obese (class 1), 35 to 39.9 is moderately obese (class 2), and 40 or higher is extremely or "morbidly" obese (class 3).

According to a study by researchers at the Rand Corporation released in April 2007, the proportion of Americans with a BMI of 30 or more increased by 24 percent from 2000 to 2005; those with a BMI of 40 or more increased by 50 percent; and those with a BMI of 50 or more increased by 75 percent. A more recent assessment by Harvard Medical School researchers indicates that BMI may not be the best indicator of future health problems. Waist size, they say, serves as a much more accurate predictor of hypertension, diabetes, and elevated cholesterol—all factors related to the increased risk of heart disease (Levitan et al. 2009; Lee et al. 2008).

The morbidly obese are candidates for antiobesity surgery. The American Society for Bariatric Surgery reported that 177,600 weight-loss surgeries were performed in 2006, quadruple the number performed in 2000.

Obesity is spreading across all age groups, races, and educational levels; it affects both sexes; and is occurring regardless of smoking behavior. Some researchers have determined that the health effects of obesity are roughly comparable to twenty years of aging, which greatly exceeds what smoking and problem drinking do to a person's health (Sturm 2002). The morbidly obese have a two-fold greater risk of all-cause mortality than those who are less obese. In fact, according to the CDC, being obese or overweight increases the risk of many diseases, including the following: high blood pressure, type 2 diabetes, coronary heart disease, stroke, gallbladder disease, sleep apnea and respiratory problems, and osteoarthritis (degeneration of cartilage and underlying bone). The link between obesity and cancer is now well established.

A review of all existing studies—a meta-analysis—of the relationship be-tween obesity and cancer concludes that there is no question that increased BMI is directly associated with the increased risk of cancer (Renehan et al. 2008). These conclusions are consistent with the findings of a 2003 study which was considered to be the most comprehensive assessment prior to this time. In that case, researchers tracked a population of nine hundred thousand adults who were free of cancer in 1982 for sixteen years (Calle et al. 2003, 1634). They concluded that current patterns of obesity and over-weight "could account for 14 percent of all deaths from cancer among men and 20 percent of those in women." They report that the heaviest men had a cancer mortality rate 52 percent higher than men of normal weight; the heaviest women had a 62 percent higher mortality rate. They estimated that ninety thousand deaths due to cancer could be prevented each year if people maintained a normal weight.

Where a person carries excess fat is an important consideration. Abdomi-nal fat is more closely associated with heart disease and colon cancer than lower-body fat, which accumulates on the hips (Steptoe and Wardle 2005). Men tend to have more abdominal fat, and have a higher incidence of both heart disease and colon cancer. Women tend to have lower-body fat, which is apparently less detrimental. At the same time, at least some of the weight gain that occurs during adulthood for both sexes tends to accumulate in the abdominal region and does pose a risk factor. According to an article in the online American Academy of Neurology journal, those who have larger stomachs during their forties are also more likely to have dementia in their seventies (American Academy of Neurology 2008). Not surprisingly, those whose BMI is over 30 are also more likely to be burdened by disability (Gregg and Guralnick 2007).

So who determines the standards for what is considered overweight and obese? Who created the weight standards to begin with? Would you be surprised to hear that the standards have historically been set by insurance companies? The initial standard was set by the Metropolitan Life Insurance Company in 1959. It was revised in 1983 and again in 1990. The most re-cently promulgated standards, announced in 1998, come from the NHLBI. Does everyone go along? Not at all. Researchers used the Alameda County database to test the proposition that keeping weight down to NHLBI stan-dards would result in lower mortality levels. (This is the same database used by John Knowles to develop the seven basic health habits that we discussed earlier in this chapter.) The latter group of researchers concluded that the NHLBI set standards that were too extreme and too stigmatizing. Spokesper-sons for various organizations that have reason to be interested in weight, including the AHA, ACS, and Weight Watchers, have also made it clear that they reject the NHLBI's standards. The debate has not had the effect of altering the NHLBI's announced standards.

Deciding What to Eat

There is plenty of advice on eating to achieve a range of objectives—to lose weight, reduce the risk of various potential diseases, prolong life, and so on. Sorting out the advice is not so easy.

A bit of advice that most people heard when they were growing up was that it was important to eat breakfast. Of course, during the 1950s everyone was advised to eat meat for breakfast as well as for lunch and dinner. Now the advice is to eat fiber-rich foods, and there is some evidence that this actually makes a difference. Apparently children and adolescents who eat such a breakfast put on fewer unwanted pounds (Bakalar 2008).

The question of how much fat we should have in our diets is a constant point of debate. If Americans are cutting down the amount of fat that they are eating, and we cannot be sure they are, they are apparently responding to the unceasing admonition to eat more low-fat products by eating a lot more of those products. Maybe eating a low-fat diet is not the answer. While it may bring about weight loss, that is not the same as saying an unbalanced diet such as this is good for one's health.

Similarly, some popular diets such as the Atkins diet, while they do allow fats, recommend very low or no consumption of carbohydrates. The essence of the argument for maintaining a low-carbohydrate, high-protein diet is that carbohydrates are absorbed quickly, meaning that carbohydrate calories turn to body fat unless they are used up quickly. Protein takes much longer to absorb, and makes us feel full during that time, meaning that the calories that come from protein are less likely to turn into body fat.

Many experts say that promotion of both high-protein and low-fat diets must be tempered. They say that eating a little more fat (as the high-protein diets recommend) or more carbs (as the low-fat diets allow) would be okay if we would only consume a lot less in total of everything we eat. Does this perspective explain why the French, who eat all that rich food, but only in small amounts, do not get fat? Of course, they too, as is true of all Europeans, have been getting fatter in recent years, according to the International Obesity Task Force, a coalition of European researchers and institutions.

The whole point of reducing one's consumption of fat is to reduce the risk of heart disease, cancer, and other diseases. However, things get complicated when we find that reducing one's consumption of fat is not the simple solution that we thought it was. According to researchers who followed the health status of forty-nine thousand women over eight years, those who were assigned to a low-fat diet had the same rates of breast cancer, colon cancer, heart attacks, and strokes as those who ate anything they pleased (Prentice et al. 2006). The matter has not been settled to the satisfaction of the scientific community, since other researchers find that severe caloric restriction does confer a reduction in risk of breast cancer (Michels and Ekbom 2004).

Animal research consistently reveals that reduced total caloric intake not only prolongs life but reduces the risk of disease over all those extra years. People who have chosen to follow a similar regimen end up being the subjects of TV specials because they are so unusual as to be exotic. Thus far, we know they expect to live a very long time, but, of course, we don't know if their expectations will be fulfilled. In fact, given recent findings, not only are these people living with the discomfort of being hungry a good bit of the time, they may actually be decreasing their chances of longevity. A recent study tracking the association between BMI and mortality reveals that it is not only the obese who have a greater risk of dying. The researchers reported finding that those who are underweight, that is, have a BMI of 18.5 or under, are also at higher risk of dying (Flegal et al. 2007). It is just that those who are underweight are less likely to die from cancer than those who are overweight or obese. The majority of researchers agree that maintaining a normal weight offers the best chance of good health.

There is also some evidence to indicate that people are more likely to become obese when their friends and relatives become obese (Christakis and Fowler 2007). Can this be seen as a kind of unconscious willingness to share what is generally considered to be an undesirable trait? The same researchers told us that people quit smoking in clusters. It seems that close ties to others are generally considered to be a good thing, but—nothing is perfect—and in this case we find close ties having negative health consequences.

The Dietary Approaches to Stop Hypertension (DASH) diet has been receiving more attention from researchers in recent years because the evidence of its positive impact on health keeps growing. The diet, which is low in animal fat, moderate in low-fat dairy products, and high in plant protein, has been shown to reduce blood pressure and "bad" cholesterol, thereby reducing the risk of both heart disease and stroke (Fung et al. 2008). Those with high DASH scores also have lower C-reactive protein and interleukin 6 scores, which are markers of inflammation that have been associated with a number of different diseases. Almost everyone who studies the impact of diet on hypertension notes that people who have high blood pressure are generally not following a healthy diet.

Another finding that has been receiving greater attention over the last few years concerns the value of vitamin D. It seems that the "sunshine vitamin" (you get vitamin D from sunlight) may serve as a cancer preventive, particularly in the case of lung cancer. According to a 2004 NIH conference of experts, we should be getting increasing amounts of vitamin D as we age. The conference concluded that vitamin D may also be a player in preventing autoimmune diseases including type 1 diabetes, multiple sclerosis, arthritis, and persistent, nonspecific bone and muscle pain (Landers 2004).

Then there is the mystery of why there are people who can eat all kinds of rich and fattening foods and not gain weight. Based on the Framingham Heart Study findings, the "participants who possess the APOA5-1131C gene did not gain weight if they had more fat in their diet. Thirteen percent of the population carries this variation" (Elliott 2007, 32). So the other 87 percent of us have finally had our suspicions confirmed and can now trot out the explanation that it is our genes that are causing us to be a little chubby, right?

Further evidence that being overweight is a matter of inheritance comes from a study initiated in 1959, designed to determine whether losing weight shrinks the size of fat cells or reduces their number, which revealed a lot more—namely, that fat cells shrink but do not go away (Kolata 2007). It also revealed that the subjects whose diets were being severely restricted so they would lose weight did lose weight at the cost of having their metabolism react as if they were starving. Their fat cells shrank but did not decrease in number. Once the study ended, most went back to their previous weight. Those who maintained a lower weight did so only by tolerating the discomfort of feeling starved. By contrast, people of normal weight who agreed to eat enormous amounts of food to see if their fat cells increased in number did gain a lot of weight but lost it within a short time after the study, with no increase in the number of fat cells.

Our attitude about obesity may be best expressed in the fact that liposuction is the most popular form of cosmetic surgery. According to one estimate, "doctors vacuum out something like two million pounds of fat from the thighs, bellies, buttocks, jowls and man-breasts of 325,000 people a year" (Angier 2007, D1). After doing this procedure for so many years, doctors have recently been surprised to discover that instead of being merely a dumping ground for the excess calories, the fat or adipose tissue that is being removed apparently operates as an endocrine organ secreting "at least 20 different hormones." Whether interfering with the functions that fat performs by removing it is more detrimental than leaving the fat in place is not clear. Even more interesting is finding that fat tissue begins to resist additional growth by releasing inflammatory hormones once one is about twenty-five pounds above one's ideal weight even if one continues to overeat. This function operates as a regulatory mechanism in the short run. However, if the inflammatory hormones continue to be released, the function becomes detrimental to one's health in the long run.

A small number of commentators have become concerned about all the attention being devoted to the rise of the prevalence of obesity. They note that obesity is certainly a problem, but the level of concern about being overweight has gone too far. Image, they say, is the primary concern, not health status. We, as a society, are exhibiting intolerance of whatever is currently deemed to be nonacceptable weight and stigmatizing those people as lacking in self-control. That induces stress. The culture supports the obsession with thinness, especially among young women, which can lead to other kinds of unhealthy behaviors, such as anorexia and bulimia.

Considering the standards of beauty young women are presented with in our society, it is not surprising to find that anywhere from 50 percent to 75 percent of adolescent girls are dissatisfied with their bodies. A study of Miss America pageant winners from 1922 through 1999 indicates that winners' height increased by less than 2 percent while weight decreased by 12 percent. The authors of the paper on this study concluded that the imagery is promoting an "ideal of female undernutrition" (Rubenstein and Caballero 2000).

The Economic Implications

Obesity at the individual level is clearly predictive of a range of health problems that will not only detract from the person's quality of life but from his or her pocketbook too. The economic implications for society have not received much attention until the last ten years or so. Thus when the estimates on cost started coming in, it was something of a surprise. The most comprehensive assessment of the cost of treating people whose illnesses are the result of excess weight was estimated to be $78.5 billion in 1998; translated into 2002 dollars, the estimate was or $92.6 billion (Finkelstein, Fiebelkorn, and Wang 2003). According to a report by the Agency for Healthcare Research and Quality (AHRQ), "the nation could save nearly $2.5 billion a year by preventing hospitalizations due to severe diabetes complications" (AHRQb 2005). Since the proportion of people becoming overweight and obese continues to rise, the amount that we are spending continues to increase as well.

According to the Government Accountability Office, uninsured children treated for obesity are approximately three times more expensive to treat than the average insured child (GAO-07-260R 2006). Those who are uninsured and presumably not being treated are of course at much greater risk of developing illnesses as adults, which will certainly make the costs of treating them much higher. Some states have begun to tax soft drinks since soft drinks are thought to be one of the primary culprits in childhood obesity, apart from lack of exercise (O'Reilly 2006a).

It seems that while weight loss may be good for us as individuals, it is not equally good for the bottom line of the country's health-care dollar. The irony is that people who watch their weight will live longer and that will result in higher expenditures for health care as they age and develop chronic illnesses that are unrelated to being overweight (van Baal et al. 2008).

Since we collect data on the basis of race and ethnicity, let us look at how much race matters. For persons twenty years and over, the percentages of overweight and obese persons are as follows for 2003–2006 (*Health, United States*, 2008, table 75).

- 57.4% of white females   72.1% of white males
- 74.4% of Mexican females   77.3% of Mexican males
- 80.5% of black females   72.0% of black males

When we look at how much socioeconomic status matters, we find that the measure being used is poverty status (under 100 percent, 100 to 200 percent, and 200 percent and over) reveals very little difference and even a reverse relationship to obesity compared to what most of the literature we have discussed so far would lead us to expect, that is, that poorer people are more likely to be overweight. This is undoubtedly due to the fact that the measure of socioeconomic status is not very precise. Studies that use a more exact measure do find a clear relationship between poverty and obesity. Researchers who tracked weight gain over a thirty-four-year period in the Alameda County study confirm this. They also found that lifetime poverty has a cumulative effect that is associated with excess weight regardless of race and ethnicity (Baltrus et al. 2005). We have no data on obesity by educational level for all Americans.

Exercise

The topic of exercise has been overshadowed by the concern about the rising rate of obesity. Of course the two topics are related, it is just that we are not hearing nearly as much about exercise as a separate topic as we did a decade ago. Statistics on leisure activity for 2006 are as follows (*Health, United States*, 2008, table 74). Among men ages eighteen to forty-four, about 35 percent say that they engage in regular leisure exercise; about 32 percent of females of the same age say that. Using race and ethnicity as the distinguishing variable, we see the following rates of exercise:

- whites at about 32%;
- American Indians or Alaskan Natives as well as Asians at about 30%;
- blacks at about 25%;
- Hispanics at about 23%.

By poverty status, we find that only 20.6 percent of those who fall under 100 percent of poverty engage in exercise, but that 34.8 percent of those who are over 200 percent poverty exercise. The differences by educational level reveal a clearer gradient—rising level of exercise with rising level of education.

- 16.5% of those with no high school diploma exercise;
- 23.5% of those with a high school diploma exercise;
- 37.6% of those with some college or more exercise.

The evidence that exercise has a positive impact on cardiovascular health is overwhelming and well established. Not only does a high level of physical fitness reduce the risk of heart disease, it reduces the risk of mortality from all causes (Stofan et al. 1998). The results of epidemiological studies, as well as experimental studies, have established the benefits of exercise in reducing the risk of heart disease, osteoporosis, and certain cancers.

While most researchers have found a strong relationship between "all cause mortality" and exercise, there was less agreement on how much exercise is necessary to benefit health until 1995 (Blair et al. 1989; Paffenbarger et al. 1993; Lee, Hsich, and Paffenbarger 1995). The question was largely settled when the CDC together with the American College of Sports Medicine issued a combined statement on guidelines for physical activity, saying that significant benefit could be achieved through moderate exercise for thirty minutes per day (Pate et al. 1995). The following year, the NIH issued a consensus statement based on an extensive literature review and discussion among a panel of twenty-seven experts also recommending thirty minutes of moderate exercise per day. The panel noted that additional benefit would be gained from more vigorous exercise (NIH 1996).

There has also been some debate about the extent to which reduction in smoking contributes to the reduction in heart disease regardless of level of exercise (Lee, Hsich, and Paffenbarger 1995; Paffenbarger et al. 1993; Blair et al. 1989). Much of that research reflects findings on men's health. This was followed up with research on women's health. The researchers concluded that light to moderate exercise is associated with lower risk of heart disease, and what is especially surprising is that this is true even for those who smoke, are overweight, and have a high cholesterol level (Lee et al. 2001). The literature on women's health generally also emphasizes the psychological benefits of exercise, which have been found to produce increased self-confidence and lower levels of anxiety and depression (Fletcher et al. 1996).

What about all the exercise that some people get doing manual labor and most of the rest of us, especially housewives, get doing routine chores? Isn't that enough? The literature on exercise distinguishes between *exercise* and *fitness*. It focuses on the benefits of leisure exercise. In part that is because relatively few people now do the kind of manual labor that would keep a person fit. Making it all more complicated is the fact that those who are engaged in manual labor do not follow a middle-class lifestyle. They are more likely to engage in behaviors that increase risk, like smoking and eating too much fast food. This makes it hard to separate out the effects of healthy from unhealthy behaviors.

More than that, it seems that the context in which physical activity takes place matters. Women who do more household work, which involves a considerable amount of movement, have worse health than those who do less (Ross and Bird 1994). Doing household chores is obviously burdensome, which detracts from its fitness benefit.

Other Risky Behaviors

There are clearly many behaviors that affect health. We will only touch on two of these: drug abuse and alcohol abuse. Obviously risky sexual behavior causes a range of health problems; however, we cannot do it justice in a few paragraphs. So we will simply not try.

Going on to consider drug use and abuse, let us look at an editorial in the *American Journal of Public Health*, which puts this topic into a perspective that may come as a surprise to you. Rather than paraphrasing it, I will quote a portion of the final paragraph.

> Psychoactive drug use is strongly related to a large number of important health problems, including overdoses, psychoses, interpersonal violence, cardiovascular disease, and infectious diseases. Psychoactive drug use can also alleviate symptoms of many psychological disorders, contribute to physical health, and undoubtedly contribute to a sense of well-being for the very large number of drug users who control their drug use. (Des Jarlais 2000, 337)

The author of this statement advocates regulating psychoactive drug use. However, he also wants to see a policy that would focus on developing more scientific knowledge about the effects of drugs, including potential benefits. Furthermore, he advocates a policy that would stress prevention, and focus on treatment rather than arrest. He outlines the obstacles that stand in the way of adopting what he sees as a more rational and humane approach. He says that our society is "euphoriphobic," that is, has a fear of pleasure. He says that Americans are also "xenophobic," meaning that we fear the strange or different. Some members of our society engage in misplaced moralism by opposing anything that appears to condone drug use, for example, syringe exchange programs. Finally, he argues that the whole enterprise engaged in the control of illicit drug use is a multibillion-dollar industry that does not wish to see the status quo altered.

You may disagree with everything said in this editorial. Many scholars also disagree with such a benign attitude toward the use of psychoactive drugs (Levy, Stephens, and McBride 2000). In my view, the value of considering such a radical perspective is that it is thought provoking. It challenges what has become the politically correct response to drug use, which many people repeat without having to give much thought to the effect drugs have on society and the factors that make those effects as problematic as they are. The debate about the medical use of marijuana serves as a good example. For example, those who favor using marijuana for such purposes say that there is clear evidence that it reduces nausea that occurs with chemotherapy. Opponents argue that giving it to one category of people, such as chemotherapy patients, simply opens the door to increased pressure to legalize it. Legitimating its use for any purpose may make it more accessible to those who are likely to misuse it and that is too great a risk to take.

Turning to the use and abuse of alcohol, the problem is not that the findings are controversial but that they bring mixed messages. Alcohol consumption patterns are clear. Consumption continued to increase on a yearly basis from Prohibition through the early 1980s (Greenfield, Midanik, and Rogers 2000). Consumption declined slowly but steadily through the early 1990s and has been stable since the mid-1990s. The researchers who study this phenomenon interpret this to mean that there has been a shift in norms with regard to excessive drinking and drunkenness. In other words, the social costs of excessive drinking have been recognized and social pressure is being applied by friends and relatives. That has had a moderating effect on alcohol consumption.

According to the CDC, the problems associated with alcohol consumption are far from being eliminated. There are seventy-five thousand deaths attributable to excessive use of alcohol, which makes it the third leading lifestyle-related cause of death.

The controversy comes when we look at the findings on the health benefits and risks associated with alcohol consumption. Over the last decade or so, we have been hearing that light to moderate drinking can reduce the risk of heart disease. According to a report in *Lancet*, the leading British medical journal, one to seven alcoholic drinks per week may be associated with a significant decrease in mortality (Mullan 2000). In fact, those who never drink have a higher risk of mortality than those who drink more than two drinks per day. These results are based on a long-term study of the health behaviors of over eighty-nine thousand American doctors. However, more recently we have begun to hear that while drinking may be good for one's heart, it may increase the risk of cancer. The evidence is particularly strong in the case of breast cancer (Morch et al. 2007; Zhang et al. 2007). The evidence is only beginning to accumulate on the relationship between drinking and other forms of cancer, so we will have to wait to see the extent to which consensus develops on this.

Religion

The relationship between religion and health is another topic that was receiving a good deal of attention a decade or so ago, but seems to have been attracting far less interest of late. When it was receiving more attention, researchers were consistent in finding religion to have a salutary effect on health (Wallace and Forman 1998). This does not come as a surprise to sociologists. Sociologists are all familiar with Emile Durkheim's study of suicide first published at the end of the nineteenth century—in 1897. Durkheim found that suicide rates in France in the years just before the beginning of the twentieth century varied depending on religious affiliation among Protestants, Catholics, and Jews.

Durkheim's explanation is still considered to be central to the explanation of the role religion plays. He argued that religion provides social connections, but some religions offer a richer set of connections than others, and it is these connections that provide protection against suicide. In this case, it is not so much the belief system that matters as much as the benefits that come from belonging to a social group that cares about its members and is willing to help with practical assistance when it is needed. It seems that the Jewish religion ties people into a social network to a greater extent than the Catholic religion and far more than the Protestant religion. Protestants in France at the time that Durkheim was making these observations were not admonished to worship communally. They were expected to communicate with God directly, which could be done at home, or anywhere else, without anyone else being present. That may have produced a closer connection to God, but it produced a looser connection to society.

The association between better health and greater religiosity has been repeatedly rediscovered throughout the twentieth century (Levin 1994). A comprehensive review of the literature on the relationship between religion and health can be found in a tome of nearly seven hundred pages (Koenig, McCullough, and Larson 2001). In the end, exactly how religion interacts with any one individual's health is still not entirely clear, although a large number of possible explanations have been explored. This includes the relationship between religion and health behavior or lifestyle, social integration and support, psychological resources, coping behavior, and various positive emotions and beliefs (Sherkat and Ellison 1999).

There is no question that religion protects against destructive behavior by imposing sanctions against particular behaviors. This is especially true in the case of adolescents. Research indicates that religious youth are less likely to engage in risky behaviors. They are less likely to carry a weapon, to use drugs, binge drink, and more likely to use seat belts, thus reducing the risk of motor vehicle injury (Wallace and Forman 1998).

Religion may offer solace in the face of serious and debilitating disease. In this case, the spiritual dimension matters most. Those who feel that their pain and suffering has a larger spiritual meaning and explanation indicate greater satisfaction with their health even when they are experiencing serious health problems (Idler 1995). It is important to note that the evidence is not consistent. Some researchers report finding no relationship between religiosity and health outcomes (King, Speck, and Thomas 1994). Possible explanations that account for a positive correlation between religiosity and health revolve around the emergence of a "sense of self" among those who are experiencing illness. Those who come to believe that their illness brings them a connection to something more important than temporal life on earth, and while it lasts, a life which has special meaning and purpose report feeling better about themselves and their health status (Idler 1995). Those who define illness as a test of faith imposed by God feel special and chosen to bear a unique burden, which has the effect of reducing stress and ultimately producing a health benefit (Sapolsky 1998, 316).

Religious involvement has been found to be particularly advantageous to African Americans. The health benefits are probably due to all the reasons mentioned thus far, but because African American mortality and morbidity rates are higher to begin with, the effect is even more salutary.

There is also some evidence to show that belonging to more conservative religious groups has a negative effect on health. This is generally interpreted to mean that the more conservative religious groups recruit persons of lower socioeconomic status. Their social-class status provides a much more powerful explanation for poor health than their religious beliefs or practices (Ferraro and Albrecht-Jensen 1991).

You might be interested in hearing about what was apparently a short-lived interest in the curative power of "intercessory prayer," which refers to prayers being said on behalf of sick persons, generally without those persons knowing that they are being prayed for. Studies reporting the benefits of intercessory prayer were being published in highly respected medical journals such as the *British Medical Journal* (Leibovici 2001). *Consumer Reports* found more than three hundred such studies to review when it turned its attention to the topic in 1998 (Consumers Union of the U.S. 1998). A number of factors related to the rising level of interest in the topic can be identified. For one, the growth of alternative medicine and complementary medicine, which sometimes links spirituality to those treatment modalities, has given further impetus to the potential link between spirituality and health. The trend has inspired medical schools to introduce courses on spirituality.

While the question of the relationship between prayer and improved health has inspired a certain amount of interest, it remains highly controversial because of the problems associated with measurement (Chibnall, Jeral, and Cerullo 2001; Sloan, Bagiella, and Powell 1999). For example, it is difficult to ascertain who is being prayed for and who is not. It is difficult to know how effective prayer is when the patient is also being treated through other, more traditional modalities. The research that has been carried out has been criticized for ignoring a whole range of related variables. Other criticisms focus on the ethical ramifications of praying for some patients and not others (Cohen et al. 2000). The topic promises to continue attracting attention, but perhaps not funding, which some researchers argue is scarce and should be directed to addressing issues that will result in more practical findings.

Poor People and Risky Health Behavior

We now know that there is a great deal of evidence showing that poor people tend to be sicker and die younger. We find that people with less education and lower income are more likely to engage in behavior that increases the risk of mortality and morbidity. They are more likely to be overweight, less likely to engage in regular exercise, and more likely to smoke and drink to excess (Lantz et al. 1998; Lynch, Kaplan, and Salonen 1997). The question is why.

Poor people may not be able to join a health club, but they could certainly get more exercise by walking. It turns out that they do walk, and many say they would walk more if they did not fear being victimized on the street (Ross 2000). However, we know that they do not benefit from this as much as the nonpoor. We know that poor people are more likely to smoke but again cannot really explain why. A clue comes from a recent study of residents of Harlem who were interviewed about their smoking habits. The researchers found that those who witnessed more violence and perceived their neighborhood to be unsafe were also more likely to smoke (Ganz 2000). We will return to these observations when we discuss policy implications. For now, let's just say that giving people more information about the risks associated with certain behaviors may not be the answer if the reason people engage in those behaviors has to do with factors that are not addressed and are outside of their control, like neighborhood safety.

Summary and Conclusions

This chapter shows that lifestyle choices have an important effect on health. Virtually all researchers agree that smoking, obesity, and lack of exercise are directly associated with an increased risk of mortality. However, more often than not, they end up saying that variations in mortality are due to multiple factors. They are especially likely to say this in connection with one of the most troubling conclusions that is steadily gaining support from researchers, namely, that a shift to more positive health behaviors among disadvantaged populations would not significantly alter the difference in their mortality rates (Lantz et al. 1998). Those multiple factors apparently have an even more powerful effect on morbidity and mortality than the kinds of behaviors we have been discussing. That is hard to believe, I know. Researchers consistently find that mortality and morbidity vary with income, education, and social class; we will bring together the evidence that attempts to explain why that is so.

After everything we have discussed in this chapter, what has become increasingly obvious is that we need to consider more carefully to what extent we believe that individuals must bear primary responsibility for their own health, which is in turn largely determined by their behavior, or whether we should focus greater attention on how health status is related to social structural differences. We need to know this to determine whether we should support health policy addressed to changing the behavior of individuals or policy aimed at altering social structural features. We will devote far more attention to this topic in the final chapter where we address policy.

For now, we can say that one of the most comprehensive long-range assessments of the relationship between socioeconomic status and increased risk of death comes from the Alameda County database. The study we referred to at the end of the discussion on excess weight that concluded that lifetime poverty has cumulative negative effects on health, one of which is weight gain, was based on this population (Baltrus et al. 2005). The original study, designed by the Human Population Laboratory, California Department of Health Services, began in 1965. The initial findings provided the basis for the seven health habits recommended by John Knowles that we discussed earlier in this chapter. Researchers have continued to compile statistics on an extensive list of variables in addition to lifestyle or health behavior, starting with specific health practices in this population. They have gone to consider depression, insurance, connection to social networks, and health outcomes, to name a few of the topics addressed. The factor that researchers kept finding to be most consistently related to variation in mortality is the poverty income level of the neighborhood (Balfour and Kaplan 2002; Yen and Kaplan 1998). As of the late 1980s, 37 out of 102 census tracts in which this population resides were classified as poverty areas (Haan, Kaplan, and Camacho 1987). While health behavior—like smoking, heavy alcohol consumption, and weight—mattered, analysts concluded that these factors were not nearly as powerful in explaining differences in mortality rates between census tracts as low socioeconomic status.

Not surprisingly, poor people involved in the Alameda County study also reported having difficulty getting health care because they could not afford it and lacked health insurance. Maybe they could overcome their health problems in spite of poor health habits if they could have only seen a doctor when they needed to. How much access to high-quality health care affects one's health is the subject of the next chapter.

CHAPTER SEVEN

~

Medical Care

According to the conventional wisdom, we should all be getting physical exams every year. Also, we should not wait to see the doctor until our symptoms are so advanced that the problem becomes hard to cure. In fact, we should be able to see the doctor whenever we need to, which many people are convinced health insurance companies are making every effort to prevent us from doing. As far as poor people and medical care are concerned, the conventional wisdom says that the reason they are sicker than other people is that they can't afford to go to the doctor; and, when they do go, they end up going to doctors who are not very good. This is, of course, after we agree that poor people are undoubtedly causing many of their own problems by engaging in all that bad behavior that we discussed in the preceding chapter. Does that sound about right?

There are some interesting half-truths buried in all of this. The basic message, however, is that medical care constitutes one of the big differences between those who are healthy and those who are not. The purpose of this chapter is to review the evidence on the extent to which medical care is the most important factor responsible for the variation in morbidity and mortality that we have discussed in each of the preceding chapters.

There is no question that medical science has developed an awesome capacity to diagnose and treat diseases over the last century. That is substantiated by the fact that we have experienced a thirty-year gain in life expectancy over that time period. Would you be surprised to hear that the experts in the field say that very little of that gain can be attributed to medical care? Some highly regarded experts calculate that about five to ten years are due to medical care (Tarlov 1996; Fuchs 1974). Other equally well-known researchers say it is less than five years (Bunker, Frazier, and Mosteller 1994; McKeown 1976).

One of the most commonly cited pieces of evidence to back up this assess-ment comes from an analysis of trends of some of the leading causes of death, more specifically, ten leading infectious diseases, from the beginning of the twentieth century through to about 1970 (McKinlay and McKinlay 1977). (These include: tuberculosis, scarlet fever, influenza, pneumonia, diphtheria, whooping cough, measles, smallpox, typhoid, and poliomyelitis.) For each of these diseases, a vaccine was introduced that was effective in preventing the onset of the disease, but it was introduced at a time when the rate of death from the disease was already on the decline. (It is not clear whether there could have been a resurgence of polio after 1955 if the vaccine had not been introduced at that time.) In short, the effect of medical science cannot be credited with decreasing the incidence of the leading infectious diseases if the diseases were declining anyway.

At the most basic level, why the incidence of certain infectious diseases declines is not difficult to explain. In part, it is attributable to the fact that viruses undergo change. They become weaker. They can also become more treacherous. New strains can emerge that are more resilient and resistant to current medications. The HIV and antibiotic-resistant TB viruses illustrate this phenomenon. Both viruses continue to evolve so that new pharmaceu-ticals and combinations of pharmaceuticals must be developed to counteract them. We will return to this topic shortly.

Another reason that explains why the eleven infectious diseases to which we just referred became less virulent in the past is that people became stronger and healthier and better able to resist infectious disease. Remember the discussion on demographic and epidemiological transition in chapter 3? When people don't have enough food, they are more susceptible to infection. When they have enough to eat they can fight off infection better. It helps to have clean water, adequate shelter, and more nutritious food. These are the factors that the public-health community says deserve most credit for the increase in life expec-tancy over the last century. There is little dispute about this observation.

As the epidemiological transition discussion in chapter 3 made clear, the kinds of diseases that affect us have changed. We are in the stage of epide-miological development characterized by a higher prevalence of chronic illness. We are also encountering newly emergent infectious diseases that have devastating consequences; to date, the rate at which we die from these diseases is still comparatively low in contrast to the rate of death from the leading chronic diseases, namely, heart disease and cancer. And, as we noted in the chapter on behavior, the rising interest in health behavior stems from the fact that modern medicine generally cannot cure chronic illness but behavioral change can have an ameliorating effect. Observers have been saying much the same thing periodically throughout the twentieth century, namely, that with all the scientific progress medicine has achieved, the medical profession still directs most of its resources to treating diseases only after symptoms appear (Barsky 1988; Powles 1974). The application of medical science is considerably less effective when it comes to *preventing* the onset of disease than treating it once we are afflicted.

Our Health-Care Arrangements

This is not to discount the importance of medical care. It is very important to us on an individual basis. The point is that it may not accomplish what people think it can accomplish for the society at large. Mainstream medical researchers do not question the relationship between medical care and health. They proceed from the assumption that effective medical care is valuable. There are also a few medical researchers who disagree with the mainstream account of why we are living longer. They say that the decline in mortality from heart disease that we experienced over the last few decades is not due nearly as much to such factors as better nutrition and lifestyle, but to improvements in diagnosis, prevention, and treatment of heart attacks. A more recent and widely accepted version of this observation offers an important clarification—the rate of heart disease is not really dropping; what is happening is that the drugs that physicians have at their disposal, namely statins, are preventing those who have heart disease from dying, which is not the same thing as saying that the rate of heart disease has dropped or that it is being cured. In short, the prevalence of heart disease continues to be high but is masked by the efficacy of the drugs. No one really disputes this.

To argue that medical care matters, there is an obvious point to be made. Medical care must be available, affordable, and of high quality. Health-policy experts consistently refer to the three basic objectives that our care system strives to achieve, namely, *access, cost containment,* and *quality* (Budrys 2005). There is no single formal document in which these goals are recorded because our health-care arrangements are not considered to be a national health-care system in any sense. Nevertheless, health-services researchers and policy makers regularly refer to the three concepts in discussing health-care reform proposals. Let's consider how the three goals interact with the kind of health care we receive.

The question of *access* to care has been a central concern of health-services researchers throughout the twentieth century (Kasper 2000). Two basic public insurance programs were introduced during the 1960s. The 1970s brought us health maintenance organizations (HMOs), which were supposed to encourage people to seek health care before their health problems became more serious. There has been a lot of discussion about the impact of HMOs on our health as well as the health of our pocketbooks since then. A major effort to bring about universal health insurance coverage, that is, increase access, surfaced during the first years of President Clinton's administration but collapsed once the details of the plan began to take shape. Interest in the topic has again gained ground during the first decade of the twenty-first century in response to the steady increase in the number of uninsured Americans, as well as the unremitting increase in the cost of health insurance, which most policy experts say is connected to the inexorable rise in the cost of medical-care treatments.

Medical care has gotten so expensive because it is now so technologically sophisticated that people generally do not pay cash for medical care services, especially hospitalization, which is why the focus of attention has turned to the topic of health insurance. The main question is whether having no insurance is detrimental to health. We will get to the research on that question after we consider the ways we get health insurance in this country.

There is also growing reason to believe that we are receiving too many tests and procedures that are being carried out because medicine is an art, not a science (Brownlee 2007). In other words, there are treatment trends that are not grounded in evidence that they produce superior outcomes over the long term; plus, there is doctors' interest in avoiding malpractice suits.

Although a sizeable proportion of Americans have no health insurance—a topic to which we will return shortly—the majority of people in this country do have the cost of their health care covered through health insurance. Health insurance comes in two forms—public and private. *Public* means that it is a government-supported program. *Private* means that it operates in the private sector, which may be further distinguished into organizations that operate on either a nonprofit or a profit making basis. (For a basic introduction to health insurance, see Budrys 2005).

Let's consider public insurance first. To do this, we need to go back about four decades. Remember this is when the country was acting as if we had just discovered that there were poor people in this country. Perhaps more to the point, we were living in a society where President Kennedy's admonition—"Ask not what your country can do for you, but what you can do for your country"—was being taken to heart. A range of programs aimed at overcoming social disadvantage came into existence shortly thereafter, during the Johnson administration, including housing assistance, food stamps, support for education, and so forth. A great deal of money was put into the health-care sector. Medical and nursing schools were told to increase enrollments as a condition of receiving government funding. Health-planning legislation was enacted to encourage hospitals—in consultation with members of the community—to build new facilities (Budrys 1986). Two major public insurance programs, Medicare and Medicaid, were enacted in 1965 with the expectation that expansion would result in increased availability of medical care for all who needed it, that is, *access* to care and eventually better health for all.

A third public health insurance program, the State Children's Health Insurance Program (S-CHIP), was introduced in 1997. It is insurance for children whose families have income that is under 200 percent of the current poverty line. The children are eligible for this insurance even if their parents are not eligible for government-supported health insurance. S-CHIP funds come from the federal government, but the state must enroll the children who are eligible. In some states S-CHIP is a separate program; however, in other states the same agency administers Medicaid and S-CHIP. The program was reauthorized in 2009 and renamed. It is now known as the Children's Health Insurance Program (CHIP). We will return to consideration of CHIP after we look more closely at the Medicare and Medicaid programs.

Medicare

Medicare is a federal program, primarily for people who are over age sixty-five, meaning the rules are the same across the country and people sign up with a single federal agency. Medicare has four parts. The hospital portion, Part A, is free to enrollees. The way the program was originally set up requires all of us to pay 6.2 percent out of every paycheck to support this portion of the plan; employers put in another 6.2 percent. The medical portion, Part B, which covers doctors' charges, is funded as we go; in other words people must sign up for it, which results in a monthly charge that comes out of the person's monthly Social Security check. The charge increases every year. In 2007, the federal government introduced a five-level graduated payment scale, meaning that people with a higher income pay more. According to Medicare projections, 96 percent of the population was expected to pay the basic charge of $96 per month in 2008; the remaining 4 percent was expected to fall into one of other four levels, which go up to $238 per month.

The amount a person is charged is based on income reported to the Internal Revenue Service.

Medicare does not cover all costs. Part B, which covers doctor's visits, requires a 20 percent copayment for each visit. Accordingly, many people buy additional insurance called *Medigap*. Private insurance companies sell Medigap policies, but these are not like other private policies. There are twelve different plans, labeled A through L, that vary in how much they cover and how much they cost. Any insurance company can sell one or more of these plans and charge whatever it wishes, as long as the plan described under that particular letter is identical to all other plans identified by the same letter. The plans are clearly described by the Medicare administration; the information is available in free publications and on the Medicare website. It is also true that many people over sixty-five do not buy Medigap insurance because they cannot afford it, which puts them at risk of very large medical bills.

Medicare Part D, the drug bill, was passed in 2003. Before this time, Medicare enrollees paid for their drugs out of pocket. Part D is not voluntary; Medicare recipients must enroll or be penalized. The drug-insurance plans, of which there are multiple versions, are sold by private companies at varying prices and levels of coverage. Medicare Part D has a unique feature that applies to everyone who is enrolled—drug purchases are subsidized by the drug plans up to a certain cutoff, $2,700 in 2009; then there is a "doughnut hole" and there is no subsidy until the person runs up a drug bill of $4,350, when the plan kicks back in and pays 95 percent of the cost. If you think there is something irrational about this, you have a lot of company.

There is also a Medicare Part C, which we will not discuss because the legislation is not only complicated but controversial and requires a little more discussion time than we can afford here. Suffice it to say that Part C is total Medicare coverage sold by private insurance companies, meaning that people are choosing to opt out of the government-run Medicare plan. It is also worth noting that insurance companies are being paid more than the average Medicare patient costs the government. In other words, private health-insurance companies got a lucrative deal from the government to offer these plans.

Medicaid

You might wonder why people who can't afford health care and private health insurance don't apply for Medicaid, which is, after all, health insurance for the poor. That is because it was never intended to cover all poor people. Originally it was meant to cover single parents—women whose income falls under the poverty line and their young, dependent children. That has changed. Let's look at what has happened over time.

The Medicaid program is administered by each respective state in cooperation with the federal government. The intent was to give states the right to determine what proportion of poor people the state was prepared to cover, or to put it another way—the amount of money the state would be willing to raise to pay for approximately half the cost of Medicaid with the understanding that the federal government would match that amount. The result is that there is a great deal of variation across states in the proportion of people who are deemed to be eligible for Medicaid and the criteria used to determine that. In all cases, eligibility is based on income as well as assets, which generally includes such items as savings accounts, land, and cars in some states, but generally not the house the applicant lives in.

Federal guidelines outline the categories of persons who are considered eligible at present, namely, mothers and their underage children, pregnant women, and "dual eligibles." Dual eligibles are persons who qualify for Medicare because they are over sixty-five or are blind or disabled in addition to being poor. You will notice that able-bodied adults without dependent children are not among the eligibles. It is true that an increasing number of states are finding ways to provide health insurance to this population, but that still leaves forty-seven million people without health insurance as of 2009.

As part of the welfare reform of 1996, states were given greater flexibility to broaden eligibility rules, including the option to eliminate the asset test for some categories of enrollees. As of 2008, only seven states require pregnant women to meet an asset test. The ceiling on assets that states allow ranges from $3,000 in Montana to $30,000 in South Carolina (Kaiser Family Foundation 2008). States were readier to eliminate the asset test in determining the eligibility for children but not for their parents. The passage of S-CHIP in 1997 complicated things.

S-CHIP provided states with funds to insure all children under 200 percent of poverty. However, some states were slow to enroll all the children who would qualify, while other states raised the cutoff (as high as 350 percent of poverty in at least one state) and were able to obtain the extra funds that other states were not using to enroll poor adults. Congress passed legislation in 2007 preventing states from enrolling any children whose family income is over 250 percent of poverty and all adults regardless of income. Some states are continuing to expand coverage for those whom Congress has defined as ineligible but are now having to do it through other programs and having to find other sources of funding.

Rules for enrolling the third category of eligibles, the "dual eligibles," vary even more from one state to another. This includes individuals who are over sixty-five or are blind or disabled and are therefore eligible for Social Security as well as Medicare insurance. Some people may also qualify for SSI—which requires proof that the person's income is below the poverty threshold, that their assets fall under $4,000, and that they are unable to hold down a job. If the person is not eligible for SSI, then the state may have a separate application process to qualify for Medicaid that may be more or less restrictive than the guidelines issued by the Social Security Administration.

As you can see, there is a lot of emphasis on determining eligibility for Medicaid and CHIP. How this is accomplished is known as "means testing." Something like the "welfare" or social services department in each state carries out this assignment. People who apply for Medicaid and CHIP must bring in various kinds of documents to prove that they are poor enough to qualify. Medicare, by contrast, is an "entitlement" program, meaning that everyone who has reached age sixty-five (and has paid into the program, which most, but not all, people have done), is blind, or disabled (of course this must be established as well) is entitled to it and can simply sign up.

The Medicaid program is now the largest public insurance program in the country. Many people continue to believe that it is a public health-insurance program that is primarily serving poor women and children. Although the majority of enrollees continue to be poor women and children, the other categories of recipients have been enrolling in steadily increasing numbers. As of 2005:

- 69 percent of the enrollees are either children or adults in families with dependent children.
- 22 percent of the enrollees are in aged, blind, and disabled categories (the remainder belong to an "other" category).

When you look at who receives the services, the profile looks quite different. We find that

- 29 percent of the expenditures cover women and children.
- 66 percent of the expenditures cover the aged, blind, and disabled.

There is an interesting anomaly here. Remember that the data on poverty in chapter 5 show that the poorest members of this society are children. A far smaller proportion of those over sixty-five are poor (less than 10 percent as of 2005) compared to the proportion of children who are poor (17 percent of all children and 43 percent of those in single-parent households). So how is it that we are spending so much in Medicaid funds on the elderly, blind, and disabled? The answer is that the care required by the latter often requires that they go into a nursing home. According to the American Association of Retired Persons (AARP), the daily rate for nursing-home care in 2009 is averaging $67,000 to $78,000 per year depending on location. It can be much more if people require additional assistance to feed and care for themselves. Knowing that nursing-home care is free for those who qualify for Medicaid presents its own solution. It doesn't even take much creativity. The way many middle-class families handle it is by transferring all of grandma's (because women live longer than men) wealth to her children. Without any income beyond Social Security and no wealth, she instantly becomes poor enough to qualify for Medicaid. Fair or unfair, this is the way it is done by increasing numbers of people.

Private Insurance

Then there is the matter of private insurance—who gets it and who doesn't. Private insurance is generally obtained through employment. The employer selects and contracts with one or more insurance plans on behalf of the organization's employees. The employer may pay for part of the policy and require employees to pay for the rest. In a growing number of instances, employers are making the plans available without covering any of the cost. Also, some employers may offer insurance to the employee, but not the employee's family. Finally, the majority of small businesses provide no insurance for their employees.

Employers are under no obligation to offer insurance. It is a benefit they can choose to offer voluntarily. The rising cost of health insurance, which increased at the rate of 87 percent from 2001 to 2005 (by comparison wages went up by 20 percent) makes clear why employers have been dropping the generous health-insurance benefits they were willing to offer in the past (Kaiser Family Foundation 2006). In fact, the proportion of Americans who receive their insurance coverage through their employers has dropped to 59 percent as of 2006, compared to 69 percent in 1984, when the rate of employment-based coverage was at its highest. Estimates indicate that the steadily rising cost of health insurance has been the basic reason for this trend—for every 1 percent increase in insurance premiums, as many as three hundred thousand individuals lose employment-based coverage (Emanuel 2008). The downturn in the economy that occurred as of 2007 caused some people to lose their jobs and to lose their health insurance as well.

The Uninsured

According to the Census Bureau, the number of uninsured persons in 2005 was 46.6 million, or 15.9 percent of the population. Other estimates indicate that the number is much larger because the government only counts those who were uninsured for the whole year (Schoen et al. 2008). According to FamiliesUSA, which contracted with a highly respected research organization, the Lewin Group, asking them to count everyone who reported being uninsured for either all or part of the year to the Census Bureau in 2007–2008, the count is 86.7 million, or about one of every three Americans (FamiliesUSA 2009).

The plight of people who cannot get insurance through their employers but make more than the poverty threshold is especially challenging. Consider the fact that working on a full-time basis at even the lowest wage can put a person's income just above the poverty line. This means that a person who works at a minimum-wage job could not qualify for Medicaid even if that person was otherwise eligible. Low-wage workers clearly cannot afford to buy private insurance on their own. (The average cost of a family policy obtained through an employer was $12,700 in 2008 [Keehan et al. 2008]. It is difficult to estimate the cost of family policies sold privately because private insurance is risk rated, meaning that it varies with the health of the individuals and it varies by the size of the deductible involved.) Politically conservative policy makers have been proposing to give poor people a tax rebate to help them buy their own insurance. That gets us into debate about the amount of money that poor people would have to be given, about the fact that poor people don't pay taxes so a tax rebate is of no value, and the fact that insurance purchased on an individual basis is not only expensive but is typically limited and almost certainly excludes preexisting conditions. Since the federal government has not been willing to deal with the issue of the rising numbers of uninsured throughout the first eight years of the twenty-first century, an increasing number of states have taken steps to provide health insurance for their uninsured residents.

Getting back to the question of who does and who does not have insurance—the answer may surprise you. Roughly 80 percent of those who were uninsured as of 2007 were members of families in which there is at least one full-time worker (Kaiser Commission on Medicaid and the Uninsured 2007). They are disproportionately self-employed—for example, farmers and small-business owners. Another sector of the uninsured are engaged in risky occupations, which insurance companies are unwilling to insure, like construction, fishing, and logging. People in their early twenties who are no longer covered by their parents' policies, but are not employed on a full-time basis, are especially likely to be uninsured. What it comes down to is that you have a much greater chance of being insured if you are at one end of the economic spectrum or the other, either desperately poor or in a well-paid and steady job. If you are working but not making very much money, you have a much higher chance of being uninsured. The problem is that these are exactly the kinds of circumstances that make people vulnerable to even greater risk of serious illness.

Does Health Insurance Matter?

Does health insurance matter is a question that has been debated for some time. The RAND Corporation launched the first major effort to answer this question about thirty-five years ago (Newhouse 1993; Brook et al. 1983). At that time, RAND set up an experiment to determine whether having access to totally free health care would improve health. Groups of people were randomized into several insurance categories, one with a rather high copayment (for each visit to the doctor), one with a low copayment, and one that received totally free care. The essence of the question was whether providing free care would make a significant difference in people's health status. The answer to another question—whether the availability of free health care would create a "moral hazard"—was of even greater interest to economists. Economists maintain that people are susceptible to the moral hazard of succumbing to the temptation to take advantage of anything that is free, even if they do not really need whatever it is—in this case health care.

The conclusions were as follows. Only poor people suffered worse health when there were additional costs. Everyone else's health was not much affected. And, yes, some people who had access to free care services did succumb to moral hazard. There was a lot more to this research that captured the attention of the health-services research community, including arguments about the measures of health used in making these determinations. However, the study's primary conclusion, namely, that free care did not improve the health of those who are not poor, received considerably more attention than the other findings, including the conclusion that the health of the poor did suffer. The conclusions and their effects on policy may have been debated, but there were few objections to the methodology that led to those conclusions until recently. The primary criticism is based on the observation that the reason that the health of those who had to pay additional costs was not affected is that they dropped out of the study, so the impact of their insurance arrangements was not included in the analysis (Nyman

2007). Since then, the researchers who carried out the study and the critics have entered into a vigorous debate about both the methods and the results of this research (Newhouse et al. 2008; Nyman 2008).

The reason the debate is important is that the series of RAND studies focusing on this topic became the basis for arguing that people should be buying their own health insurance because they would then be more sensitive to the cost of health care and would be less susceptible to moral hazard, that is, the risk of using health-care services just because they have insurance. In fact, this is the logic that brought us to what is currently known as "consumer-driven health care" insurance—low-cost, high-deductible plans. According to conservative policy makers, the primary advantage of low-cost, high-deductible insurance is that it allows people to choose the kind of insurance that best meets their needs. There should be no surprise in finding that those who are most likely to buy such insurance are in excellent health (read that as young) and do not worry about the high deductible (meaning that you pay for all the care you receive until you exceed the deductible, which may be anywhere from $1,000 to $5,000; it works like car insurance) because they have no reason to think that they will need to seek care. Consumer-driven health plans are particularly appealing to those who are wealthy in addition to being healthy, because such plans are generally linked to Health Savings Accounts (HSAs), which allow people to set aside a certain amount of pretax income for health care in interest-generating accounts. Critics of such plans consider these two categories of subscribers to be "free riders." The critics go on to say that to the extent that more healthy people can be persuaded to buy this form of private insurance, all the other insurance plans will become more expensive, which will further discourage employers from insuring their employees and force people to buy their own insurance and this is, of course, exactly the objective that conservative policy makers who value private enterprise, that is, the opportunity for the insurance companies to make more money, believe to be the desirable outcome.

As of 2008, only 5 percent of the population had purchased insurance on an individual basis, either low-cost, high-deductible or more conventional plans. Why more people do not buy health insurance on their own is clear. Most people are not interested in high-deductible plans because they know that they will have some medical expenses, they just don't know what kinds of illnesses they will face and the expenses they will encounter, which is why people want insurance in the first place. As to conventional private insurance, people don't buy it because it is not readily available; it is very expensive; and it excludes preexisting conditions—anything that you have been diagnosed with previously. In effect, people don't buy it because it is not a good value.

While policy advisors on the conservative side of the divide emphasize the benefits of reducing moral hazard, those on the liberal side raise questions about the wisdom of employing mechanisms aimed at discouraging people from using medical-care services. The latter contingent of policy makers point out that patients are often not the best judges of which aspects of their care are essential and which are not. They cite research indicating that it is the chronically ill who are most likely to cut back on health services. Thus, they say that increased "cost-sharing" required by the high-deductible plans has the potential of negatively affecting health in the long run even though patients may feel that they are monitoring their own health well in the short run (Wong et al. 2001). Those who do buy high-deductible insurance are essentially buying catastrophic insurance. The same researchers warn that forgoing preventive care, even if one is young and healthy, is not something that can be done without consequences.

While we generally do not hear many people saying that health insurance is unnecessary, we do still hear the most adamant opponents of universal health insurance saying that access to health-care services in this country is not really a problem. They continue to argue that people who need health-care services can get care and not have to pay anything. They say that free care is available to those who really need it—through free clinics and hospital emergency rooms. A more careful look reveals that, yes, Americans can in fact get free, easily accessible care during an acute episode or accident. However, they are not nearly as likely to get continuing care, so that the problem is not really resolved. Furthermore, according to the Kaiser Family Foundation, access to free care is not as certain as it was in the past. A report entitled "Growth in Uninsured Americans Outpacing Federal Spending on the Health Safety Net," notes that as the number of uninsured

> increased by 4.6 million from 2001 to 2004, federal safety net per uninsured person fell from $546 to $498 during the same period. After adjusting for inflation, total federal spending for care for the uninsured increased by 1.3% from 2001-2004 while the number uninsured increased by 11.2 percent. These trends resulted in an 8.9 percent decline in spending by the federal government (Kaiser Family Foundation 2005).

The result is that community health centers have been confronting an increasingly uncertain future and public hospitals across the country have been closing down. The recent downturn in the economy is, of course, exacerbating the situation. Thus, medical care traditionally delivered by private-sector nonprofit hospitals, that is, charity care, is less available as such hospitals succumb to pressure to compete through cost cutting while the number of people requiring free care continues to increase.

This should not be interpreted to mean that the uninsured are not receiving care when they have acute health-care problems. It is meant to draw attention to the fact that the care they do receive is not really free. This is known as uncompensated care. According to one estimate, hospitals and doctors contributed a substantial portion of uncompensated care, but the government paid the largest share, amounting to about $30.6 billion in 2001 through a patchwork of payments and programs (Hadley and Holahan 2003).

How Much Does Health Insurance Matter?

There is obviously a lot more to say about the way that health insurance is obtained in this country, but let us now turn to the question to which we have been referring throughout this discussion—how much does it really matter? The fact that the country is willing to tolerate a growing level of uninsurance has stimulated a great deal of attention to the question, so there is now an overwhelming amount of evidence indicating that it matters a lot (Rice 2003). The most comprehensive statement on the matter comes from the Institute of Medicine (IOM), which issued six book-length reports between September 2001 and January 2004. The 2002 report, "Care Without Coverage: Too Little, Too Late," states that committee members reviewed the results of the "best-designed research studies investigating the health of working-age adults with and without health insurance" (IOM 2002a, 5). The resulting report focused on the relationship between insurance and (1) use of preventive and screening services; (2) cancer treatment and survival; (3) chronic illness, including diabetes, cardiovascular disease, end-stage renal disease, HIV infection, and mental illness; (4) hospital-based care; and (5) general health status. The executive summary statement is as follows:

- Having health insurance is associated with better health outcomes for adults and with receipt of appropriated care across a range of preventive-, chronic-, and acute-care services. Adults without health insurance coverage die sooner and experience greater declines in health status over time than do adults with continuous coverage.
- Adults with chronic conditions and those in late middle age stand to benefit the most from health-insurance coverage in terms of improved

health outcomes because of their high probability of needing health-care services.

- Population groups that most often lack stable health-insurance coverage and that have worse health status, including racial and ethnic minorities and lower-income adults, would benefit most from increased health-insurance coverage. Increased coverage would likely reduce some of the racial and ethnic disparities in the utilization of appropriate health-care services and may also reduce disparities in morbidity and mortality among ethnic groups.
- Health insurance that affords access to providers and includes preventive and screening services, outpatient prescription drugs, and specialty mental-health care is more likely to facilitate the receipt of appropriate care.
- Broad-based health-insurance strategies across the entire uninsured population would be more likely to produce these benefits than would "rescue" programs aimed only at the seriously ill (IOM 2002a, 14).

Another review of the literature carried out by the Commission on Medicaid and the Uninsured, which is a program sponsored by the Kaiser Family Foundation, resulted in a similar set of findings (Hadley 2002). This report is based on a review of 9,000 citations in 230 distinct sources over the previous twenty-five years with the aim of identifying the costs of not covering the uninsured. The following represents a selected and limited sample of the results found in the report.

- Insurance was estimated to reduce the risk of mortality by about 10 to 15 percent.
- The uninsured were found to receive less preventive care, to be diagnosed at more advanced stages of illness, and once diagnosed tended to receive less therapeutic care, including drugs and surgical interventions.
- Reports related to specific diseases indicated that the uninsured had higher mortality rates, were less likely to receive surgery for treatable diseases, and more likely to die in the hospital.
- Uninsured infants and children were at higher risk of adverse outcomes, avoidable hospitalization, and mortality.
- In general, the uninsured were 30 to 50 percent more likely to be hospitalized for an avoidable condition. It is worth noting that such hospitalizations have increased over the last twenty-five years, estimated to be about 12 percent of all hospitalizations as of 1998.

- The fact that the cost of hospitalization increased over this time period is also not to be ignored. The cost of an avoidable stay was estimated to be about $3,300 in 2002.

One more dimension of this report that has not been widely disseminated is the effect poor health has on earnings. While it is not surprising to find that poor health is linked to lower income, it is more troubling to be confronted with concrete evidence substantiating it.

- The researchers point out that poor health has negative effects on educational attainment, ability to work, and productivity. In combination, poorer health was estimated to reduce earnings by between 10 and 28 percent depending on race and gender. The poor health of one member of the family could also cause another member to reduce work hours or stop working entirely to become a family caregiver.

An extension of the latter observation comes from a 2003 press release issued by the IOM, which reported "the value of what the United States loses because of the poorer health and earlier death experienced by the 41 million Americans who lack health insurance . . . to be $65 billion to $130 billion every year" (IOM 2003).

The 2007 updated report on the effects of uninsurance issued by the Kaiser Commission on Medicaid and the Uninsured reinforces conclusions presented in earlier reports. "The Uninsured: A Primer, 2007" makes the following observation:

> Health insurance makes a difference in whether and when people get necessary medical care, where they get their care, and ultimately, how healthy people are. Uninsured adults are far more likely than the insured to postpone or forgo health care altogether and less able to afford prescription drugs or follow through with recommended treatments. The consequences of reduced access to care can be severe, particularly when preventable conditions go undetected. (Kaiser Commission on Medicaid and the Uninsured 2007, 7)

The report follows up with eight specific points (which I quote in part):

- About one-quarter of uninsured adults say that they have postponed or forgone care in the past year because of its cost—compared to only about 5 percent of adults with private coverage. Part of the reason for this is that nearly 60 percent of uninsured adults do not have a regular place to go when they are sick or need medical advice.

- Nearly one-quarter of uninsured adults say they did not fill a drug prescription in the past year because they could not afford it. Uninsured persons who have been injured or recently diagnosed with a new chronic condition are less likely than the insured to receive all the services that were advised.
- Uninsured children are much more likely to lack a usual source of care, to delay care, or to have unmet medical needs than children with insurance. Uninsured children with common childhood illnesses and injuries do not receive the same level of care. As a result, they are at higher risk for preventable hospitalizations and for missed diagnoses of serious health conditions.
- Access to health care improves after an uninsured person obtains health insurance; similarly, losing coverage, whether it is private insurance or Medicaid, substantially decreases access to care, because care is too expensive and people are worried about medical bills.
- Lack of coverage, even for short periods of time, results in decreased access to care. As the period lengthens, more of the uninsured face problems of having unmet needs for medical care or prescription drugs.
- Because the uninsured are less likely than the insured to have regular outpatient care, they are more likely to be hospitalized for avoidable health problems and experience declines in their overall health. When they are hospitalized, they are more likely to receive fewer diagnostic and therapeutic services and also are more likely to die in the hospital than are insured patients. Middle-aged adults who are continuously uninsured are much more likely to experience a decline in their health and/or develop problems with their mobility over a four-year period than continuously insured adults.
- The uninsured are less likely to receive timely preventive care. Insured nonelderly adults are at least 50 percent more likely to have had preventive care such as pap smears, mammograms, and prostate exams compared to uninsured adults. Consequently, uninsured cancer patients are diagnosed at later stages of the disease and die earlier than those with insurance.
- Having insurance improves health overall and could reduce mortality rates for the uninsured by 10 to 25 percent. The number of excess deaths among uninsured adults aged twenty-five to sixty-four was estimated to be about eighteen thousand.

A 2007 report by FamiliesUSA makes reference to the finding reported by the IOM in 2003 —that eighteen thousand deaths are attributable to lack of health insurance—by pointing out that this makes lack of insurance the sixth-leading cause of death (FamiliesUSA 2007).

It is hard to miss the fact that evidence on importance of having health insurance just keeps mounting as a review of findings over the last couple of decades ago clearly shows (IOM 2004; Hadley 2008). The observations made in earlier reports continue to be salient. For example: as the illnesses of the uninsured progress, their illnesses become more expensive to treat, which results in longer hospital stays and use of more resources (Epstein, Stern, and Weissman 1990). The poor and uninsured have worse health-care outcomes because they delay getting care (Weissman et al. 1991). When they suffer acute injuries, they are more likely to die in the emergency room (Haas and Goldman 1994). They get less care, care of poorer quality, are more likely to die when they are hospitalized, and are less likely to receive procedures that are "subject to [the doctor's] discretion" (Altman, Reinhardt, and Shields 1998). Not surprisingly, the research shows that not having insurance over a long period of time is more detrimental to a person's health than not having it for a short period (Sudano and Baker 2003; Baker et al. 2001; Schoen and DesRoches 2000). Then there are all the financial problems that mount when a person does not have health insurance, which only exacerbates the problem people have getting the care they need. If they could not pay for the care before they went bankrupt, they are even less likely to be able to pay for it after they are bankrupt. About half of all bankruptcies are the result of medical bills (Himmelstein et al. 2005).

This is not to say that having health insurance alone is likely to overcome health inequalities. A number of researchers have found that having health insurance does not reduce health disparities as much as they expected (Lille-Blanton and Hoffman 2005). They find that having a regular source of care has the biggest effect, which is, of course, far more likely for those who have health insurance and are not forced to fall back on emergency-room visits when their health problems become more severe.

Those who take up this topic invariably conclude that being poor and being uninsured go together and that these two facts in combination explain a major share of the variance in people's health. We also know from the NHIS data collected by the government that socioeconomic status correlates with self-reported health status. In other words, poor people are more likely to report that their health is "poor" and that such an assessment is highly correlated with a higher risk of mortality. Finally, there are social-psychological costs in being poor and unable to get medical care that have only begun to be explored in recent years. We will return to this observation in the final chapters of the book.

A final note on how much health insurance matters to people who don't have it comes from Oregon. Oregon has often taken positions regarding health-care issues that few other states in the country would consider—legalizing physician-assisted suicide, for example. Its most recent innovation is a lottery in which health insurance is the prize. At the beginning of 2008, six hundred thousand people in Oregon were uninsured. Ninety thousand of those people entered the lottery in the hopes of winning one of the ten thousand health-insurance plans the lottery is prepared to award.

Quality of Care

As we see, there is ample evidence to indicate that inadequate access and high cost of care constitute two major obstacles to good health. Let us now turn to the third goal that policy makers refer to in debating health-care reform—the *quality* of care. Discussions about the quality of care are demanding because agreement on appropriate measures is difficult to achieve.

While efforts to improve the quality of medical care in this country have a long history, the report issued by the Quality of Health Care in America Committee of the IOM in 1999, *To Err Is Human*, galvanized attention to the problem in a way that had not been true before. The report stated that at least forty-four thousand to ninety-eight thousand people die in hospitals of medical errors (Kohn, Corrigan, and Donaldson 1999). The report made clear that most errors are not due to "individual recklessness" or "bad apples" but to faulty systems and processes. On the fifth anniversary of that report, an updated analysis supported by the Commonwealth Fund gave the U.S. health system an overall grade of C+ (Wachter 2004).

The same year the National Committee for Quality Assurance (NCQA) reported that between forty-two thousand and seventy-nine thousand avoidable deaths are caused by gaps in health-care quality (Robeznieks 2004). The NCQA reached this conclusion on the basis of information gathered from 563 managed-care plans covering sixty-nine million people. The NCQA relies on a set of standardized measures—the Health Plan Employer Data Set (HEDIS), which has gained wide acceptance but which continues to be the subject of criticism—to rate managed-care plans. The NCQA report did say that more doctors were following generally agreed upon guidelines and that quality was steadily improving. However, as critics point out, this approach rates managed-care organizations, not doctors. Since doctors may be affiliated with more than one managed-care plan, these ratings don't tell us who is a good doctor and who is not.

It is true that patients don't have enough information about individual doctors to make a judgment about a doctor's abilities, but it may be even more interesting to find that the majority of doctors do not have access to data about their own clinical performance (O'Reilly 2006). Given that such data are not readily available makes it difficult to move to the next step, which many policy makers continue to press for, that is, establishing a pay-for-performance system to reward doctors for improvements in the quality of care they deliver. Even apart from arguments about measures, pay-for-performance plans require a major investment in costly technology, which smaller medical practices have not been able or willing to purchase. The IOM, which has endorsed twenty-six pay-for-performance measures, has gone on to say that developing additional measures that everyone would agree on would best be accomplished by a federal office created to coordinate and fund the development of quality measures (Glendinning 2005).

The impetus behind the quest for more information on quality is in large part due to the research on medical practice patterns, which has been a topic of interest since the 1970s when John Wennberg first documented the differences from town to town in Vermont (Mullen 2004). It was around this time that Wennberg pressed for and succeeded in creating the AHRQ, which funds research that aims to distinguish treatments that are efficacious from those that are ineffectual. AHQR now operates under the auspices of the U.S. Department of Health and Human Services. The agency has turned from attempting to explain why there is so much geographic variation to assessing which medical treatments are more successful and to research focusing on problems related to racial and ethnic disparities.

As you know from our discussions thus far, the basic question is why certain groups of people are more likely to experience higher mortality and morbidity rates than others, and as far as this chapter is concerned, the extent to which this is explained by access to medical care. Because the differences in morbidity and mortality rates are so readily apparent by race and ethnicity with far less information on differences by socioeconomic status, the focus of attention has turned to the question of whether the disparities are due to differences in the quality of medical care. The evidence seems to be remarkably consistent—minority patients receive care that is of lower quality. However, what accounts for that remains unclear. The search for answers led Congress to request the IOM to study the problem, issue a report, and provide recommendations leading to the elimination of health-care disparities. The findings were published in the form of a report entitled *Unequal Treatment* (Smedley, Stith, and Nelson 2003).

Attempts to explain the fact that blacks experience higher levels of morbidity and mortality but tend to receive less intensive medical treatment are unceasing. The range of potential explanations that have been examined include cross-cultural miscommunication, lack of trust, differing preferences, discrimination, and of course, lack of access (Kasper 2000). According to the Institute of Medicine, it is also true that minority patients are more likely to refuse recommended services (Smedley, Stith, and Nelson 2003). While no single factor explains why that occurs, poor communication between doctor and patient provides a partial explanation for noncompliance and refusal of care. The IOM notes that refusal rates are, however, too small to explain health-care disparity.

One persistent hypothesis, namely, that the explanation might be related to the race of the physician, is also apparently not a significant factor, at least not in the treatment that patients who have experienced a heart attack receive. Researchers who explored this topic found that the race of the physician did not explain variation in quality of care, since both black and white physicians make similar clinical decisions with regard to care of their black patients (van Ryn and Burke 2000). This is not to say that the race of the physician does not matter. African American patients who see same-race doctors consistently indicate a higher level of satisfaction with the care they receive (Cooper-Patrick et al. 1999). This is largely due to greater patient involvement and better doctor–patient communication. There is reason to believe that this can lead to better outcomes.

Other researchers have considered the extent to which the patient's ability to pay might influence doctors' decisions. Research carried out at Veterans Administration (VA) hospitals is especially striking because veterans are entitled to free care for as long as they live. Researchers consistently find that blacks are less likely to undergo life-saving cardiac procedures even though ability to pay is not a consideration (Whittle et al. 1993). The VA continues to try to identify the factors that explain variation in outcomes. An issue of the journal *Medical Care* published thirteen articles focusing on this question, but ended up concluding that there is no significant racial disparity in access, it is what happens after that that matters (Demakis 2002). However, the evidence on outcomes is more complicated. For example, researchers found that black patients were more likely to have amputations while white patients had less disabling surgery.

Nor does the availability of primary care physicians, who are thought to be better at providing basic care than specialists, make much difference. In a study of 273 metropolitan areas, the lack of primary care physicians was found to be more closely associated with mortality among whites than blacks. In the case of blacks, socioeconomic status explained more than access to primary care physicians (Shi and Starfield 2001).

Studies of race differences in utilization of Medicare benefits, which are obviously available to almost all people over sixty-five years of age, indicate that whites are more likely than blacks to receive services for twenty-three procedures and more likely to receive services requiring high technology (Escarce et al. 1993). Researchers repeatedly find that Medicare coverage is not enough to promote effective use of medical-care services among enrollees, nor does it equalize health outcomes (Gornick et al. 1996).

Most researchers agree that it is important to understand better the process of care seeking and care giving. The emerging consensus is that although blacks are more likely to be poor, it does not prevent them from receiving high quality of care at the point of crisis. It does affect everything that happens before and after that. The problem begins with the fact that they seek care at a later stage of disease because they lack insurance and the funds to seek care earlier. They lack the funds to buy the necessary medications and follow the prescribed treatment regimen after the critical event, such as taking more time off from work to recover. Then there are all those mundane access problems that might discourage poor people, regardless of race, from seeking care, which can be summed up as cost in time and money to get to the doctor.

Receiving health care at the point of crisis in a hospital outpatient department or emergency room rather than from a personal physician who knows their medical history is what explains why poor blacks are more likely to lack continuity of care (Konrad et al. 2005; Kasper 2000). There is strong evidence to indicate that having a regular source of care, that is, a relationship with a primary care physician, is related to better health outcomes for everyone, even more so for the elderly (Rosenblatt and Wright 2000).

Researchers do not necessarily come up with the same answer to the question of whether the quality of care minorities are receiving has gotten better or worse in recent years. The report by David Satcher, the former surgeon general, and his colleagues, to which we referred in the chapter on race and ethnicity, concluded that 83,570 excess deaths "could be prevented if the black-white mortality gap could be eliminated" (Satcher et al. 2005). The "2005 National Healthcare Disparities Report," supported by the AHRQ and using 179 measures of health-care quality and fifty-one measures of access to care, found that care for African Americans was better than it was for Hispanics (AHRQ 2005a). The authors stated that the findings should not be surprising given that 21 percent of Hispanics under sixty-five reported being continuously uninsured for two years, compared to 10 percent of blacks, and 7.2 percent of both Asians and whites. This is consistent with the results of a study supported by the RAND Corporation which concluded that quality of care is much closer to equal when access is equal (Asch et al. 2006).

In the end, the problem of racial disparity is not going away and according to some may have gotten worse in some instances (LaVeist and Isaac 2008). The AHRQ created "Excellence Centers to Eliminate Ethnic/Racial Dispari-ties" (EXCEED) in 2001. The IOM continues to press for an answer to the question of "where do we go from here?" (IOM 2005).

Summary and Conclusions

The question this chapter raises is how much difference does *access* to, *cost* of, and *quality* of medical care make in explaining differences in health status. In the view of the experts who have considered this question, the answer is that it is of utmost importance to the individual. At the same time, the same experts generally say that there is more to it than just being able to get health care when it is needed. How do you align these two seemingly contradictory arguments? One way to interpret it is to say that everyone should have the same opportunity to obtain medical care because this is such a basic need. However, making health care available does not mean that the vast disparities in health status and risk of death across population groups will disappear.

That is true in part because we know that there are a whole host of rea-sons to explain why people do not get health-care services when they need them—because they do not recognize the symptoms, they do not want to admit that their symptoms mean that there is something seriously wrong, that friends and family have said that the symptoms are not worth worrying about, because the person does not believe that taking care of health issues is the worth the effort, and so on.

We will be exploring many of these factors in more detail in later chap-ters, especially the last factor we just mentioned. Consider the impact of realizing that society does not value one enough as a member of society to provide something that is so essential as health care. Is it reasonable to think that people who are left out of the insurance pool might see it as a reflection on their worth to the rest of society? In that way, it is not so much having access to quality health care that matters, but the fact that one is excluded from the privilege that matters. To the extent that this might be true, it is not hard to imagine that kind of thing taking on a life of its own with negative consequences for a person's overall sense of well-being, which has implications for physical health status.

Sound like this is too far a stretch? Medical sociologists have long been interested in the circumstances surrounding performance of the "sick role." Do you know people who explain their failures by invoking sickness? College students provide an excellent illustration of this phenomenon. Have you heard students who fail a test say that it happened because they had a cold or did not get enough sleep? Even saying that they partied too much the night before is better than admitting that they studied and still did not do well. The function of using sickness as an excuse is meant to suggest that one really has the ability to succeed at whatever the task might be, but something outside of oneself simply stood in the way, something that is clearly alterable. That is very different than admitting failure. It is certainly much better than letting the thought enter one's own consciousness that one failed because one does not have the ability, and probably never will. Not having health insurance works very much like this. Recognizing that society does not care enough to provide one with such an essential commodity and believing that there is not very much one can do to change that—is obviously enough to make a person extremely discouraged.

These observations move us away from medical care and bring us closer to the topic of stress, which we take up in chapter 9. Before we get to that, let us consider whether genes have anything to do with it.

CHAPTER EIGHT

~

Genes

In February 2001 two articles, one published in *Science* and the other in *Nature*, announced that scientists affiliated with Celera Genomics of Rockville, Maryland, a private company, and the International Human Genome Sequencing Consortium, a group of academic centers largely financed by the NIH and the Wellcome Trust of London, had succeeded in mapping the human genome. The contribution at the level of science was monumental. The impact on clinical practice continues to be far less clear. Since then, a steady flow of new reports has appeared identifying the exact location of genes implicated in the onset of specific diseases. That is not the same thing as saying that we have come closer to understanding how to apply such information to prevent the onset of disease.

We are moving at a much faster pace in understanding the role that genes play in the production of the proteins that determine which functions newly created cells will be performing. The study of proteins, "proteomics," is of particular interest to pharmaceutical companies, which consider proteins to be excellent targets for drug intervention. Pharmaceutical companies are developing a new field called "pharmacogenomics" with the aim of personalizing pharmaceuticals in response to an individual's genetic profile. How broadly applicable this approach to treatment turns out to be is not entirely clear.

Let me make my position with regard to genetics clear at the outset. I will argue that genetic science offers tremendous potential for understanding inheritance and its impact on the risk of developing disease. As things stand, however, genetics is moving faster on the diagnostic than the curative front—in fact, moving at astonishing speed on the diagnostic front. According to GeneTests, a genetic information repository funded by the NIH, as of 1995 tests for about three hundred diseases were available; by 2008, tests for over 1,500 diseases had become available (Hansen 2008).

Representatives of the medical establishment keep telling us that genetic testing holds great promise but that there are many issues that must be addressed before test data can be translated into medical practice—greater assurance of accuracy and protections from possible misuse of the information, for example. Given how fast this field is moving ahead, I do not wish to get caught up in the debate about what genetic science will be able to accomplish in the future or when that will happen. Instead, this chapter focuses on what we have learned about the relationship between genetic inheritance and health and illness to date.

Let's consider the facts. How much do we really know about the role that genes play in the development of disease? And more to the point, exactly what can be done about diseases that have a genetic basis? While these two questions are on the surface perfectly reasonable and straightforward, the answers are not. This is a very complex field of study. It is developing so quickly that statements made months, even weeks, ago are already out of date. There is a considerable degree of debate regarding what is known. We will be skimming the surface. Furthermore, we will be doing so from the perspective filtered through my interpretation of the subject matter, which is grounded in social science rather than basic science. With that admonition, let us begin with a bare-bones overview of the evolution of knowledge that explains how heredity works and how genes fit into the big picture.

Principles of Heredity

It all starts with Gregor Mendel, the monk who, in 1866, identified the basic patterns of inheritance in the garden peas he was experimenting with. Peas were good candidates for these experiments because they are "true" breeds, meaning that each new generation is identical to the last because peas are self-pollinating. What Mendel did was to cross-pollinate different strains of peas to see how they would change in succeeding generations. He observed seven traits, but for purposes of illustration we will focus on the trait that is mentioned most often in the literature—the smooth or wrinkled characteristic of the peas. When he crossed a strain of smooth with a strain of wrinkled peas, he discovered that the smooth-skinned peas predominated in the next generation. He assigned labels and letters to these traits using a capital letter (**A**) for the dominant trait and a small letter (**a**) for the recessive trait. Designated this way, the traits are known as "alleles." With this simple labeling arrangement and observation of the distribution of the traits in succeeding generations of peas, he established the basic mathematical formula that explains patterns of heredity. Scientists still use the same labeling formula.

Mendel found that in the first cross-bred or hybridized generation, all the offspring looked the same (had the same phenotype) and carried the same genetic make up (genotype). This happened because each of the offspring inherited 50 percent of their genetic makeup from each respective parent, resulting in an **Aa** genotype. Mendel found the smooth characteristic to be dominant, which meant that all the offspring were smooth skinned but carried the wrinkled trait. The second hybridized generation was different. It would follow what has become known as Mendelian principles of inheritance. For every four individuals in this generation, the results, or genotypes, were as follows: **AA, Aa, Aa, aa.** This meant that three of the four had smooth skins (phenotype) but there were three distinct genotypes represented among the four. This is exactly the way that inheritance works in humans for any single trait.

Mendel's findings did not attract wider interest until the beginning of the twentieth century. By then scientists already knew that cells were the building blocks underlying all life forms. They had also concluded that the nucleus of the cell contained rodlike structures known as chromosomes. They knew this because they could see these structures using relatively early techniques for preparing slides and the microscope lenses available at the time. By 1920, scientists had determined that chromosomes were composed of two biochemical substances—proteins and DNA (deoxyribonucleic acid). In 1956, scientists determined that humans have twenty-three pairs of chromosomes or a total of forty-six chromosomes.

It was, however, the 1953 discovery of the components and structure of the DNA molecule that was the biggest breakthrough in genetics. Two scientists, James Watson and Francis Crick, determined that DNA consists of two intertwined strands (the double helix) and that the two strands could replicate themselves by separating. In addition to describing the structure of the DNA molecule, Watson and Crick identified the four chemical components involved: adenine, thymine, guanine, and cytosine, that is, A, T, G, and C. All of this is important because it also revealed that the DNA molecule is the location of the genetic code that determines an organism's essential characteristics. DNA does this by specifying how the amino acids, which are the building blocks that form the protein, are to be joined.

(Remember, the chromosome is composed of DNA and protein.) The amino acids define the functions the protein will perform.

The concept of "new genetics" now appears regularly in discussions that revolve around the promise of genetic science. However, this concept is not as new as the label suggests. Furthermore, it has a more specific definition than one might guess. It refers "to the body of knowledge and techniques arising since the invention of recombinant DNA technology in 1973" (Cunningham-Burley and Boulton 2000, 174). It was not until geneticists were able to produce and manipulate DNA in the laboratory that the new genetics made possible the identification of specific genes as markers for particular diseases.

It was during the second half of the twentieth century that we began learning much more about genes and discovering more about their role in promoting protein synthesis. Protein synthesis is the extremely complex process that translates DNA code into different kinds of protein that, in turn, determine the functions that the resulting cells are to perform. (RNA [ribonucleic acid] is involved as well, but to understand more completely how it contributes to this process, you will need to refer to genetics texts.) For purposes of this discussion, you need to know that proteins perform a wide range of functions. For example, one class of proteins, called hormones, is responsible for growth. Another class, called structural proteins, produces connective tissue responsible for holding the body together. There are protective proteins that produce antibodies in response to foreign substances, and so on.

That brings us back to what genes do. Genes are discrete sequences of DNA arrayed on chromosomes. Genes contain the DNA code for synthesizing proteins. What differentiates us from other organisms is the complexity of the code that directs proteins to combine in certain ways, which produces different kinds of cells, which results in different kinds of tissues, and ultimately different organs.

The researchers who mapped the human genome said they were surprised to find that humans had about thirty thousand genes, which is only about twice the number of the fruit fly. More recent estimates indicate that we have about twenty thousand genes.

When the members of the two groups of geneticists who mapped the human genome originally reported their findings, they noted that about 75 percent of human DNA sequences are repetitive, or as they put it, made up of "junk." In other words, those DNA sequences do no coding. They estimated that about 1 to 1.5 percent of the total pool of genes is involved in coding. This means that only a small portion of human genetic material is still active and evolving. Initially the inactive genes were compared to an archeological site that researchers said was providing us with information about our genetic origins. Subsequent research, just a few months later, found that the inactive genes can become activated. When and how is obviously a matter of great interest to researchers. We will get back to that in a moment.

What are we to conclude about the significance of having a map of the human genome? Geneticists say that there is no question that the ability to locate genes on a map of the human genome is a tremendous accomplishment. However, they go on to say that the genetic code that is responsible for inheritance is enormously complex. They add that it is important to recognize that the map of the human genome has not come with instructions on how it can be altered, even by those who have the knowledge to interpret this map.

That explains why proteomics (the study of proteins) has gained ground so quickly in spite of the complexities involved. According to some geneticists, mapping proteins is a challenge because proteins act like a moving target. It is estimated that there are three hundred thousand to one million proteins, each composed of twenty different amino acids, which change over a person's lifetime. They change through interaction with sugars or oxygen and through interaction with other proteins. The effect of this is that proteins may act to turn off gene functions or make them produce great amounts of the same protein.

If genetics is so complex at the level of basic science research, it is no wonder that translating it into applied medical science is so uncertain.

Practical Implications of Genetic Theory

One well-known geneticist, Steve Jones, notes that his colleagues and other medical scientists have been promising that cures based on genetic breakthroughs are just around the corner for the last twenty years. They have yet to deliver on those promises. The problem is not that advances in genetic research are insignificant, but that patterns of inheritance are much more complicated than some people would have us believe.

The fact that twelve thousand distinct genetic conditions were listed in the Online Mendelian Inheritance in Man (OMIM) database maintained by the NIH as of 2009 begins to explain why the chances of finding cures for even a small portion of inherited susceptibility to disease are low. At the same time, diagnosing disease by pinpointing the genes involved in any one individual's illness holds considerably more promise. The disease may not be curable, but, under the best of circumstances, its effects may be better contained through the use of targeted drugs.

How difficult this is and how long it might take can be illustrated by two conditions—first, sickle cell anemia and second, Down syndrome. Sickle cell stands out as the most commonly used illustration of how much or how little power we have over inheritance. Sickle cell disease, which is often mentioned to support the idea that there are genetic differences between races given that blacks are far more likely to have it, was identified in 1910. It was apparent from earliest years that those affected were severely anemic. They had cells that were smaller or sickle shaped rather than being round. Eventually the "sickled" cells were found to be carrying insufficient oxygen to sustain the life of other cells in the body. The genetic inheritance pattern was not completely understood until 1956, when it became clear that sickle cell disease is transmitted as a single recessive trait. Going back to Mendelian heredity law, this means that both parents either have to be carriers of the recessive gene (**Aa**) or have the disease (**aa**).

Sickle cell anemia is a prime example of single-gene inheritance. In other words, there are no other genes involved. The inheritance pattern is clear and predictable. Yet reasonably complete understanding of the inheritance pattern and of the disease itself has not led to a cure. Therein lies the problem.

Down syndrome is a far more common condition (Landers 2008). In fact, it is the most common chromosomal condition that we know of. It affects one in every eight hundred children born in the United States. It results from an extra copy of a single chromosome, chromosome 21, in either some or all cells. In a few cases, individuals carry portions of material from chromosome 21 on other chromosomes. Down syndrome is linked to a range of physical and mental disorders. So it is curious, according to some researchers, how little attention has been devoted to studying Down syndrome and how poorly understood it is.

There is no question that we are learning a great deal more about inheritance patterns—for example, we know which diseases result from one mutated copy of a gene, as in Huntington disease, and those for which two mutated copies must be present, as in sickle cell and cystic fibrosis. We know which diseases are linked to the X chromosome, that is, transmitted by the mother. However, as I have already said, expansion of the knowledge base underlying genetic theory is not being translated into application at the level of medical practice at anywhere the same speed as genetic discoveries are unfolding.

Given that the number of diseases that are passed on via a single gene is relatively small compared to diseases that involve multiple genes (i.e., is multifactorial), many geneticists do not expect things to change very quickly. They may be altering that assessment in light of the speed at which genes are being identified that are linked with particular diseases, but the number of skeptics does not seem to be dwindling. The challenge inherent in interpreting the role played by multifactorial gene inheritance is that it cannot be said to cause disease. It is better understood as a process that permits diseases to develop in combination with external environmental and individually adapted health behaviors. Generally, all three must be present—genetic susceptibility, environmental support or tolerance of certain contributing factors, and individual participation in certain behaviors that foster development of that particular disease. Even that sounds well understood and predictable. It is not.

There is no single test that will predict the onset of disease from multiple gene inheritance because different populations of people have developed mutations that are represented in a long and complex series of genes. In other words, there is no single test that can identify the indicators for diseases, which are connected to multiple genes, which differ from one population to another.

To illustrate, cystic fibrosis may arise from one thousand mutations or errors that have evolved in a particular gene over a long period of time. As a result, 70 percent of the cases in Western Europe are due to one such mutation, but "2,000 miles to the east, that mutation causes only a small fraction of cases. In Jewish populations in the United States it is involved in only about a third of cases, but among North African Jews quite a different mutation is most common" (Jones 2000, 8). The result is that it is impossible to develop screening tests that will identify with any certainty all those at risk for even the most common genetically linked diseases.

There is also a predisposition to heart disease that runs in families. One link is the tendency toward high cholesterol levels that runs in families. However, about two hundred different genetic combinations are implicated. In short, it makes much more sense to rely on a blood test than striving to develop a sophisticated genetic test, especially since we already know some of the best predictors of heart disease—smoking and diet. As to the prevalence of diabetes, which is also known to run in families, Jones prefaces what he considers to be the most effective treatment by saying that detection is extremely complicated because "no single gene accounts for more than a tenth of individual susceptibility" (Jones 2000, 9). Because "genetics has little relevance to treatment . . . banning cheeseburgers would do far more" (Jones 2000, 10).

There has been a great deal of excitement surrounding the possibility of identifying the genes that predispose a person to cancer. The Harvard Center for Cancer Prevention published a report in 1996 focusing on prevention that concluded that cancer is a preventable illness, which is far from the way others in the field would characterize it (Begg 2001). By the beginning of the twenty-first century, inherited forms of cancer were thought to account for about 5 percent of the total (Weitzel and McCahill 2001). The problem is that, while inherited gene susceptibility may be high, onset still cannot be predicted. It can only be monitored to detect onset at the earliest stage.

There has been a great deal of progress in finding the relationship between genetic predisposition to lung cancer and behavior, namely smoking, in recent years. In 2006 we learned that chromosome 10 was implicated in nicotine addiction in the African American population and that there were suggestive linkages on chromosomes 9, 11, and 13 (Li et al. 2006). Two years later, we were told that nicotine dependence among persons of European descent is linked to a variation in a portion of chromosome 15 (Thorgeirsson et al. 2008). The results of this research indicate that nonsmokers without the variant have less than 1 percent chance of lung cancer; for a smoker who does not have the variant, the risk is 14 percent. Smokers who had one copy of the variant were found to smoke an average of one more cigarette per day than those who had no variant. Smokers who had two copies of the variant smoked two more cigarettes per day. The researchers concluded that genetics plays a role in how the brain handles nicotine. The consensus seems to be that genetic factors account for at least 50 percent of the risk of nicotine dependence across the populations that have been studied. Because about one-third of the global population smokes, there is an urgent need to understand the impact of genetics on smoking behavior. Most researchers go on to say that even though they are coming closer to identifying who is at greater risk of smoking-related disease, especially lung cancer, the best advice doctors can give, with or without genetic testing, is still the same—that people should not smoke.

Testing for genetic predisposition to breast cancer provides another topical example of what can be expected when a great deal of effort goes into fighting a particularly dreaded disease. Two genes are known to be implicated in one case out of twenty: BRCA1 and BRCA2. This means that most cases are not attributed to the genes known to be involved. Only about 2 percent have a specific family history that puts them at risk of BRAC mutations. The U.S. Preventive Services Task Force, sponsored by the AHRQ, recommends that only those women who have a family history undergo genetic testing (U.S. Preventive Services Task Force 2005).

As to the relationship between genes and environment, the difference in rates of breast cancer among women who share the same genetic background makes the point very effectively. The rate of breast cancer of Asian immigrants is similar to the rate among women in their homeland, but increases by 80 percent among third-generation Asian American women (Hoover 2000). What causes this dramatic increase is not at all clear. Commentary on this particular piece of research by a representative of the National Cancer Institute reinforces the point with an observation about research on identical twins. Given that identical twins are assumed to share an identical genetic code, one would expect them to develop the same diseases. In actuality, identical twins have about 15 percent chance of both developing breast cancer.

The reason that identical twins may not develop the same disease is that researchers now say that identical twins do not actually have an identical genetic profile (Bruder et al. 2008). The fact that twins can develop differences in response to environmental factors has been known for some time. What is new is the finding that unique changes can occur as a result of "epigenetic factors." Chemical markers can slow down or shut off some genes completely and speed up others. In short, variations do occur and they may offer either greater protection from certain diseases or contribute to their onset.

Another indicator of the relationship between genes and the environment came with the discovery of a gene linked to violent behavior, which attracted a great deal of attention a few years ago (Caspi et al. 2002). A team of scientists, led by clinical psychologists, discovered that a particular gene that provides the code for an enzyme (MAOA) that metabolizes neurotransmitters in the brain was linked to aggressive behavior in persons who were maltreated in childhood. The critical finding was that maltreated children who were unable to produce a sufficient amount of this enzyme were far more likely to turn to violence than maltreated children who were able to produce large amounts of the enzyme. Yet children in the study with a low level of the enzyme, who had not been maltreated, were not any more likely to exhibit antisocial behavior than those with a high level of the enzyme. The study again reinforced the fact that environmental influences are critical to the expression of behavior linked to this genetic flaw.

For now, let us conclude this portion of the discussion by saying that while our understanding of how genes and the environment interact is limited, there are a number of truisms that most people in the field can agree on. One, genes have intrinsic properties that respond to extrinsic signals. Two, genes are overwhelmed by a hostile environment. And, three, disease that can be linked to multiple gene causation is invariably the result of some combination of environmental insults and genetic predisposition.

We have already considered examples of the hostile physical environment internal to the body created by behavior such as overeating and smoking. Although we will not be exploring such matters here, it should not be difficult to imagine how a hostile external environment, such as air or water pollution, could overwhelm genes. The research on the impact that a hostile social environment might have is in its earliest stages, as illustrated by the discovery of the "violence gene."

The Relationship of Genes, Age, Sex, and Race

A little more background on when genes come into play and age may clarify the relationship between genes and genetic susceptibility. Genes have their greatest impact on human beings during the earliest stages of development. (The following is based on Baird [1994].) Accordingly, the impact of genes between conception and birth is especially important. Over half of fertilized eggs fail to produce babies. About 40 to 60 percent of zygotes are lost before the woman realizes she is pregnant. About 15 percent of pregnancies are lost prior to twenty weeks' gestation. In about half of spontaneous abortions, there are chromosomal abnormalities. Of fetuses carried to term, nearly 7 percent of stillbirths and neonatal deaths involve chromosomal abnormalities. The general interpretation is that nature is preventing lethal and abnormal genes from developing further.

Genes have a greater impact during early years of life than during later years. Moreover, genetic causes have become more apparent at this stage over the last century because other causes, such as infectious disease and nutritional deficiencies, have declined. At the beginning of the twentieth century, the infant mortality rate was about 150 per one thousand live births. Only about five out of one thousand of these deaths were considered to be due to genetic causes. When the infant mortality rate fell to less than ten per one thousand live births by the last decades of the century, genetic causes were implicated in one-third of the deaths. It is not that death from genetic problems increased. It is that as deaths from other causes declined, the deaths from congenital and genetic abnormalities grew as a proportion of the explanation.

In one study of over twelve thousand admissions to a pediatric hospital, 11.1 percent were clearly due to a genetic issue, 18.5 percent were for congenital malformations, and 2 percent were suspected of possibly being genetic. In short, over 30 percent were due to genetic disorders or birth defects. Other studies confirm this finding, concluding that the majority of pediatric patients with multiple admissions to pediatric hospitals are there due to problems that they were born with.

The impact of genes declines as people age. The least adaptive genes are lost first because the individuals who are the carriers are less likely to survive. The pathological genes that survive into adulthood contribute to disease only in combination with particular environmental factors. The proportion of cases in which genes play a role in early onset of disease during adulthood, for example, chronic heart disease before age forty-five, is small; much earlier mortality is far more likely in such cases. Apart from instances in which the indicators are this obvious, there is little we can be sure about when it comes to which individuals will become ill or how many of them will become ill.

Moving on to the topic of genes and sex, it is clear that of the twenty-three pairs of chromosomes that characterize human beings, only one is sex linked. Men are characterized by an XY chromosome and women are characterized by an XX chromosome. The Y chromosome is special for a number of other reasons. It is the smallest one, about one-third the size of the female X chromosome. The X chromosome contains about one hundred times more genes than the Y chromosome. However, the Y chromosome is one of the few that continues to change—it is continuing to degenerate, losing much of its active genetic material. At the same time, it is accumulating mutations. There are two sides to this. The negative side is that men are responsible for something like two-thirds of genetic disease. The positive side is that the Y chromosome is also responsible for introducing beneficial mutations.

One of the leaders in the international research project responsible for sequencing the human genome, Eric Lander, made the observation that the human genome is a "fossil record" of the last billion years of evolution (Nelson 2001). He noted that we will be able to learn a great deal more about human evolution than we knew before the genome was mapped. He also stated that geneticists could make a number of startling observations already: (1) that human complexity appears to lie in the diversity of proteins, not genes; and (2) that the DNA of any two people is 99.9 percent identical. That assessment has since been revised, with the figure dropping to 96 percent (Connor 2006).

The latter observation has implications for the use of race as a distinguishing category in any kind of research. Prevailing thought is that the genetic differences across racial groups appear as variations in the number of copies of particular genes (Connor 2006). It is also becoming clear that people's response to particular drugs has some relationship to racial genetic inheritance. Thus, some observers say that genetic differences, even if they are not well understood but are somehow related to race, should continue to be a focus of research because the findings promise to have a positive effect on treatment decisions. Others argue that focusing on racial differences will have negative social consequences.

With these basic facts in mind let us go back to the question this chapter opened with, namely: how much will increased understanding of the composition of the human genome either revolutionize medical care or explain variations in mortality and morbidity?

Gene Therapy and the Search for Cures

Gene therapy is at its earliest stage of development. In fact, the first step is obtaining a full sequence of people's genetic code. At this writing only two people have had their genetic code sequenced (Harmon 2008). One is James Watson, the codiscoverer of the structure of DNA. He had his genome sequenced in 2007 by a company that donated $1.5 million to demonstrate its technology. The other is Dan Stoicescu, who was the first customer of Knome, a company based in Cambridge, Massachusetts. A number of others, who can afford the $350,000 price, are in the process of signing up. Efforts to reduce the cost are being actively pursued by a number of competing companies.

There are also companies offering to identify a person's racial heritage based on a mail-in test for about $400, which some geneticists have labeled "recreational genomics." People who have used these services and have been interviewed by journalists say they are surprised to find that their heritage is not exactly what they thought it was. A few have had so much doubt that they went through the process with another company and did end up with different results. Clearly, such enterprises are still at an early stage of development.

The main problem facing those who are interested in going beyond recreational genomics to therapeutic genomics is that even when the location of genes linked to particular diseases is identified, there is so little that can be done to intervene. Altering genes is too risky because there is no assurance that all of any particular gene's functions have been fully identified. Genes that do not appear to have any function may in fact become activated when something happens to activate a related gene. The risk of making a mistake is simply too great.

A 1998 conference of experts convened by the NIH to explore the risks of conducting gene therapy experiments on fetuses ended up focusing on two issues (Gianelli 1998). One concern was that the technology would permit the creation of "designer babies." Depending on how you define this phenomenon, it is already happening. Human embryos are being created in the laboratory by prospective parents who provide eggs and sperm, and then decide which embryo to implant in the uterus. (What is done with the remaining embryos has evolved into a major battle over the use of the "stem" cells, which can be used to replace diseased tissues and regenerate organ growth, remarkably even in unrelated persons.)

In a small number of cases, which received national attention, parents wanted to be assured that they would produce an infant who was genetically matched to an older sibling who was suffering from a fatal illness. The infant's cells would be used to help the older sibling. Whether or not that is an ethically acceptable route to help save the older sibling continues to inspire debate. However, this kind of genetic selection was not the primary concern raised during the NIH conference. The greater fear under discussion revolved around the risk that the genetic manipulation associated with being able to choose from an array of embryos would cause genetic mutations in future generations.

It is fair to say that any discussion of gene therapy that takes place at the present time very quickly moves to discussion of ethical issues involved. For example, is it reasonable to advocate prophylactic surgery (Weitzel and McCahill 2001)? This refers to surgical removal of healthy tissue before it becomes diseased in the expectation that it will become diseased as predicted by genetic screening. As you might imagine, there are a number of problems associated with this solution. To begin with, there is the issue of accuracy of predictive tests. There is also the trauma and risk associated with surgery. Some forms of surgery, breast surgery for example, have serious psychological consequences for self-esteem, sexual relationships, and so on. You already know that predicting the risk of breast cancer is far from a sure thing. On the other hand, what else is there that can be done when there is no cure? The only other thing to do is careful monitoring. That in and of itself is very likely to have psychological effects. No wonder some people do not want to know what their risk is even as others are willing to undergo surgery to avoid even an uncertain level of risk.

Genetic Testing and Ethical Questions

Genetic testing and manipulation invariably touches off discussion that raises the specter of eugenics, that is, genetic engineering with the goal of eliminating the weak to improve the population. Even though everyone who is engaged in genetic research and the search for cures is quick to reject any connection to eugenics, the suggestion is difficult to shake off.

Let's look more closely at what it is about genetic tests that makes the whole issue so emotionally charged. How are they different from the medical tests that we have all been undergoing all along? The statement by the Committee on Bioethics of the American Academy of Pediatrics considered these questions (2001). They came up with a set of recommendations on genetic testing in response to the concerns they identified. They identified three potential risks: (1) genetic testing has implications for genetically related persons in addition to the individual being tested; (2) there are psychosocial risks, not only anxiety, but guilt, impaired self-esteem, and social stigma—plus, there are practical risks such as loss of insurance and employment discrimination; and (3) the value of genetic information is limited because it is not likely to alter medical treatment. The Academy acknowledges that none of these factors makes genetic testing that different from any other kind of medical testing. It is the cumulative effect that imposes a greater burden given that the benefits are so uncertain.

The Academy's position is to always advocate what is best for the child. Accordingly, it considered the benefits to the child of three types of screening tests—of newborns, of carriers of particular genetic traits, and predictive tests for late-onset disorders. The Academy agreed with the 1994 IOM report (the organization that advises government, identified in chapter 5), which recommended that tests performed on newborns be done only if the following criteria are upheld: (1) that identification of the condition provides a clear benefit to the child, (2) a system is in place that can confirm the diagnosis, and (3) treatment and follow-up is available. These are not abstract concerns. Various kinds of tests are already being conducted, in some cases mandated by states and performed on a voluntary basis in other states. Which tests are performed and whether the benefits outweigh the costs are questions of continuing concern and actively being monitored by the Academy.

The American Academy of Pediatrics agrees with the IOM that screening of adults to determine whether they are carriers of genes that are clearly implicated in particular diseases has both benefits and costs. The greatest benefit is that the results are available and important for those making reproductive decisions. The Academy is opposed to screening newborns to obtain carrier status, because that will not come into consideration until much later, when they are themselves ready to bear children.

Testing for late-onset diseases is more complicated. There are a number of diseases for which genetic tests now exist that can predict onset with a reasonable degree of accuracy. Tests for others are being developed. The question is whether knowledge of future risk is desirable if there is no cure. The Academy's position is that this decision should be left to the child when the child is old enough to make that choice.

Prenatal screening is even more controversial. The reason is obvious. At present, there is only one remedy available if and when a genetic flaw is identified during pregnancy. That is abortion. If abortion is objectionable to the parents, then why do prenatal screening? On the opposite side of the same coin, some geneticists worry that parents are too often ready to terminate pregnancies for trivial reasons.

This brings us back to the problem of designer babies. The phenomenon has been aptly named "unnatural selection" by one observer (Silverman 2001). Medicine has been ready to intervene to overcome the natural selection process through assisted-reproduction technology and technological intervention to save increasingly smaller premature infants. From this perspective, medicine is already altering the natural selection process. What is not yet clear is whether such interventions will have negative long-term effects on future generations. That will become clearer as this generation, which is the first to have relied on reproductive enhancement technology, begins to reproduce. The question that troubles some observers is—to what extent is the technology that makes it possible to engage in genetic engineering through embryo selection to produce designer babies increasing the rate at which "unnatural selection" is proceeding?

Commercial Interests and Law

Coming from another direction is a very different set of ethical concerns that have, thus far, received relatively little public attention even though commercialization and gene patenting have been hot topics within legal circles for at least two decades. Indeed, much is being translated into law before we have a chance to absorb it all (Buchanan et al. 2000).

One of the earliest and most interesting cases to attract the attention of lawyers involved in health law was the John Moore case (Kaufert 2000). John Moore was a patient whose physician patented his blood cells without his knowledge in 1984. When he discovered this, Moore became extremely upset for several reasons. He thought he had been going back to the doctor month after month to have his blood "tested." In actuality, his doctor was drawing his blood "to culture" or grow more of the cells he was interested in propagating. The doctor ultimately sold the patent for the product he developed using Moore's blood to a Swiss pharmaceutical company for $15 million. Moore sued. The court determined that he was not entitled to any profits stemming from his blood because it might set a precedent that would destroy pharmaceutical companies' incentive (read that as monetary incentive) to do medical research. Complicating matters further, the lawyers who took a favorable view of Moore's complaint were quick to point out that giving Moore part ownership of the "product" would introduce certain risks that he might not wish to accept. Being part owner would make him legally liable for any mishaps that might occur in using the product.

Because this case attracted so much attention, a legal/ethical remedy has evolved. There are now entire populations that have become the subjects of genetic research because they have been largely isolated for generations, such as the Amish, Icelanders, and some Pacific Islanders. The groups are now being fully informed about the nature of the research and being asked for permission to use any byproducts. All of this is a matter of predetermined contractual agreement, generally including some form of compensation.

The ultimate ownership of genes and cells stopped being a matter of debate once it became clear that the courts would side with those seeking patents. In 1994, Myriad Genetics obtained the patent for the BRCA1 gene, the first gene linked to breast cancer. Furthermore, it survived court challenges of its right to hold the patent. Accordingly, it is now in a position to charge a considerable fee for every genetic test that involves this gene. Other corporations have followed the same path.

There is also considerable discomfort in medical circles about the fact that companies doing genetic research are offering physicians and hospitals considerable amounts of money to obtain any biopsy tissue they collect from patients with genetic diseases. True, the tissue would otherwise be discarded. However, the companies are using this material for the purpose of developing tissue banks for expanded genetic research that they hope will lead to discoveries for which they can eventually charge large fees.

The rising number of tests being offered directly to consumers is the topic that is most troubling to geneticists, and for good reason. According to the Genetics and Policy Center at Johns Hopkins University, the Federal Drug Administration, which is responsible for evaluating the quality of drugs and medical devices, regulates "test kits" that it considers to be medical devices. However, it does not monitor genetic tests made in the laboratories that use them. It states that the Federal Trade Commission, which is responsible for protecting consumers against unfair or deceptive trade practices, has taken no action. It issued a fact sheet in 2006 warning consumers to be skeptical of claims and advising them to discuss results with a health provider. The center goes on to say that as of the first few months of 2009, thirteen states have passed laws prohibiting direct to consumer testing; twelve states permit specified tests to be offered; and twenty-five states permit testing with no restrictions.

As we already noted, there are now about 1,500 tests available to the consumer. Some of the most common are tests for breast cancer, which run about $2,800. Other commonly mentioned tests include tests for Down syndrome, Huntington disease, cystic fibrosis, albinism, and Alzheimer's disease. Those who are interested in ameliorating the risk of developing particular diseases through diet can turn to nutritionists who practice "nutrigenomics" and offer to prescribe an individually designed diet (Pollack 2002). The level of concern about the sudden rise in the number of tests and related services being offered to consumers is reflected in the statements advising caution being made by experts, for example, the American College of Medical Geneticists, the American Society of Human Genetics, the Genetics Alliance, and the National Human Genome Research Institute, to name a few.

These experts warn that it is not only that many of the tests are not sufficiently sensitive to provide accurate results; it is that individuals need to treat the whole matter of testing more carefully. They advise people to get genetic counseling before going through screening and discuss the results with health-care providers. However, there is no lack of consumers or investors interested in "consumer genetics" and "recreational genomics"—clearly commercialization in this field is alive and well.

Privacy and Genetic Discrimination

Apart from the quality problems that may be connected to direct-to-consumer genetic-screening products, there are added concerns about privacy. There is the risk that employers and insurance companies might get access to the results of the genetic reports, which could result in loss of health insurance, or worse, loss of people's jobs. Medical privacy legislation is working its way through Congress.

Fear of losing health insurance is not limited to those with genetic diseases. In fact, it was the fear on the part of persons diagnosed with HIV that gave rise to talk about the need to insure privacy of medical records. Not only is there obvious emotional trauma associated with being diagnosed with a fatal disease or the potential of developing a fatal disease, but the social stigma that follows is also enormously burdensome, as is the potential that this information will have economic consequences.

People offered the opportunity to go through genetic testing often refuse if they believe there is a risk of employers getting access to the results. Given all the talk in this country about the rising cost of health insurance and the rising number of people who are losing their health insurance, there is enough reason to fear loss of insurance without giving employers or insurance companies added reason to drop insurance coverage.

The list of concerns about the use and misuse of genetics is only beginning to surface in the public domain. The discovery of the "violence" gene is a case in point. Now that we know that a genetic defect is responsible for the expression of violence in some cases, should the courts treat those persons differently, akin to the way we treat persons with diminished capacity? Should we inform schools and social service agencies of the risks presented by children with this genetic profile?

Society has not had enough time to resolve questions regarding whose interests we think should be protected—those of individuals or those of society? Should the public be involved in defining what is an undesirable trait? Should research aimed at eliminating undesirable traits be supported? By the same token, should there be public support for research that aims to enhance genetic inheritance—for example, increased intelligence? Talk about the use and misuse of genetic knowledge is certain to create controversy. That is undoubtedly why there seems to be so much more emphasis on its potential to bring about a vast number of benefits to individuals and far less emphasis on its potential costs to society.

Summary and Conclusions

In the end, with so much that is still unknown about the relationship between genes and disease, why do so many people keep saying that the human genome is the breakthrough that will revolutionize medical care? The assessment made by Barbara Hanson in 1995, well before we knew as much about genetic inheritance as we do now, has not lost its authenticity:

> Genetic attributions emerge where issues are socially troublesome and biologically inexplicable, giving them a social life separable from their connections to physical biology. Their clarity and perceived simplicity give something to blame for troubles and in so doing provide relief from either individual or collective responsibility.
>
> Genetic attributions are a perfect icon for a process for dealing with troubles which shifts responsibility. Bio-medical research localizes troubles in individual bodies, shifts responsibility away from the system, and justifies pain and expense.
>
> We are either hapless victims or valiant warriors fighting valiantly for control of something. Our fight is noble. Our failures are not our fault. We must fight. We will probably fail. But the fight is what is important. We need bigger microscopes to fight! (Hanson 1995, 1, 3)

In short, to the extent that we can convince ourselves that investing our money and hope in genetics will provide solutions, we can avoid thinking about factors that might offer more complete explanations but are far more difficult to resolve. As Steve Jones puts it:

> Ill health runs in families. Usually, this has rather little to do with genes. The best predictor is simple: class. . . . Wealth and poverty are inherited, and most people born poor stay that way. In Britain, the difference in life span between the most and the least affluent is 11 years, which dwarfs anything that DNA might do. (Jones 2000, 4)

The latter is an observation that deserves a great deal more attention. It is at the heart of the subject matter that we will take up in chapter 9. Before we do that, we will deal with the tenth variable mentioned at the beginning of the book: stress.

Before turning to stress, it is worth mentioning that the link between genes and stress is the latest research frontier to attract researchers' interest. This has happened as researchers began to find that the genetic material that some were quick to label as "junk" a short time ago is actually composed of inactive genes that can be activated by stress. I should note that the field of stress-induced genetic change is still in a very early stage of development and very far from the kind of material that people like me are accustomed to reviewing. However, the fact that researchers are now able to document the link between stress and genetic change is significant. To illustrate, the expression of inactive genes appears to explain why some people do not respond to drugs as they are expected to do. Multidrug resistance to anticancer agents, for example, appears to be a genetic response to "cyto-toxic" stress, which is stress at the cellular level rather than stress that occurs at the level of the mind and body (Chano et al. 2002).

CHAPTER NINE

Stress

A sociologist by the name of W. I. Thomas presented us with a definition of stress in 1931 that, in my view, really captures the essence of stress (Thomas 1966 [1931]). He said it can be best understood as the "definition of the situation." In other words, if a person defines the situation as stressful, then it is stressful. Let me explain by asking you to consider how you would feel about being invited to go skydiving. That involves jumping out of a plane and going into free fall for about fifty seconds before you open your parachute. Many people would only do it if they were forced. But there are also those who think it would be fun and are eager to try what they see as an exciting challenge. If the large number of Internet sites showing people grinning and laughing while they skydive is any evidence, there are enough people in the second category to make it worthwhile for somebody out there to advertise this service.

See what I mean about definition of the situation? As unpleasant and embarrassing as this may be, you will probably agree that if people in the first group were being suited up to jump knowing that they would be floating around in the clear blue sky for a while, they would very likely break out into a sweat, possibly get a sudden headache, feel like they might have diarrhea at any moment, or develop an urgent need to urinate. The worse the perceived threat, the worse the symptoms. How do you feel prior to making a presentation in front of an audience? Many people experience sweaty palms and possibly some of the other symptoms I just listed. Of course, there are also those who are eager to try skydiving and those who love being on stage and experience only elation on those occasions. So there you have it. Just as W. I. Thomas said, stress is in the eye of the beholder of the situation. Admittedly, the beauty of this definition does not hold up very well once you try to turn it into a standardized measure.

Coming up with a measure is exactly what makes identifying who is stressed, and exactly how stressed a person is, so problematic. As you know, unless you can measure stress, you can't compare its effects from one person to another. If you can't do that, then you can't say much about its relationship to health except to say that it matters somehow and that some people seem to be more stressed than others. That opens the doors to speculation and misrepresentation. It allows unsubstantiated ideas to take hold, such as—top executives have very stressful jobs so they must be at greater risk of illness or death. The conventional wisdom says that executives must make major decisions that affect the future of whole companies and large numbers of people and that is what makes their jobs so stressful. Maybe. But you have to ask yourself, how is it that they seem to cope with all that responsibility so well? Top executives are a lot healthier and tend to live a lot longer with what is generally assumed to be high stress—in fact, a lot longer than their employees, especially their lower-level employees. (I hope you are not tempted to say that it must be genetic!) But that is getting ahead of the story. We will return to the issue of stress that those at the top are experiencing because understanding how that works provides some basic insight into this whole topic.

This chapter is devoted to examining what researchers have discovered about the relationship between stress and health that might contribute to our understanding of the variation in mortality and morbidity. Before we proceed, I should tell you that we will be emphasizing the physical consequences of stress. In other words, we will not be examining the relationship between stress and mental health in any depth. The study of mental health is a separate discipline with a tremendous amount of research and literature of its own. It is complex. We simply cannot address it with any degree of accuracy as an aside to a discussion primarily devoted to variations in physical health.

There is an enormous body of literature that focuses on stress per se. Moreover, the topic has been attracting the attention of researchers from entirely separate disciplines for quite some time. However, their work has not been integrated until relatively recently. Social psychologists focused on measuring people's psychological reactions to particular events and sought to identify factors that might ameliorate the negative effects of stress. In the meantime, biomedical researchers were working on identifying objective measures of a person's physical response to stress and epidemiologists were exploring the pathways between social networks and health status. Let's consider the work produced by social psychologists first.

Stressful Life Events

The scale developed by T. H. Holmes and R. H. Rahe in 1967 was considered to be a major breakthrough in the effort to link life events, stress, and health consequences. The researchers assigned weights to particular life events, starting with death of a spouse at the top of the list amounting to 100 points, divorce 73 points, marital separation 65 points, to things like change in number of family get-togethers 15 points, vacation 13 points, and minor violations of the law 11 points. The idea was to review events in a person's life, count the points, and predict the risk of illness over the next two years. The more points, the more likely one would come down with an illness. The reasoning went like this: any change in one's life requires making adjustments—the greater the adjustment or adaptation that is required, the more stress is produced.

Sound like a logical step forward? What do you think the criticisms might be? One of the first things that critics found troubling was the lack of differentiation between negative events and positive events. Shouldn't negative events have qualitatively different effects? Some critics clearly subscribed to W. I. Thomas's view of stress, even if they did not attribute that insight to him. For example, wasn't it possible that the death of a husband who had been abusing his wife could come as a relief to the wife? Wouldn't her stress response be very different and a lot lower than that of a wife who had a wonderful relationship with her husband? Could you really assign a set number of points to events without taking into consideration the context within which those events took place, that is, the definition of the situation the persons involved were placing on it?

Other critics pointed out that stress might have preceded certain life events. In some instances, stress could contribute to, even cause, negative life events rather than be a response to negative events. For example, stress due to severe chronic illness of a child could be a major contributing factor leading to divorce. Moreover, critics noted that ongoing stress is certainly different from resolved stress. That is, a long-term serious illness of a spouse may be more damaging to a person's health than the sudden death of a spouse.

A review of psychological literature indicates that the field of health psychology began to broaden its focus some years ago, devoting far more attention to physical health as a factor related to mental health. In fact, about one-third of the articles published in psychology journals between 1990 and 1992 examined physical health issues (Adler and Matthews 1994, 230). The objective of such articles was to explain who gets sick by identifying the diseases that have a stronger link to variations in psychological dispositions. The paradigm that has taken hold over the last decade states that it is the combination of social environment and individual dispositions that leads to certain health behaviors that are mediated by psychophysiological mechanisms. In short, it is the interaction between mind and body that causes stress and ultimately produces disease.

The challenge that continues to motivate researchers is explaining how psychological mechanisms produce health-damaging effects at the physiological level. Two sociologists, Bruce Link and Jo Phelan, are generally credited with being the first to suggest that we need to understand the "pathways" that explain the causes of disease (Link and Phelan 1995). While those pathways are far from being fully mapped out, each new effort to examine the link between the reality each of us experiences and the impact this has on our health status has become considerably clearer than was the case even a short while ago. We will consider some of those findings shortly.

The "Coping with Stress" Literature

Debates about the value of assigning points to life events did not continue to occupy the attention of psychologists and social psychologists. Researchers turned to studying *stressors* without trying to standardize stress effects. Indeed, stress research turned to the exploration of factors that account for the variation in how well people cope with stress. Thus we find that enormous effort has been devoted to the study of coping behavior and advantages associated with social support. When Peggy Thoits surveyed the social-psychological literature on stress and health in 1995, she identified approximately three thousand articles published over the preceding ten-year period. A review of this body of work produced a number of consistent findings, plus persistent unanswered questions, which led Thoits to comment on the policy implications associated with this work.

Thoits determined that the social-psychological literature had, until that time, devoted greater attention to stress effects related to mental health but less to physical health. She found that observations about mental health could not be generalized to physical health because, from the perspective found in this literature, the connection between the two was still not well understood. Most disappointing was finding that there was no consensus regarding which coping strategies were most effective in either case—for mental or physical health.

One of the persistent questions pursued by researchers in this field has to do with the role of social networks and social integration. To some extent this reflects the conventional wisdom regarding women's readiness, in contrast to men's reluctance, to talk about their problems with their friends and relatives. The idea is that women benefit from being able to release stress because they can rely on social-support networks composed of persons to whom they can unburden themselves. Reality turns out to be a little more complicated than that. For a start, more recent research indicates that high levels of stress in men are linked to heart disease, but high levels of stress in women are linked to cancer (Ferraro and Nuriddin 2006). Clearly there is a lot more work to be done in understanding what accounts for that.

Returning to Thoits's survey of the literature, researchers consistently reported finding that men have more "extensive" networks but that women have more "intensive" networks. It was, however, the presence of a "significant other" that was most important in both cases. (This is the person with whom one has the closest and most valued connection.) Researchers repeatedly found social integration to be a positive factor and social isolation to be a negative factor. The perception of support was consistently correlated with better mental health. But what turned out to matter most was whether the individual believed that support, either psychological or practical, would be forthcoming. In other words, it was not the actual receipt of support, but the belief that it would be there if needed that was most important.

Researchers find that certain demographic variables are consistently linked to greater levels of stress. Would you be surprised to hear that lower-status persons, those who are unemployed, women, and minorities were all more likely to have higher stress levels? According to Thoits, it is curious that the sociologists involved in this research did not emphasize or examine further the significance of findings related to these very basic demographic variables. Sociologists and social psychologists might have been expected to pay more attention to how much social class or status matters for a number of reasons. First, there is the economic dimension of social class. Having the resources, most notably money, to overcome some problems that cause stress would help overcome some basic sources of stress, such as having the money to pay for various services; for example, having enough money to pay for "respite" help in the case of those who are primary caretakers of a severely ill relative. Second, there is the fact that social structure imposes structural barriers to coping with and resolving problems in some cases, most notably for women and minorities, meaning they typically make less money, have less job security, do not enjoy the benefits of membership in "old boy networks," and so on.

Thoits concluded with the following observation after reviewing this immense body of work—that it tells us that a person's place in the social structure exposes the person differentially to stress. While damage is moderated by an individual's coping ability, it is also true that psychological resources and particular strategies are patterned in ways that may leave disadvantaged groups more vulnerable. Beyond reaffirming the fact that demographic variables matter, the research reported in this enormous body of literature explains relatively little that would help us to understand why people experience varying levels of stress. Nor does it point to any interventions that could be counted on to counteract stress with any certainty. This is probably due to the fact that the interventions that were attempted typically did not affect the normal course of events over which the person could impose little control. In other words, getting support from a counselor or therapist does not overcome all the practical, real-world problems that are causing the stress in the first place.

We sometimes hear about individuals who experience exactly the same intolerable conditions and end up successfully overcoming the odds and going on to live out fulfilling and satisfying lives. There are always arguments about how this happens grounded in competing conventional wisdom explanations—some people say it is genetic, while others argue that it just shows that everyone could have overcome those problems and simply did not strive to do so for a whole host of other reasons on the conventional-wisdom list.

Social psychologists have only recently become interested in understanding why people in similarly stressful situations are more or less "resilient." Although they knew that some people exhibited better "personal coping resources" than others, they did not go on to investigate the source of those resources (Pearlin and Schooler 1978). There was little reason to go beyond what had become generally understood—that coping resources were unequally distributed by social status. It is also worth noting that some researchers have argued that "personal agency" may be responsible for the differences. In other words, it is possible that people with "better mental health self select themselves into social contexts that reduce their chances of experiencing stressful events" (Thoits 2006, 317). However, Peggy Thoits makes the following observation regarding this proposition.

> People do not usually select themselves purposefully into states of misery and confusion; they are *socially* [sic] placed, *socially* [sic] channeled, and *socially* [sic]

shaped, sometimes despite their best efforts to meet and overcome threats and misfortunes. (Thoits 2006, 318)

In other words, we need to know a lot more about why some people have better mental health to begin with; why they are able to define situations as positive or negative and build on those observations; and how they engage in something that some have labeled "structural amplification," that is, participate in constructing a more rewarding social environment that brings more social and psychological benefits (Mirowsky and Ross 2003).

Does this leave you with the impression that a lot of people have devoted an enormous amount of time and effort to investigating stress reactions, coping responses, social support systems, and individual competence or resilience and that none of it produced clear answers that can be effectively applied? That is certainly true in my view. In the end, according to Thoits, the findings do not offer policy makers much to go on either. There is no basis for arguing that any of the findings can be translated into interventions that promise to lower the incidence of disease, reduce costs, improve work performance, and so on.

While this body of research seems to have hit a wall, another category of researchers, those who focus on measuring physical indicators of stress and responses to stress, have been coming up with some exciting discoveries. In fact, they can now tell us a great deal about how physical effects are linked to psychological effects and how all of that leads to clearly identifiable diseases like heart disease (Dimsdale 2008), diabetes (Golden 2007), addiction (Cleck and Blendy 2008), plus a lot of other less well known diseases.

Epidemiology and the Link between Social Networks and Health

Throughout the 1970s and 1980s, epidemiologists were consistently finding that absence of social ties was related to almost every cause of death. Indeed, this body of research is now known as *social epidemiology*. (The following is based on Berkman and Glass [2000].) While the findings on the power to predict health outcomes using measures of connectedness (in contrast to isolation) were indisputable, it is also true that the explanation for this phenomenon was not clearly understood. A new wave of research, which really took off during the late 1980s, resulted in a model showing the links between social structure, social networks, and psychosocial support mechanisms, each contributing to the creation of specific pathways that directly affect health. The latter include the following three dimensions—health behavior, psychological resources, and, ultimately, physiological responses. We will return to the topic of social isolation and its opposite—embeddedness—in a network in the final chapters of the book.

The same researchers determined that social isolation causes chronic stress, which leads, in turn, to accelerated aging and functional decline. This body of literature, which is now extensive, is important because it focuses on the link between social experience and physical response, that is, the pathways that are responsible for physiological effects, which lead, in turn, to disease and early death. The measures used to carry out this research are considered to be objective and well established. That has allowed the application of the accelerated-aging hypothesis to be linked to a far broader range of social experiences, including the relationship between chronic stress and racism, which we will get back to a little later.

The Physiological Response to Stress

Any in-depth discussion of the physiological response to stress invariably begins with the work of Hans Selye, who began reporting his findings on stress in the 1930s. Robert Sapolsky, a professor of neuroscience involved in stress research, provides us with some insider information on how Selye came upon his discoveries (Sapolsky 2004). It seems that Selye was working with laboratory rats, testing to see how a particular extract would affect them. He needed to give them daily injections. However, he wasn't very good at handling them. So he would drop them, have to chase them around the lab, flail at them with a broom to get them out from wherever they were hiding, and so on. After a few months, he discovered that the rats were developing ulcers and had enlarged adrenal glands and shrunken immune tissue. Unfortunately, the rats he had been using as control subjects, which he had been injecting with saline, were developing the same symptoms. So the test extract was obviously not responsible. What was producing these effects only became clear after Selye studied the phenomenon in much more detail. His work, which he named the "general adaptation syndrome," laid the foundation for the study of the physiology of the stress response.

Remember the skydiving illustration and mention of the physical response that might be expected of those who do not think skydiving would be very enjoyable? The sweaty hands, the need to go to the bathroom, and so on? That describes what Selye identified as the "flight-or-fight" response, which is characteristic not just of humans, but of all mammals. The difference is that mammals, at least those in the wild, unlike the lab rats that Selye was handling, deal with fight or flight situations better than we do. According to

Sapolsky, that is exactly *Why Zebras Don't Get Ulcers*. (That is the name of his book [2004] and the basis of the following discussion.)

The difference between humans and zebras is not in how the two species respond to feeling threatened. That is pretty much the same. In responding to a stressful situation, all mammals ready themselves to fight or run away from the source of threat. The physiological response to stress involves mobilization of energy, shutting down of routine physiological processes, and elimination of anything that will get in the way of running or fighting. Thus, the body responds with a rush of hormones to provide energy where the energy is needed—to muscles. To concentrate energy, the body inhibits other routine processes such as digestion, growth, immune responses to disease, reproduction (the sex drive), and so on. The body strives to eliminate dead weight that might reduce the efficiency of the fight or flight response by signaling that the body should eliminate excess fluids and waste (meaning we have the sudden urge to run to the bathroom). It alters some other functions that might be useful in the struggle by sharpening cognitive and sensory skills while blunting pain.

This set of bodily changes is highly adaptive if you actually need to fight or flee. The problem is that most of the threats human beings experience are not the kind that require a physical response. The kinds of threats that most of us are exposed to are symbolic rather than physical. Being "told off" and threatened with being fired by one's boss is a good example. Neither fighting nor running away are considered to be appropriate responses. However, people also do not take such encounters in their stride. They respond to the threat with the same set of physiological reactions that are designed to facilitate fight or flight. These physical adaptations then go unused. That is the core of the problem that leads to stress-related disease. The likelihood of stress-related disease is greater for those persons who find themselves in such circumstances often and/or have difficulty turning off the fight-or-flight adaptive process.

The explanation sounds pretty simple at one level. The hormones that provide energy are used up in either fight or flight. After that, things mostly go back to normal. It is when hormones are not used up that damage occurs. Some hormones are more damaging than others. In actuality this is a very complicated process, not completely understood by experts. To learn the specifics about how the process operates, I refer you to Sapolsky's book. The following is a brief synopsis of what Sapolsky tells us about stress and how it produces bodily harm.

Certain glands (if you think of the brain as the major controlling gland, you are right on target) are responsible for releasing stress hormones. The hormones that are released immediately in the face of threat are epinephrine and norepinephrine (called adrenaline and noradrenaline in some English-speaking countries). A second set of hormones, released minutes or hours later, are called glucocorticoids, or more specifically, cortisol. It is this second set that is implicated in stress-related disease. Problems occur when cortisol is not used up or absorbed during the fight-or-flight episode. The buildup of cortisol damages organs, which is what ultimately causes stress-related disease. In short, it is not the stress itself that causes illness. It is that stress causes hormones to be released, which are not absorbed, and it is the build-up of those hormones that causes illness.

There is some evidence to indicate that the way many of us learned to cope with stress may be causing health problems for Americans. It explains why an increasing proportion of Americans are becoming overweight and why poor Americans are at even greater risk of obesity than those who are not poor. The fact that we pick up the habit of indulging in comforting high-fat snacks when we are stressed out provides an important piece of the puzzle. Ads for high-fat snacks certainly suggest that we will feel better after we eat them. Unfortunately, researchers are finding that fat ingested when a person is experiencing stress does not burn off (Stoney et al. 2002). One result is weight gain. The other even more troubling result is increased risk of heart disease, which is associated with the high levels of total cholesterol, triglyc-erides, and low-density lipoprotein cholesterol (LDL, or what many people know as bad cholesterol) that make all those fatty foods so tasty.

We are not alone in registering a preference for sweet, fatty food when we are stressed out. Animal research indicates that in the case of subordi-nate monkeys, consumption of such foods helps to tamp down the release of stress hormones. High-status monkeys express less interest in such snacks. Researchers say that the behavior of the low-status monkeys amounts to a coping strategy to deal with stressful situations that is detrimental to their health just as the same kind of behavior is detrimental to human health (Tierney 2008).

Why Some People Manage Stress Better than Others

The question that has long puzzled researchers is why stress causes higher levels of *distress*, with all its detrimental health consequences, in some people more than in others. We have just learned that people who have close con-nections and benefit from belonging to a supportive social network are less likely to succumb to disease and early death. Researchers who focus on the physiological precursors that lead to disease kept trying to come up with an answer. A number of possibilities present themselves.

For example, sleep deprivation has been found to be responsible for the onset of stress-related disorders based on both human and laboratory animal studies. Since the body requires sleep to repair itself, restricted sleep results in changes in both brain systems and neuroendocrine systems (Meerlo, Sgoifo, and Suchecki 2008; Sapolsky 2004, 233–38).

The nonphysiological precursors of stress are far more difficult to capture. One intriguing hypothesis is that people who have a greater sense of control over life events are less stressed. Back to skydiving—the people who think skydiving might be a fun thing to do are defining it as an exciting challenge and are choosing to do it. You can see how being forced to do it would cause distress, but choosing to do it would be a voluntary act under the person's control. It is the definition of the situation that matters, which is where control by the individual comes in.

Virtually all researchers involved in stress research agree that control over much of what happens in one's life largely depends on one's ultimate status or position in society. Remember the reference to executives who have to make all those important decisions and how stressful people say that must be? The idea that executives are highly stressed and at risk of developing an ulcer is probably due to all the attention the "executive monkey" experiment, conducted in 1958, received (Sapolsky 2004, 268–69; Cook et al. 1981). In this experiment, half of the monkeys were in a position to press a bar that would delay or avoid electric shock. The other half received the shock when the executive monkey did. The "executive" monkeys got the ulcers. That experiment gave credence to the idea that there is an "executive stress syndrome." But like what sometimes happens when the details of research projects are revealed, this study came under criticism when the selection process that produced the "population of research subjects" was more closely examined. It seems that the researcher selected monkeys who were readier to press the bar to serve as the experimental executive monkeys. Yes, they got the ulcers, but perhaps it had to do with their innate temperaments or personalities—not the executive role they were playing.

Researchers find that personality does indeed matter. People really can be classified as having Type A or Type B personalities. Cardiologists have long connected Type A personality with heart disease. Some time later, researchers discovered that being Type A plus having a hostile streak is an even better predictor of the onset of heart disease. The most recent refinement of this connection involves one more aspect linked to personality differences.

It seems that repressing the expression of strong emotions has the effect of exaggerating the physiological responses connected to the stressful events.

To illustrate, in a study focusing on how people's blood pressure levels are affected by negative experiences, researchers found that blood pressure rises when people feel that they are being treated unfairly (Kreiger and Sidney 1996). However, it goes down if they are able to do something about it. Researchers in one study found that black working-class adults had higher blood-pressure levels in comparison to the whites and middle-class blacks in the study. They interpreted this to mean that people who feel powerless to do something about adversity deny that it is happening. They even begin to accept such treatment as "deserved." The fact that they cannot do anything to alter the situation when such events occur results in a steady state of elevated blood pressure or hypertension. What makes this observation particularly noteworthy is that, if you recall from chapter 5, we found that blacks have higher levels of hypertension. In fact, they have levels that are four times higher than that of whites (Young and Gaston 2000). We also found in chapter 5 that society has been less likely to attribute any lack of success on the part of blacks to racial discrimination during the late 1990s than it was several decades before that (Schuman and Krysan 1999). In other words, society has been saying that blacks who are not successful can blame no one but themselves even as they experience unfair treatment and racial discrimination. It should not be difficult to understand how this can lead to chronic stress, which, in turn, leads to accelerated aging. In short, stress provides a better explanation for why blacks have higher rates of hypertension than whites than most of the other variables we considered thus far. Of course, this may change. We will have to see the extent to which attitudes change in light of the fact that two major changes have occurred in American society: the election of an African American president and the economic downturn that occurred at around the same time—and whether this has any impact on hypertension rates among blacks.

Even though the volume of research on the relationship between psychological stress and physiological stress has been steadily increasing, we are still unable to predict who is most likely to register stress and under what circumstances. We do not know enough about stress to understand why seemingly similar events affect people differently. It may be that personal agency or self-selection regarding the choices a person makes in dealing with stress has not received as much attention as it deserves, since some people facing adverse situations exhibit much higher degrees of resilience than others (Thoits 2006). Of course, that still leaves the question of why some people have greater personal agency resources. We will consider one possible astonishing answer when we get to the end of this chapter.

We do know that people operate with different priorities and opt for different ladders in striving for success and that might provide a partial answer. This insight might help to explain why a highly successful corporate executive might be more stressed about not having been selected to head the committee that will choose the architectural plan for the new city library than he is about losing out on plans to take over a competitor's business.

The reaction, which many people in this country would see as irrational, may not be so irrational if you look at it from another point of view. Yes, the executive and his company would miss an opportunity to make a great deal of money for which he would very likely have been rewarded with a huge bonus. However, the executive might reason that there will be other opportunities for takeovers, but only one major new city library built in his lifetime. At the same time, another executive of comparable status might view serving on the library committee as a necessary but unwelcome drain on time that could be devoted to uncovering more takeover opportunities. In other words, the individual chooses the hierarchy he wants to be on top of. And it is not always the one that brings the greatest monetary reward. Playing a significant role in creating a physical structure that will stand after one is long gone might feel like a much more lasting achievement to some.

Clearly the level of stress people experience varies because they are "defining" situations differently. That explains why some people who seem to have everything are far from satisfied, in fact, feel deprived. "Having everything" is a relative concept. The sense of deprivation is also relative. That explains W. I. Thomas's observation that the "definition of the situation" a person employs becomes "real in its consequences."

One might conclude that learning to define the situation in ways that reduce threat should, in the end, have positive effects that reduce the risk of stress-related disease. That comes close to being true. The problem is that this solution is a lot easier to advocate than it is to carry out. To illustrate, Sapolsky uses the example of a group of people who have spent years imprisoned as political hostages (1998, 311–12). Upon release, one can see that some of the prisoners have succumbed to incapacitating posttraumatic stress disorder (PTSD), suffer nightmares, and have trouble returning to anything resembling normal life. Then there are a special few who say that, yes it was terrible and they would never want to go through anything like that again, but it made them realize what is really important in life. In retrospect, they say it was an important life-shaping experience. What explains the difference? Personality is part of the answer.

Personality is affected by what the person has learned or experienced before that catastrophic event. Those who have learned that they can deal with stress, even overcome it, can be expected to do better than those who have learned that they are largely ineffectual in dealing with stress. This is where the concept of "learned helplessness" comes in. People can and do learn that nonresistance or giving up the fight is the easiest route to take in the face of stress. To what extent this is innate and to what extent it is learned is not entirely clear. However, trying and failing on a regular basis is probably an important part of the explanation. There is certainly evidence to indicate that facing challenge and learning to deal with it helps to establish a record of accomplishment that builds self-confidence. It doesn't change the level of *stress* but it does affect the amount of *distress* the person experiences. (Remember the glucocorticoid part of the story—prolonged stress or sense of stress keeps the cortisol level elevated and that is what damages organs.) Developing a sense of self-confidence based on actual experience means the period of acute distress is shorter, allowing the body to return to a more normal state more rapidly. The cortisol level does not stay elevated as it does in those persons who feel that they have little control over their environment. People who feel that they have relatively little control experience a low, but constant, level of distress, which shows up as an elevated cortisol level and leads to damaging physical effects.

On the other hand, successful adaptation to stress under some circumstances, during wartime for example, may not turn out so well in the long run either. As we learn more about PTSD, we find that the people who adapted well during the crisis period may have developed coping mechanisms that were well suited to the wartime situation but are maladaptive for civilian life (Alonzo 2000). Distancing oneself from emotional attachment to peers who might die works well at the time. Distancing oneself from others during civilian life creates problems. That is a central feature of PTSD. Even though PTSD became a diagnostic category only as of 1980, it has become clear that it comes with enormous social costs that the mental health community still doesn't know how to reduce very effectively. Persons with PTSD are estimated to experience almost one day per week of work impairment (Davidson 2001).

How much of our response to stress can be explained by personality requires untangling the relationship between traits that we are born with as opposed to traits that we acquire through experience, that is, that are environmental. The answer is not at all clear. As medical science progresses, what we mean by environment is being redefined. It turns out that much of what was long thought to be genetic is really a matter of intrauterine environment. That the prenatal environment matters has been clear for a long time (Nathanielsz 2001; Barker et al. 1989; Barrett 1981). Such obvious influences as maternal nutrition, infection, and complications during delivery have received considerable attention in recent years. The fact that maternal anxiety during pregnancy is associated with complications has also been recognized for some time (Khashan et al. 2008). However, the long-term effects on the physical and mental development of the child are only beginning to be understood (Quellet-Morin et al. 2008).

There is a growing body of research on the relationship between brain development in infants and children that focuses on how stress affects the neurobiological maturation of the brain (the discussion presented here is based on Mustard [2000]). It is becoming clear that the inability to deal with stress in adult life is due to poor "wiring of the brain," which occurs during the early stages of life. To illustrate, neglected or abused children do not develop core brain function, which is what leads to dysfunctional behavior. Children brought up in stressful home situations have difficulty coping with the challenge of school because of inadequate development of core brain functions. They are the ones who are disruptive, antisocial, and sometimes violent. By contrast, those who grow up in a favorable environment have strengthened cognitive capacity, which is manifested in higher IQ scores, achievement in mathematics, and general learning capacity. Researchers may have to reconsider these conclusions in light of the most recent findings on how genetic predisposition to violence interacts with environmental factors. They will need to identify the neurological pathways that operate to link how the genetic predisposition to violence combines with an abusive environment to affect brain development.

What is known is that neurobiological development occurs as the number of connections among neurons grows, which produces synapses. The density of the synapses is related to the size of the frontal cortex—what we think of as the size of the brain—which diagnostic imaging can show. In short, there is now ample evidence to show that early childhood stress, which occurs at the psychological and emotional level, translates into both mental and physical health problems in adult life. Even more impressive is the research on the pathways between early brain-core development and disease, that is, psychoneuroendocrinology and psychoneuroimmunology. One way to put it is: cells are doing the learning. Clearly, early brain development increases cognitive ability, which shows up in higher childhood IQ scores, which, in turn, predicts to longer life expectancy and to all the social and economic benefits that high achievement can bring (Power and Kuh 2006).

The Lessons Baboons Can Teach Us

Doing empirical studies with humans as subjects of stress research is complicated because those who fund and oversee research frown on the kind of research that would induce stress to measure the subject's physiological responses. It is also hard to follow human subjects around to observe how they respond to a range of stressful and nonstressful situations in their daily lives. However, nonhuman primates are increasingly being called upon to tell us about the physiological responses of all primates, especially humans (Capitano and Emborg 2008). That is precisely why Robert Sapolsky studies baboons. When he explains how he conducts baboon research, the constraints seem nearly as high as they would be if the subjects were human. He has to make sure he anesthetizes them without stressing them out. He has to make sure that he is working with subjects that are not sick or injured. He doesn't use females because anesthetizing them might affect their pregnancy negatively or injure an infant they are nursing and so on. From where we sit, however, the constraints are clearly worth it because his findings are awesome!

His reports on the correlations between personality and physiology among baboons are particularly revealing. Perhaps the most surprising findings have to do with the consequences of rank within the group. It is the link across these variables that makes his findings so awesome. He reports finding a cluster of behavioral traits associated with low resting glucocorticoid levels among males who have higher rank within the tribe. This is where personality intersects with health outcomes. It appears that the males who can readily differentiate threatening situations from nonthreatening situations experience less negative impact from stressful events.

This is how he explains it. How a baboon reacts when a rival approaches is the issue. The males who can accurately distinguish between threatening and nonthreatening behavior on the part of the rival are much better off. The baboons that respond by going into a fight-or-flight response when the rival is merely wandering by and making no threatening gestures are the ones who end up having stress-related disease. In other words, in the latter case, the baboon is not only producing stress hormones inappropriately, but he is not using up those hormones in either fight or flight. That means that his cortisol level is elevated unnecessarily and too often with all the negative physiological consequences that produces.

Another way that baboons differ one from another is in their ability to take control of the situation when threatened. Sapolsky finds that low-ranking baboons are more likely to give up in the face of threat. They simply do not resist when bad things happen to them. Higher-ranking baboons respond by trying to take charge in an effort to resolve the situation. Even apart from rank, those who do not respond have higher cortisol levels. Particularly interesting is the observation that high-ranking male baboons have the capacity to choose to walk away from competition. Their responses are not programmed. They have the ability to decide how they will respond to stressful situations and the amount of stress they will accept. An indicator of how much they are like us comes through in the following example. Sapolsky describes one baboon who was next in line for the top position. He opted to walk away from the opportunity to compete, that is, fight, for the top position when the occasion presented itself, choosing to spend more time with his mate and his youngsters.

Among those who stay to fight, it matters whether they are able to interpret not only the threat but the outcome of the fight appropriately. Some baboons are better at taking satisfaction in winning than others. Those who act as if they are not sure if they really won continue to have elevated cortisol levels. How about losing the fight? What is the healthier response—going off to sulk and lick one's wounds or turning around and beating up a subordinate? Sapolsky tells us that he regrets having to report that the baboons who beat up subordinates, thereby releasing their aggression, end up having lower cortisol levels.

Finally, there are social affiliation differences. Mutual grooming is considered the "social cement" that establishes strong bonds among all nonhuman primates (Wilkinson 2001). Social alliances constitute an important resource in baboon communities because an animal facing an attack can count on receiving aid from animals that it has recently groomed. The baboons who spend most time grooming females—not as sex play, just as friendly play—and get groomed by them have lower levels of cortisol. The same is true of those who spend time playing with the young.

There are clearly a range of implications about human interaction that we can take from this brief introduction to Sapolsky's findings on baboons. The fact that reciprocity operates in the life of baboons to produce a more workable basis for social life suggests that it is a universal principle, meaning it has implications for human society (Wilkinson 2001). Equally striking are Sapolsky's findings on the significance of hierarchy, status, and rank. We will have to consider what the implications are for human primates, namely us, associated with the fact that high-ranking baboons deal with stress better than the low-ranking baboons. We have learned that high-ranking baboons experience the same degree of stress as low-ranking baboons, but high-ranking baboons are much better at resolving distress. Once the threatening event is over, their cortisol level drops. The baboons at lower ranks do not respond in the same way. Their cortisol level does not drop. It stays elevated.

We must consider the implications associated with one other finding related to rank. It seems that when the top-ranking baboons are forced to leave the top spot, they lose most of the health advantages that they had while they occupied that position. The next occupant of that spot gains those advantages. This is a startling observation. The health advantages, as indicated by glucocorticoid levels, have a lot to do with the hierarchical position the individual occupies—in combination with the personality characteristics attributable to the individual who occupies that position. There is, of course, a lot more going on, but the idea that hierarchy matters so much is clearly worth reflecting on.

To the extent that humans are anything like baboons, this must mean that one's position in the hierarchy has implications for one's health. True, people, unlike baboons, have more than one hierarchy to choose from. However, we must not forget that the opposite is also true, that is, some people have far fewer options and far less attractive options than others. How much effect this observation has on health brings us to the topic of social inequality, which is the subject of the next chapter.

Summary and Conclusions

Before we get to such questions, namely, how we might explain the extent of inequality we observe in our society, we need to wind up our discussion of stress. It seems that we have not answered the basic question that this chapter started with. We have not specified the extent to which stress is related to variation in mortality and morbidity. While we discussed what differentiates those who deal better with stress from those who don't do so well, we did not get much beyond where we were when we began the chapter with W. I. Thomas's observation that it is the definition of the situation that determines whether any particular event is stressful or not.

The basic question for which we cannot seem to find an answer is: is there any evidence that people can learn to manage stress better? Given all the research that has been carried out, one would think that researchers would have been able to identify stress-management techniques that are effective and can be learned. The conventional wisdom tells us that unburdening one's self by talking about one's stress is important. The question is: is there any research to support that belief? Yes, but as we have seen, it is more complicated than that.

The one thing that researchers all agree on is that the best thing to do is be born to parents who are particularly supportive and who help one learn some very basic lessons in attribution. It turns out that "learned optimism" does make a significant difference in a person's ability to deal with stress (Seligman 1991). Here is the way it operates. When something good happens, it benefits us to define it as something that we deserve, have earned, and are justified in expecting that other good things will happen again for the same reasons. When something bad happens, it benefits us to define it as an unlucky occurrence that is unlikely to befall us again. That is the prescription for a positive response to stress. Taking the opposite stance is the prescription for increased risk of stress disease—that is, reacting to negative events as if they are only natural and to be expected and positive events as if they are unexpected, undeserved, and only happened by chance. You see that the trick is absorbing the first set of interpretations. That perception of reality is learned best when the lessons start during one's early years.

In the end, what can we conclude with regard to stress based on the research we have reviewed in this chapter? How about advice on building a support system? Yes, but it better be a caring group of people, not just more people who don't care very much one way or the other. Having a wider social network may not help to reduce stress at all and may even contribute to it. And, as we have already seen in the chapter on health behavior, it can increase our chances of engaging in unhealthy behaviors (as in those that lead to weight gain). It can also help us stop engaging in risky behavior (as in smoking).

We also learned that having an ideally suited "significant other" counts for much more. The problem is that this information, powerful as it is, does not tell us how to create a truly reliable, lasting support system or, for that matter, find a truly caring significant other.

We know that uncertainty is stressful. Information provides a measure of certainty, which translates into a greater degree of control. At the same time, getting information that causes even more stress is to be avoided because all the evidence indicates that getting discouraged is harmful. Unfortunately, there is no way to control which kind of information one will receive.

Being born to parents who are higher up the socioeconomic scale and therefore more likely able to provide a wide range of psychological and material advantages may be the single most powerful antidote to stress over the lifetime. It is, of course, the least practical piece of advice one can offer. The observation does, however, bring us to the last variable that we will be considering in the effort to understand variation in mortality, morbidity, and health—socioeconomic inequality.

CHAPTER TEN

~

Social Inequality

The variable that we will be discussing in this chapter, social inequality, has been attracting increasing attention over the last decade. Those who employ this concept identify it as the study of *population health*. That makes it clear that the focus is on differences between groups of people rather than individuals. While that is exactly what we have been considering up until now, this heightened degree of emphasis is significant because it presages policy implications that we will consider in the last chapter.

To establish the context for exploring the impact of social inequality on health, let's go back to the beginning, to the basic question that we said we would address. Our primary objective was to identify which factors provide the best explanation for enormous differences in mortality and morbidity across the U.S. population. We said we would examine the extent of the variation in health status each of the nine variables explains—starting with age, sex, race, poverty, health behavior, medical care, genes, stress—and ending with inequality.

Let's review what we learned so far. We can start by agreeing that there is no shortage of data. Early on, we discovered that the way national statistics are collected has an impact on how discussion regarding variations in mortality and morbidity rates is framed. The fact that these rates are regularly reported by race alters the way we see the data.

The way statistics have been collected to date forces us to consider why some racial/ethnic groups have higher death rates than others. However, as many observers have repeatedly reminded us—race has no biological basis.

Now that genetic mapping is becoming more common and pharmaceutical companies are finding that there are differences in how people of different races respond to certain drugs, the statement that race has no biological basis is being made with some reservations. That does not change the fact that we still cannot predict which individuals of any race will succumb to any particular disease, because, as most geneticists keep telling us, genetic differences are so heavily influenced by environmental factors that genetic inheritance ends up playing a relatively small part in explaining variations in health between different groups of people. At least that is the situation at present.

We continued to refer to racial differences throughout the discussion, noting that the researchers, who readily acknowledge that race and ethnicity are socially constructed indicators, nevertheless make the point that it is hard to ignore the existence of substantial variation across racial/ethnic categories. That explains why they, and we, have devoted so much attention to the high mortality rates among blacks. To complicate matters further, we found early on that what researchers were saying about the relationship between race and health applied to the relationship between poverty and health. The result is that many researchers end up saying that poverty explains a great deal, but not everything, about why blacks tend to have poorer health and much higher mortality rates.

According to an increasing number of researchers, there is convincing evidence that social class offers a far better explanation for the variation in mortality than race. To illustrate, a particularly striking finding emerged in a study designed to explain why the residents of Harlem exhibit an especially high rate of death from heart disease in addition to high death rates for other causes. In this case neither race nor poverty were differentiating variables because the research subjects were all poor African Americans. They all exhibited high risk factors associated with heart disease such as hypertension, smoking, being overweight, and having little leisure-time physical activity (Diez-Roux et al. 1999). However, it turns out that those who exhibited three or more of these risk factors had both a lower income level and less education. In other words, when race and socioeconomic status are held constant, the relatively small measure of social inequality that differentiates the persons in the sample population turns out to be a powerful predictor of mortality.

Social Class, Income, and Education

There is no question that the poor, especially poor blacks, experience worse health and higher mortality than the nonpoor. The challenge is to identify exactly what it is about being poor that is primarily responsible. To answer that question, a number of researchers began investigating what it is about the lives of the poor that is so different from the lives of the nonpoor that would explain variations in health. They shifted their focus from examining the effects of poverty to exploring the effects of "comparative income and/or wealth." For now let us concentrate on the relationship between the basic indicators of social class and health.

Since health statistics collected by the government in this country generally are not reported according to social class, researchers who wish to use social class to explain variation in health must find other data sources that will provide them with this information. They must explain what indicator they are using to represent social class and why they prefer it to another indicator. Social scientists identify three different components of social class—income, education, and occupation. Let us consider each starting with income, and more specifically, economic inequality.

Before we do that, it is worth remembering from previous chapters that health statistics are increasingly being reported using poverty—not income—as a distinguishing variable. As you will recall, the categories being used are: under 100 percent of poverty, 100 to 200 percent of poverty, and 200 percent of poverty and above. Clearly the cutoff is too low to provide information about those whose income puts them at more than twice the poverty threshold. We might want to know, for example, if being at four times the poverty level provides commensurate health benefits. Or how about eight or ten times the poverty level? As we shall see shortly, these amounts are not even close to the incomes those at the top of the economic ladder have been raking in. The point is that answers to such questions are impossible to get using the statistics on poverty and health status.

Economic Status

There are basically two indicators involved in assessing economic status—income and wealth. Income refers to the flow of money from wages, salary, interest earned on savings, and various monetary windfalls, like a tax rebate. Wealth refers to total assets, that is, the value of everything one owns. Let's focus on the economic inequality as indicated by income first. We will return to the relationship between economic status and health after considering the matter of economic inequality more fully.

The idea that America is the land of opportunity and that each succeeding generation can expect to do better than their parents was reflected in the reality of economic trends for the post–World War II generation of Americans who did experience a steady rise in income. From 1947 through 1973,

Americans in every income category saw their income go up from year to year. As of 1973, the rate of increase in average income seemed to stagnate. Upon closer examination, we find that this observation does not apply to everyone. Income for the top 20 percent of the population increased while falling for the bottom 20 percent over this period (Wolff 1995, v–vi).

Let us consider hourly wages of workers who work for the minimum wage, which is the basic hourly rate of pay that employers are required to pay by law. The minimum wage has gone up in spurts. In 1990, it was $3.80 per hour, which translates into an annual income of $7,904. The government increased the minimum wage by 37 percent between 1990 and 2000. Sounds like a pretty good increase in earnings, doesn't it? However, there are a couple of other facts that will certainly alter that assessment. First, inflation rose 32 percent over the same period, meaning that goods and services a person buys went up by 32 percent. In the end, the average worker increased his or her earning power by about 5 percent between 1990 and 2000.

The minimum wage remained at $5.15 per hour for nine years prior to 2006, when legislation was passed to increase it incrementally every year over the next three years. That means that in 2006 a person working forty hours per week at $5.15 per hour, for fifty-two weeks a year, was earning $10,712—not much over the poverty line for one person, which stood at $9,800 that year. In 2007, the rate went up to $5.85, meaning that a person was earning $12,168 per year. The 2008 rate was $6.55, or $13,624 annually; in 2009, the rate was $7.25, or $15,080 annually. As you may recall from chapter 5, the poverty threshold for a single person under age sixty-five in 2009 was set at $10,830. Does that mean that persons earning over $15,000 in 2009 are no longer poor and will no longer be at risk of all the problems associated with poverty? Researchers will have to find a way to answer this question convincingly if only because future policy decisions will have to consider the response.

The second point of comparison, the gain in income among CEOs (chief operating officers) as compared to the gains made by average workers puts the shift in economic inequality in perspective. (The following is based on Ruccio [2007].) On average, the earnings of CEOs of major corporations in this country increased steadily from 1990, when the pay ratio between average executive to average production work was 107, to 2000, when it peaked at a 525 ratio. At the greatest extreme, some CEOs were earning nearly eight hundred times as much as the average production worker was earning that year. The gap declined some since then to a low of 281 in 2002 but increased again to a 411 ratio in 2005. If worker pay had risen at the same rate as CEO pay, the average production worker would have been earning

$108,138 instead of $28,315 in 2005. That captures the reality of inequality pretty graphically, doesn't it?

If you think those comparisons are impressive, just wait. Income inequality, as big as it is, is not nearly as dramatic as the inequality in *wealth* in this country. The government does not collect data on the distribution of wealth very systematically because it is difficult to obtain unbiased information. Asking people what they own and how much it is worth is unreliable because people often don't know what their property is worth and those who do know may wish to hide it. Scholars who are interested in the topic end up using a wide range of sources and indicators. In other words, it is an arduous task (Keister 2000).

Focusing on financial wealth, that is, discounting the worth of the family house and car, we see the following distribution for 2001 (Domhoff 2006).

Let's consider what this table says. First, the top 10 percent of the population owns about 80 percent of the wealth. Second, and even more striking, is finding that the top 1 percent owns about 40 percent of it. Those in the bottom 80 percent not only own less, in an increasing proportion of instances, they have negative wealth. In other words, they owe more money to creditors than what their possessions are worth—their houses, for example. (As news reports kept telling us, the economic downturn of 2008 reversed the steady trend of increasing value of houses, which caused a high proportion of families to owe more on their mortgages than their houses were worth.) More troubling to many observers is the fact that the distribution of wealth has become increasingly more unequal over the last two decades (Krugman 2007). Inequality increased significantly during the 1980s. The net worth (mainly investments, but includes cars and houses) among the top 1 percent of wealth owners increased from 33.8 percent in 1983 to 37.4 percent in 1989 (Wolff 2004).

Although the rate at which inequality was accelerating leveled off some during the 1990s, the United States has become one of the most economically unequal countries in the world (Kawachi, Wilkinson, and Kennedy

Table 10.1. Distribution of Wealth Ownership

Top 1% owns	40% of wealth	Top 1% owns 40%
Next 4%	28%	Top 5% owns 68%
Next 5%	12%	Top 10% owns 80%
Next 10%	11%	Top 20% owns 91%
Bottom 80%	9%	Plus bottom 80%
Total	100%	= 100%

1999). Those who focus on this phenomenon are concerned about it because they consider the distribution of wealth to be a powerful indicator of social well-being. Before we discuss why they believe that to be the case, let's consider the relationship between education and social class.

Educational Status

The fact that education is directly related to mortality differentials was initially documented in 1973 (Kitagawa and Hauser 1973). However, it was not until the 1990s that researchers began trying to disentangle the effects of education from the effects of income (Pappas et al. 1993). Finding that income matters more up to a certain minimum level of income, and that educational differences have a greater impact after that point, was not particularly surprising (Backlund, Sorlie, and Johnson 1999; Ecob and Smith 1999). Low income has predictable negative effects on health because it limits access to the whole range of valued resources. Determining that education is associated with variation in health status independently of income required researchers to do further analysis (Elo and Preston 1996; Feldman et al. 1989).

While the salutary effects of education seem just as obvious on the surface as the advantages associated with higher income, the premise that education and income could each have an independent impact on health needed to be better understood. One particularly comprehensive analysis by Catherine Ross and Chia-ling Wu identified three ways in which education affects health (Ross and Wu 1995). First, well-educated persons enjoy certain advantages related to their work roles. They are less likely to be unemployed and more likely to work full-time. Their work is more likely to be fulfilling. They make more money, which permits them to enjoy all the advantages that higher income plus economic security can provide. Second, education results in greater social and psychological resources. It gives individuals a greater sense of control over their lives and greatly reduces the sense of powerlessness in the face of unpredictable forces. Education provides knowledge, which helps in problem solving and making life choices. All of this combines to help people feel esteemed and able to participate in a network of mutual obligation in which others can be counted on for support. Third, well-educated people are more likely to engage in positive health behaviors, in part because education provides important information about risks and in part because they feel good enough about themselves to make these choices.

Ross and Wu used self-assessed health status and physical functioning to examine the relationship between education and health outcomes. As you recall from chapter 2, where we considered measures of health status, researchers have been using self-assessed health status as an indicator because it is highly predictive of mortality. In other words, those who say that they have poor health are at higher risk of dying than those who say their health is good or excellent. Thus, it is important to recognize that researchers consistently report that self-assessed health status is invariably associated with educational level.

Focusing on the opposite side of the coin, Ross and Wu put it this way: "Stressors, hardships, beliefs, and behaviors that affect health are not randomly distributed, they are socially structured" (1995, 740). It is not accidental that people with less education are more likely to be unemployed and endure economic hardship with all the attendant practical and psychological costs. They receive less medical care and receive it at a more advanced stage of illness; they engage in more negative health behaviors; and they experience a higher level of stress because they cannot count on others who are experiencing similar deprivations to assist them if that becomes necessary. This has cumulative effects.

What about the fact that poor people with less education are more likely to engage in behaviors that are detrimental to their health? If only we could teach them to stop doing all those things—smoking, overeating, and so on—wouldn't their health improve regardless of income and education? When researchers look into this question, they find that differences in health behaviors between the poor and the nonpoor have only modest explanatory power. Paula Lantz and her colleagues looked at four health behaviors—smoking, alcohol consumption, physical activity, and BMI among over 3,600 adults for a 7.5-year period (Lantz et al. 2001). To begin with, they found that those with less than twelve years of education and incomes under $10,000 were two to three times more likely to suffer poorer health. While there was nothing surprising about that, the researchers came up with two other findings that were considerably more surprising. First, they found that the health behaviors of poor people were not sufficiently different from the behavior of the nonpoor, at least not different enough to explain the extent of difference in health status. Second, they found that education explained more of the variance than income.

The same researchers concluded that education opens up a complex network of pathways that combine to produce lifetime advantages. More controversial is the logical conclusion that one must come to about the health behavior of the poor, namely, that it does not explain poor health as much as the conventional wisdom has most people believing it does. Accordingly, altering the health behavior of the poor, that is, convincing them to stop indulging in all those bad habits, is not likely to improve their health very much. It is certainly not likely to improve it as much as those who are committed to advocating changing the health habits of the poor as one of the most important routes to improving their health had led us to expect.

The relationship between education and health became considerably more newsworthy when a group of researchers affiliated with Harvard Medical School announced that their research indicates that life expectancy gains since 1981 occurred only for the better educated (Meara, Richards, and Cutler 2008). Between 1990 and 2000, life expectancy grew 1.6 years for the highly educated but remained unchanged for the less educated. The results of this study were disturbing, given the increased focus on health disparities and programs aimed at reducing them. The researchers found that diseases of the heart, cancers, and COPD (chronic obstructive pulmonary disease) accounted for 60 percent of the deaths. They concluded that the differential rate of smoking by educational level accounted for much of the widening gap in mortality and life expectancy.

Earlier work on the relationship between smoking and mortality may shed some light on the matter. Researchers who studied the cessation of smoking after a heart attack found education to be important in predicting subsequent smoking behavior (Wray et al. 1998). Knowledge of the detrimental impact of smoking was not a factor, since all patients were given the same advice. However, those with less education did not quit smoking after a heart attack. This explains, in part, why post–heart attack life expectancy varies with social class. The same conclusion applies to the fact that fewer African Americans than whites quit smoking between 1985 and 1995. Social class proved to be a more powerful predictive variable than race alone (Kiefe et al. 2001).

Further examination of the relationship between education and health indicates that education is a more powerful determinant for some racial/ethnic groups because it differs in the extent to which it affects health behaviors (Kimbro et al. 2008). The researchers found that education has a less powerful effect on the foreign-born than native-born; and has varying effects among Hispanic and Asian subgroups. As the authors point out, education is surely destined to receive a great deal more attention because of its implications for policy intervention.

Chronic Disadvantage

The issue of lifetime advantages associated with higher levels of income, education, and social class brings us to an added dimension—the passage of time, which is reflected in age. Adult behaviors do not suddenly emerge during adulthood on a random basis. Nor are health behaviors randomly distributed across social classes. Behavior in adulthood can be traced to the circumstances that a person experienced during childhood (Lynch, Kaplan, and Salonen 1997; Kuh and Wadsworth 1993). As research advances, more has become known about the pathway between psychosocial stress and childhood biological development. According to a group of researchers at the University of Chicago, social inequalities and marginalization has greatest impact during the perinatal/early childhood and puberty/adolescent periods (Furumoto-Dawson et al. 2007). This is when developmental genes are expressed and interact with the social-physical environment. Accordingly, the researchers say that they are focusing on understanding how psychosocial stress affects gene expression via the neuroendocrine regulatory function, which is essential in understanding adult health vulnerability.

It has long been clear that there is a high degree of association between such adult behaviors/characteristics as smoking, alcohol consumption, physical activity, and obesity, and the social class of origin. The social class of the parents predicts the health-related behavior of offspring during their adult years (Peck 1994). What is particularly important about this observation is that we must face the fact that there is something beyond individual choice of behavior and lifestyle that would explain such patterns. Johannes Siegrist and Michael Marmot have turned to "habitus," a concept introduced by the French sociologist Pierre Bourdieu, to interpret epidemiological findings (Siegrist and Marmot 2006). Bourdieu uses this term to explain that individual behavior is the result of sociocultural shaping and sociostructural opportunities, that is, all the factors that characterize the social environment in which we live out our lives.

The effect of socioeconomic inequality on health status varies by age. Differences are large at the earliest stages during the prenatal period and infancy (remember this is the period during which humans are most vulnerable and susceptible to environmental influences); diminish during adolescence; grow increasingly larger during the adult years; and decrease again during old age (Robert and House 2000; Williams 1998; West 1997). Finding that the disadvantages associated with lower socioeconomic status are cumulative over the lifetime makes sense. Why they disappear in old age requires further explanation. One part of the explanation is that those who are most disadvantaged die before they reach old age (Willson, Shuey, and Elder 2007). However, there is more to the story.

The research on variation in health status among the elderly indicates that it is not what happens to people at that stage in life that determines their current health status. It is what happened to them much earlier in their lives that determines it, and that, in turn, is shaped by such factors as social class, gender, and race/ethnicity (Arber and Ginn 1993; Beckett 2000; Breeze et al. 2001). Not surprisingly, researchers find that the effects of social class, gender, race, and ethnicity overlap, resulting in double- or multiple-jeopardy situations for some (Estes and Linkins 2000). Such factors go a long way in explaining the racial disparity in the male mortality rate (Warner and Hayward 2006).

We know that the effects are both psychological and biological, because psychological stress produces physiological reactions that have measurable consequences that researchers are increasingly able to identify (Feinglass et al. 2007; Goodman 1999). We have known for some time that stress, which results in depressive symptoms that have a biomedical basis, is highly predictive of mortality (Fiscella and Franks 2000). We have also known that stress over the long term is what is the most damaging. There is now good evidence that the damage occurs at the cellular level and this is what accelerates aging as much as ten years (Herd, Schoeni, and House 2008). Persistent low income, as opposed to periodic low income, is a particularly strong determinant of mortality. The explanation is that long-term stress is closely associated with chronic deprivation (Lynch, Kaplan, and Shema 1997; McDonough et al. 1997). Food insecurity is obviously a major problem (Seligman et al. 2007).

One question that continues to receive a great deal of attention concerns the extent to which differences in the quality of health care affect longevity. There is clear evidence that chronic morbidity in later life is associated with poor childhood health (Blackwell, Hayward, and Crimmins 2001). There is also a great deal of evidence to indicate that the disparity in the kind of health care people receive at an earlier age is directly linked to social class and/or race. Is it possible that increased access to medical care at a later age can make up for that? It seems that researchers are not prepared to conclude that the availability of Medicare to everyone over sixty-five in this country is enough to explain why the variation in health status declines during old age. Some researchers do speculate that Medicare may have a greater positive effect than has been recognized in research. However, they point out that it is difficult to arrive at a conclusive determination because it is impossible to evaluate accurately all the dimensions involved—access to care, quality of care, health status—over a person's entire life course, and so on.

This is not to say that the evidence indicating that the difference in the quality and quantity of health care contributes to the difference in mortality between social classes is inadequate. A comprehensive review of the existing evidence on the topic by the IOM concluded that there is no question that racial and ethnic minorities receive lower-quality care (Smedley, Stith, and Nelson 2003). This observation is explained in part by a recent survey of physicians in high-minority practices who report struggling to deal with the restricted resources that plague their patients, which they say affects the physicians' ability to deliver high-quality care (Reschovsky and O'Malley 2008). At the same time, there is no evidence that there are differences in the quality of care minority patients and white patients receive when they are hospitalized; disparities, as we already mentioned in the chapter on the effects of medical care, appear after the patients are discharged (Gaskin et al. 2008).

One particularly powerful bit of evidence comes from examining the outcome of serious injury. There is evidence to show that persons who are lower social class, poor, and/or minorities risk a greater chance of death from injury (Kelly and Miles-Doan 1997). The researchers who reported this result identified two components, which are obvious once someone points them out—namely, less access to care plus greater exposure to more lethal types of injury.

Virtually everyone who studies the relationship between medical care and health disparities agrees that the access to health care provided by health insurance is not enough to reduce differences in health status associated with social class. One of the most convincing points to be made in this regard is that health disparities do not disappear when we look at countries that make health insurance and health-care services available to everyone in the country. Clearly, access to health care is important, but there is something more complicated going on that simply providing access to medical care will not overcome. Data coming out of England provide an excellent illustration, not only because the British have had universal health care for so long, but because they have been collecting mortality statistics for even longer.

Mortality and Social Class in Britain

The fact that mortality is inversely related to social class has been obvious to British scholars since the first census was taken in 1851 (Deaton 2002; Hollingsworth 1981). The British have been collecting mortality statistics by social class regularly since 1911(Marmot et al. 1997). The problem was explaining why higher death rates and shorter life expectancy correlated with lower social-class standing. The unexpected increase in disparity between the lower and upper classes, which had been developing since 1950, but which really gained momentum in the late 1970s, catapulted the topic to the center of attention among British scholars interested in health and the health-care system (Wilkinson 1986). What made the issue so troubling was that Britain established the National Health Service at the end of World War II with the hope that providing universal health-care services would overcome the inequality in life expectancy. The fact that universal access to health-care services had not achieved that goal puzzled researchers and health policy makers alike.

The concerns voiced by members of the medical community in the late 1970s pointing out that the health status of the population was not improving as fast as it was in some other rich countries is credited with causing the government to take notice. In fact, the UK had the eighth-lowest rate of infant mortality in 1960, but by 1978, it ranked fifteenth in World Bank rankings (the discussion to follow is based on Townsend, Davidson, and Whitehead [1992]). A working committee charged with assessing trends and offering recommendations to the government was established in 1977. The committee produced a report in 1980, known as the Black Report, named for the chairman of the group, Sir Douglas Black.

The report documented the fact that mortality rates for those at higher social-class levels had steadily declined over the last two decades, while the rates for those at the lower levels had not only not declined, but increased in some years. The authors of the Black Report concluded that availability of health care did not overcome social and economic differences, which they concluded were central to the explanation for the existence of health disparities. The fact that a Conservative Party was now in office—replacing the Labour Party, which had commissioned the report—had much to do with the government response to the findings outlined in the report. Leading government figures attempted to minimize the significance of the findings and generally tried to suppress the recommendations by refusing to distribute the report. The government could not stifle discussion about the findings and was eventually forced to establish a new committee charged with updating findings. That report, "The Health Divide," was issued in 1987. (For the inside story of government machinations aimed at quashing both reports, see Townsend, Davidson, and Whitehead [1992].)

British health researchers responded to the findings presented in the Black Report by launching a major study of factors affecting population health, known as the Whitehall studies. The conclusions presented in the Black Report and the extensive empirical evidence based on the results of the Whitehall studies are largely responsible for the spread of interest in health disparity across Europe and eventually in the United States.

Occupational Inequality and the Whitehall Studies

Whitehall is comparable to our State Department. It is where vast numbers of workers are engaged in the work of running the government in England. The Whitehall studies focused on the relationship between the health status of these civil-service workers and a variety of factors associated with their health. The data were collected in two stages. Whitehall I involved 19,019 men aged forty to sixty-nine who were observed from 1967 to 1970 (Davey Smith, Shipley, and Rose 1990). The Whitehall II study was conducted from 1985 to 1988 (Marmot et al. 1991). This time, 6,900 men and 4,314 women were involved. Whitehall employees were grouped into four employment grades in the first study and twelve grades, which were collapsed into six, for purposes of the second study.

The Whitehall studies are considered to be especially good databases for several reasons. The most important reason is that there is no room for error regarding social class. Although all British citizens willingly report their social class in filling out government forms, there is always room for error. In the case of the Whitehall studies, social status is not a matter of self-report but civil-service designation linked to the position, that is, occupational status, of the person working at Whitehall. Income and education are not used because civil-service status encompasses all three indicators of social class—occupation, education, and income. Two other variables drop out, namely, poverty and access to health-care services. All study subjects have the same health-care coverage given that England has universal health care to which all members of the society are automatically entitled. Beyond access to health care, everyone at Whitehall has reasonable job security and a steady income, which means that poverty is eliminated as a variable. Finally, the data collection process is thorough and longitudinal and there is follow-up over a long period of time. Whitehall II builds on the interpretations coming out of Whitehall I, meaning that tentative hypotheses were explored using a new set of interview questions aimed at testing the impact of particular variables identified in examining the results of the Whitehall I study.

Whitehall I Findings

How compelling are the findings? They are absolutely amazing, in my opinion. Consider the following partial review of the results obtained in Whitehall I. You should know that administrators are the highest-ranked workers at Whitehall, whose employment status is associated with the highest status, income, and level of education. While they may come from the ranks of the upper middle class, they are not aristocrats. Similarly, at the other end of this spectrum are workers who certainly earn less and have considerably less education but it is worth remembering that they have a reasonably secure job and steady income.

Table 10.2 reveals a clear gradient in the percentage of people who died and according to rank during the first ten years after the Whitehall I data

Table 10.2. Ten-Year Mortality Percentages (Number of Deaths)

Cause of Death	Administrators	Executive	Professional/ Clerical	Other
Lung cancer	0.35 (3)	0.73 (79)	1.47 (53)	2.33 (59)
Other cancer	1.3 (12)	1.7 (195)	2.2 (73)	2.2 (46)
Coronary heart disease	2.2 (17)	3.6 (399)	4.9 (160)	6.6 (128)
Chronic bronchitis	0.0 (0)	0.08 (8)	0.43 (15)	0.65 (13)
Other respiratory	0.21 (2)	0.22 (24)	0.52 (18)	0.87 (15)
Gastrointestinal diseases	0.0 (0)	0.13 (15)	0.20 (7)	0.45 (15)
Accidents and homicide	0.0 (0)	0.14 (17)	0.18 (5)	0.18 (3)
Suicide	0.1 (1)	0.15 (18)	0.15 (4)	0.25 (4)
All causes	4.7 (41)	8.0 (892)	11.7 (393)	15.6 (326)

Source: Table 2.2: Age-adjusted Mortality in Ten Years (and Number of Deaths) by Civil Service Grade and Cause of Death. M. G. Marmot, "Social Inequalities in Mortality: The Social Environment." In *Class and Health*, ed. Richard Wilkinson (London: Tavistock Publications, 1986), 25.

were first collected. The table shows that the lower the occupational rank, the higher the chances of dying from each of the major causes of death under review.

Next, we see in table 10.3 how closely smoking is associated with mortality and how that varies by occupational rank. Smoking is, of course, a major factor in both lung cancer and heart disease. As you will recall from earlier discussion, U.S. researchers consistently suggest that social class provides a better explanation for differential risk of mortality than behavior, even smoking behavior, but researchers in the United States have never been able to state that conclusion with as much convincing evidence as the Whitehall researchers.

Those at higher grades of employment are less likely to smoke, a fact that is confirmed by one of the forthcoming tables. However, a far more striking fact is revealed by the data reported in the table above. While the correlations are not perfect, there is enough evidence here to conclude that the higher the civil-service grade, the lower the level of association between smoking and the two causes of death that are directly linked to smoking. What is startling is that this holds true even for those who are current smokers. That seems to me to be a truly compelling finding—that social class has a mediating effect on the risk of smoking-related disease. In short, if you want to smoke and avoid disease, it helps to join the highest social class. Not smoking is obviously the more logical alternative.

Table 10.3. Mortality Percentages by Grade and Smoking Status

Cause of Death	Administrators	Executive	Professional/ Clerical	Other	Total
Nonsmokers					
Heart disease	1.40	2.36	2.08	6.89	2.59
Lung cancer	0.00	0.24	0.00	0.25	0.21
Ex-smokers					
Heart disease	1.29	3.06	3.32	3.98	3.09
Lung cancer	0.21	0.50	0.56	1.05	0.62
Current smokers					
Heart disease	2.16	3.58	4.92	6.62	4.00
Lung cancer	0.35	0.73	1.49	2.33	2.00

Source: Table 2.2: Age-adjusted Mortality in Ten Years (and Number of Deaths) by Civil Service Grade and Cause of Death. M. G. Marmot, "Social Inequalities in Mortality: The Social Environment." In *Class and Health*, ed. Richard Wilkinson (London: Tavistock Publications, 1986), 25.

Whitehall II

The discovery that persons in higher grade positions were at less risk of dying, even if they did engage in risky behavior, needed to be explained. The Whitehall II study focused on a wide range of factors that researchers suspected might be implicated. This time, 10,314 civil servants participated (6,000 men and 4,314 women) (Marmot et al. 1991).

The Whitehall II population was asked to fill out a questionnaire and attend a screening examination. We now have six grade levels to consider and data that are reported for males and females separately. Let's look at some of the results of the examination first. Employment categories are ranked from high to low, that is, 1 is highest and 6 is lowest.

Does any of this surprise you? Some of it should be quite surprising, at least at first glance. Let's consider the physical indicators first. The differences in cholesterol, blood pressure, and BMI are not significant. That there is so little discernible difference was surprising to those who analyzed these findings. There is a higher level of obesity among those at the lower end of the scale, but it is not a perfect gradient. More recent updates on the impact of obesity indicate that it is a factor and that it ". . . may be a consequence of the psychosocial impact of living in a more hierarchical society" (Pickett et al. 2005, 670).

The height gradient is interesting because it is a perfect gradient for men but not for women. It turns out that height has historically been considered to be a good reflection of social conditions experienced during childhood. British analysis of variations in mortality from earlier in the century had

Table 10.4. Health Examination Study Results

	Sex	Employment Category					
		1	2	3	4	5	6
Physiological measurements							
Cholesterol	M	6.05	5.97	5.93	6.02	6.00	6.00
	F	5.79	5.85	5.80	5.80	5.90	5.86
Systolic blood pressure							
	M	124.3	124.6	123.9	124.8	125.4	125.4
	F	117.6	120.5	120.6	119.2	119.7	119.5
Mean BMI							
	M	24.6	24.4	24.6	24.5	24.8	25.1
	F	23.7	23.7	24.3	24.1	24.5	25.3
% obese							
	M	4.1	3.7	4.6	5.1	6.0	10.7
	F	7.4	4.6	7.9	7.8	10.3	13.2
Height in centimeters							
	M	177.8	177.1	176.3	176.3	174.3	172.9
	F	165.5	165.1	165.3	163.1	162.8	160.7

Source: Table III: Physiological Measurements, Health Behaviors, and Family History by Employment Grade Category (Age-Adjusted). M. G. Marmot, George Davey Smith, Stephen Stansfeld, Chandra Patel, Fiona North, Jenny Head, Ian White, Eric Brunner, and Amanda Feeney, "Health Inequalities among British Civil Servants: The Whitehall II Study," *Lancet* 337 (June 1991): 1390.

Table 10.5. Health Behaviors Study Results

	Sex	Employment Category					
		1	2	3	4	5	6
Current smoker (%)	M	8.3	10.2	13.0	18.4	21.9	33.6
	F	18.3	11.6	15.2	20.3	22.7	27.5
Mean units of alcohol in last seven days	M	14.6	12.6	13.9	12.9	11.5	10.1
	F	12.1	9.8	9.3	7.0	5.2	3.6
No moderate or vigorous exercise (%)	M	5.1	5.4	4.9	7.5	16.2	30.5
	F	12.0	14.7	10.8	13.2	19.7	31.1

Source: Table III: Physiological Measurements, Health Behaviors, and Family History by Employment Grade Category (Age-Adjusted). M. G. Marmot, George Davey Smith, Stephen Stansfeld, Chandra Patel, Fiona North, Jenny Head, Ian White, Eric Brunner, and Amanda Feeney, "Health Inequalities among British Civil Servants: The Whitehall II Study," *Lancet* 337 (June 1991): 1390.

already revealed that height was inversely related to mortality. That had been interpreted to mean that early life environment is predictive of adult health. These results suggest the same interpretation.

The most dramatic differences, and the ones to which we should direct most attention, are those that appear as perfect or near perfect gradients. While you were certainly not surprised to find that fewer men smoke at higher grade levels, the picture of female smoking turns out to be not nearly as clear. As you can see, there is a higher proportion of female smokers in the top grade level. Exercise follows a similar pattern.

I expect that the gradient for alcohol intake came as a surprise to you as well. What do you think it means that there is more drinking going on at higher grade levels than lower grade levels? While we are not told this, it probably means that there is more social drinking at higher grade levels, which is very different from binge drinking and regular excess drinking, which is more typical of those at lower social class levels. Although in this case, binge drinking and regular excess drinking behavior is not likely to be common among any of the Whitehall staff, first because none are members of the lower class and second because they would not keep their jobs for very long if they did engage in such behavior.

The interview results are far more striking. Let's look at selected results.

You have to agree that the psychosocial variables presented in table 10.6 are highly revealing, even more revealing than the data reported in the health examination and health behavior tables. These findings challenge the idea that fast-paced work has negative effects. The data here clearly indicate that higher-level positions bring with them a fast work pace but that the pace is combined with high control over work and variety in the work. In turn, this is exactly the combination of characteristics that is associated with a higher level of work satisfaction.

The answers associated with questions about work are more revealing than answers to questions about life outside of the work setting, including family, friendship, and social support. However, the differences in interactional activity are still interesting to consider. The higher the grade, the less likely the associations are with family and more likely they are with friends. This is particularly interesting in the case of women. The higher the grade, the greater the difference in the pattern of association with friends versus relatives. Only 19 percent of the women at the highest grade see three relatives per month, while 45 percent of women at the lowest grade do so. By contrast, 71 percent of women at the highest grade see at least three friends a month, while that figure drops to 50 percent for the lowest grade. At the same time, when we get to emotional support we find some difference by

Table 10.6. Psychosocial Characteristics Study Results

		Employment Category					
	Sex	1	2	3	4	5	6
Work Characteristics							
Work characterized by							
high control (%)	M	59.3	49.7	43.1	31.6	24.7	11.8
	F	51.2	45.4	47.1	31.2	20.1	10.2
Work is varied (%)	M	70.5	52.1	41.9	27.1	18.2	3.9
	F	71.2	55.2	40.5	31.7	14.0	4.7
Work is fast paced (%)	M	58.0	43.6	43.7	27.9	20.8	15.8
	F	60.9	50.3	43.7	31.1	29.7	18.0
Work is highly satisfying (%)	M	58.2	38.7	34.1	29.5	29.4	29.8
	F	57.5	42.2	40.3	36.6	41.5	47.7
Social Support							
See at least three relatives							
per month	M	22.1	24.8	20.0	27.2	29.7	30.6
	F	18.9	23.7	21.1	24.1	30.4	44.9
See at least three friends							
per month	M	65.3	61.3	58.5	56.4	50.4	50.2
	F	71.2	62.8	67.1	63.6	52.9	49.0
Receiving confiding/							
emotional support	M	31.3	33.7	28.3	28.3	34.6	26.1
	F	37.3	33.8	33.0	32.5	32.9	31.8
Sometimes not enough							
money	M	7.0	12.6	21.5	26.4	34.4	37.2
	F	7.7	6.0	9.6	13.2	24.4	29.6

Source: Table IV: Psychosocial Characteristics by Employment Grade Category (Age-Adjusted). M. G. Marmot, George Davey Smith, Stephen Stansfeld, Chandra Patel, Fiona North, Jenny Head, Ian White, Eric Brunner, and Amanda Feeney, "Health Inequalities among British Civil Servants: The Whitehall II Study," *Lancet* 337 (June 1991): 1391.

employment grade, but not very much. That certainly doesn't tell us nearly as much as the question about having enough money, which reveals a much greater degree of differentiation. This is especially true for males. Only 7 percent worry about not having enough money (to pay bills), while 37 percent of those at the lowest rank report worrying about money.

More recent studies, focusing on the same population, have addressed the question of how much control over work matters. The researchers concluded that an individual's perceived control over life and work is a key concept in explaining health differentials (Steptoe and Willemsen 2004; Bosma, Schrijvers, and Machenbach 1999). In a follow-up study of mortality after retirement relative to employment grade based on the Whitehall I data, the researchers found that grade level is a more powerful predictor of mortality during employment years. Its power to predict mortality decreases after retirement. The researchers interpreted this to mean that work status plays a role separate from socioeconomic status and that work status has an independent effect on risk of mortality. In short, the sense of control over work may spill over to sense of control over other aspects of life and this is what may be responsible for generating significant health advantages prior to retirement.

For skeptics who might be ready to dismiss data on British civil servants in the assumption that a study of American civil servants would not look anything like that, the news is far worse than that. Consider the results of a study aimed at examining that exact question. The study population of American civil servants was limited to non-Hispanic whites to avoid the known negative influence of racial disparity on the findings. The results revealed that both higher social-class Brits and Americans were healthier than their respective middle and lower social-class counterparts. However, higher social-class Americans reflected a disease pattern similar to lower social-class Brits—in each of the following categories of disease: hypertension, heart disease, diabetes, cancer, lung disease, heart attack, and stroke (Banks et al. 2006). In other words, even though the hierarchical pattern of illness is the same within the two countries, there is a big overall difference between the two countries—Americans experience a higher rate of illness than Brits at all socioeconomic levels. So would you agree with the American experts who interpreted this to mean that it is something about the stress of living in this country that accounts for that?

Why people in this country are suffering from a greater burden of poor health than people in other countries appears to confirm what we learned about social inequality in the last chapter. The research on pathways between environment and physiological effects has taken an interesting turn as psychobiologists begin to find clearer links between psychological reactions and biological outcomes (Chandola et al. 2008). One group of researchers has been collecting saliva samples over the course of the workday to establish the amount of cortisol (this is the hormone that we discussed in relation to the baboons in the chapter on stress) output over the day (O'Donnell et al. 2008). The researchers concluded that cortisol output was inversely related to the approach subjects used in coping with stress. Those who reported most stress were higher socioeconomic status (SES) individuals who said that they were experiencing low job control and were not able to do much about it.

Even more intriguing is the entry of "neuroeconomists" into this research arena. In one study, they established that they can influence people's economic decision making by spraying a neuropeptide, oxytocin, into a person's nostrils (Damasio 2005). The spray increases a person's trust, thereby encouraging greater cooperation in a range of activities from intimate friendship to financial investment decisions. What does that tell you about the impact that cultural background, human nature, and any number of other factors have on our behavioral choices? Obviously, this research is raising more questions than it is answering. The researchers do not ignore the potential for misuse of this chemical by dishonest persons interested in influencing the behavior of others.

The Question of Natural Selection

Before ending this discussion it might be well to address the question of whether we have not missed something and should consider a reverse causation explanation. Is it possible that poor health causes people's social status to drop and that is what explains the link between poor health and lower social class status? This question and the small body of research related to it are known as work on the "selection" issue. As you recall, the Black Report, which documented the existence of clear disparities in mortality by social class in Britain, stimulated debate on this point. The authors of the Black Report anticipated this. They reviewed research that specifically addressed the question and determined that reverse causality did not explain the association (Townsend, Davidson, and Whitehead 1992, 105). Additional research reviewed in the later report came to the same conclusion (Townsend, Davidson, and Whitehead 1992, 312–15).

A number of investigators have considered the question since then (Robert and House 2000). Researchers have found little or no evidence to support the idea that poor health is the cause of a lower income level over an individual's lifetime. (This is not to ignore the fact that poor health does have an impact on income in the case of the elderly, which we noted in chapter 4 in discussing age and sex.) Researchers have consistently found that poor health results from low income rather than the reverse (Mirowsky and Hu 1996; Blane, Davey Smith, and Bartley 1993). A study specifically designed to compare the health of upwardly versus downwardly mobile males in England and Wales provides further support for this conclusion. The researchers found that the upwardly mobile reported more illness than the members of the group toward which they were moving; by contrast, the downwardly mobile reported less illness than the group to which they were moving (Bartley and Plewis 1997).

Summary and Conclusions

This chapter began with a review of what we learned in previous chapters. If we had concluded the discussion before considering the evidence presented in this chapter, we would have been forced to conclude that all of the variables we reviewed to that point were important, but the picture was not complete. Many of the studies we reviewed earlier suggested that income or education or social class would provide a more complete answer. But since the United States does not use these variables on a regular basis in collecting health data, gathering evidence on the impact of social class on health is not as systematic as it might be. To determine just how important social class and/or any of its components might be, we turned to the studies that have come to stand as the foundation from which other researchers have proceeded, namely, the Whitehall studies.

In considering the big picture painted by the Whitehall studies, we must conclude that, all things considered, being at the top of the heap is a lot better than being at the bottom. The question is, to what extent can this interpretation be generalized? Is hierarchy the major explanatory factor that operates across social settings? Can the same be said of all circumstances and of all people, that is, people in most other societies? Maybe the health problems of persons lower down on the scale are primarily due to money problems, that is, income. There probably is no criticism or question you could raise that has not been explored by researchers. For us the challenge is how to organize the results of the enormous body of research that has been stimulated by the Whitehall studies. It all amounts to an information explosion. We will devote the following chapter to information that builds on the Whitehall studies with the aim of explaining health inequalities.

CHAPTER ELEVEN

~

Population Health

There has been an explosion of research related to social class and health status showing that social class is a powerful, and arguably the most powerful, predictor of health. New research on the relationship between the main indicators of social class—income, education, and health status—is reported every week. In this chapter, we aim to organize some of these findings in an attempt to create a more complete and clear picture. We will be doing so using the following headings: (1) the "relative income hypothesis" and criticisms of its application in health studies; (2) international evidence on inequality; (3) work and its effects on health; (4) the relationship between community or place of residence and health; (5) spillover effects. And finally, we'll conclude the chapter with some comments on age, sex, and race in connection with inequality.

The Relative Income Hypothesis

"Relative income" is how we see our income in comparison to the income of others. If I can see most people making a great deal more than I make, then I am likely to be dissatisfied with my income. It is also relative in comparison to what I expect to use it for—for purchasing essential goods and services or what I have come to believe are essential goods and services. It is interesting to note that the "relative income hypothesis" concept was apparently introduced by James Dusenberry, a Harvard economist, in 1949, but was rejected by mainstream economists who were firmly committed to the idea that people's views of their income and purchasing decisions were grounded in economic rationality. In spite of a steady stream of contradictory evidence, the rational choice model prevailed until quite recently when maverick economists began to build reputations by publishing clever accounts of economic irrationality. Most people would now agree that what one believes is a "good" income is relative and that whether people perceive themselves to be poor is also relative. Furthermore, there is now lots of evidence to indicate that our purchasing decisions are heavily influenced by the symbolic meanings that become attached to various products rather than rational estimates of the value of those objects. Why else would people want to buy extremely expensive cars, jewel-encrusted watches, diamond rings, and other luxury items that must be insured, kept in secure places, not mentioned to the wrong people for fear of theft, and so on?

For a while there was a good deal of debate on the question of whether perceptions of one's relative income can have any impact on one's health status. Three strands of criticism of the "relative income hypothesis" emerged: (1) that the relationship between socioeconomic inequality and health is a statistical artifact and that the primary link is between individual income and health; (2) that the measures used are flawed; and (3) that the hypothesis is inconsistent with international trends. The proponents of the hypothesis were apparently able to satisfy the critics because the debate seems to have ended (the criticisms and responses are discussed in Kawachi, Wilkinson, and Kennedy [1999]).

Although the six different measures of income distribution currently used by economists are highly correlated with one another, Kawachi and Kennedy say that the *Gini coefficient* is the preferred measure, as it allows researchers to measure variation in levels of inequality (Kawachi and Kennedy 1997b). The Gini coefficient divides income of whatever population is being studied into deciles (10 percent each). This way the income of the top 10 percent can be compared to the income of people at lower levels. The Gini coefficient is related to the *Robin Hood Index*, which is used to specify the proportion of total income earned by the bottom 50 percent, 60 percent, or 70 percent of households in a society—whichever percentage the researchers decide to use. What is significant about the Robin Hood Index is that researchers consistently report finding a strong inverse relationship between the proportion of income going to the bottom and the mortality rate for the population as a whole. For a more extensive discussion of the Robin Hood Index and inequality in general, I recommend Wilkinson's book, *Unhealthy Societies* (1996).

International Evidence

As you must agree, we have spent a fair amount of time in preceding chapters examining the factors that are associated with mortality in the United States without finding any that have greater explanatory power than social class as measured by two of its primary components—education and income. The evidence that social class, using occupational rank as an indicator, has profound consequences came through very clearly in the Whitehall studies. Do you think we would find similar results in other countries? Remember that one of the startling facts we confronted at the beginning of the book was finding that the richest and most highly developed countries, most notably the United States, do not necessarily have the longest life expectancy. If the countries that enjoy longest life expectancy are not the richest countries, what do you think explains their advantage?

There is clear evidence that an increasing level of income has an enormous effect on population health up to a certain stage of economic development in developing countries. A higher income level is crucial for the reduction of mortality in the early stages of a country's industrial/economic development (Wilkinson 1996; Kim and Moody 1992). Once industrialization, and its counterpart, epidemiological transition, are achieved, further economic development, as indicated by a higher level of personal income, does not necessarily bring improvements in health. That is why we could not see a strong relationship between a country's wealth and life expectancy in chapter 3 where we examined comparative life expectancy among highly developed countries.

It is logical to think that rich countries have healthier populations because they can afford to spend more on the health and welfare of their citizens. Scholars who have tested the proposition that increased public spending on health would make a difference in the health status of the population across the countries for which the World Bank collects data discovered that it explains less than one-seventh of one percent of the variation in mortality across all those countries (Filmer and Pritchett 1999). Thus, the idea that socioeconomic inequality may provide the best explanation for the variation in health status continues to find support, if only because so many other logical possibilities have been tested and discarded.

There are a number of countries that merit special attention as we explore the relationship between inequality and health outcomes. I focus on the following countries because these are the ones mentioned most often in the literature to illustrate how economic development and inequality affect population health. We begin with a brief look at China, which is a developing country that is rapidly moving toward becoming a fully developed, modern, capitalistic society. However, it is still considered to be in the process of developing because it has such a huge rural population that has not benefited very much from ongoing economic development. Next, we turn to Japan, which became a highly developed country during the decades immediately following World War II. The question we aim to explore is—why did the health status of its population improve so much in a relatively short period of time? After that, we focus on Russia, whose status as a highly advanced society is no longer so certain, precisely because it has experienced a sharp decline in life expectancy while its socioeconomic arrangements undergo enormous change and disorganization. Finally, we return to the United States and Britain.

According to the 2008 World Development Indicators profile of countries compiled by the World Bank, in 2006 China had a life expectancy of seventy-two years and annual per capita income of $4,660. (It is worth noting that per capita income in 2000 was $930 with a life expectancy of seventy, which obviously indicates a very rapid rate of economic advancement without a comparable effect on life expectancy.) By contrast, in 2006 U.S. life expectancy was 77.8 years and per capita income was $44,070. (All the figures on per capita income are based on the value of the U.S. dollar.) How is it that China's far lower income is not reflected in life expectancy that is substantially lower than that of people in the United States? The answer seems to lie in understanding the difference between *relative wealth* and actual wealth or the reverse—*relative poverty* and actual poverty (Sen 1998). It provides a powerful illustration of the "relative income hypothesis" we discussed earlier.

Living in a society where what you have is not that different from what others have means that you are not poor. Living in a society where some people have a great deal more than you do makes it obvious how deprived you are. After all, most poor people in the United States have TVs, refrigerators, cars, telephones, hot running water, and so on. Until relatively recently most people in China did not. What is important is that the Chinese did not feel disadvantaged *in comparison* to their immediate neighbors; people living in rich countries were too far away to matter. Will that change as those Chinese who have been left behind discover the pleasures of increased wealth enjoyed by their countrymen living in the fast-growing and modernizing Chinese cities? That remains to be seen. Whether any changes in life expectancy occur and whether those changes can be attributed to the sudden realization among the Chinese that there is a great deal of inequality within the country will have to be determined in retrospect. Again, we shall have to wait to see if someone asks such questions and identifies data that provide answers.

A comparable interpretation has been applied to the finding that immigrants who come to the United States have better health than their counterparts born in this country. When people from less-developed countries come here they are more often than not a lot poorer than the average American. However, most enjoy a more advantaged health status, as indicated by lower mortality, than persons of the same racial/ethnic background who are born here (Singh and Siahpush 2001). The difference is especially striking in the case of many black and Hispanic immigrants, whose health status drops sharply with succeeding generations. (The pattern for Hispanics is not as clear; more on that shortly.) It is unlikely that there is something special about immigrants, such as genetic superiority, that might explain their advantage as indicated by mortality rate, particularly low infant mortality, since the advantages vanish with succeeding generations. It is important to recognize that what happens goes beyond the obvious lifestyle changes—diet, patterns of exercise, and so on. The change in the person's standing vis-à-vis other persons in this country constitutes a far more dramatic change.

Moving on, let's consider Japan. Prior to World War II, Japan was an underdeveloped country with a life expectancy lower than any of the industrialized countries to which Japan's rate is now compared. What accounts for the fact that Japan's life expectancy increased over the next thirty or forty years and that it is now consistently the highest or second highest in the world (Marmot and Davey Smith 1989)? In 2006, Japan's per capita income was $38,630 and life expectancy was 82.3. Obviously, they live considerably longer than Americans at a lower per capita income. How is this possible?

Don't even think of saying it's their diet. Their diet did not get "better." In fact, if anything, it got worse because we so generously introduced them to all that tasty, high-fat, high-calorie food available at fast-food restaurants. Fortunately for them, diet does not change very quickly. The Japanese still prefer to eat what they were eating all along on a regular basis while adding an occasional hamburger to their diet. They also smoke a lot, at least the men do. They take relatively little time off from work, which sometimes leads to early death from overwork. Their cities are crowded and polluted. You think that it might be their health-care system? Yes, Japan has universal health-care insurance. At the same time, their surgical rate is very low because the culture discourages cutting into the body. So, while the Japanese go in for a lot of high-tech diagnostic testing (they have far more high-tech machinery than the United States), this does not lead to nearly as much surgery as we undergo in the United States. All of this presents a confusing picture when we compare ourselves to the Japanese. There is obviously more to this story—a story that the American business community is especially eager to understand.

American businessmen became interested in the Japanese style of management a few decades ago in an effort to figure out how the Japanese achieve such high productivity levels. It appears to me that U.S. businessmen, and the gurus they listen to, missed seeing some of the most basic characteristics of Japanese culture in and outside of the workplace. Anybody who sees Japanese tourists in this country must notice how they dress. They prefer to look alike, which makes income differences less apparent, rather than look as distinctive as they can, which is what we prefer. That is just the tip of the iceberg of comparisons we can make with regard to social class in the two countries. While we deny the existence of social-class differences, our behavior belies our rhetoric. The Japanese simply do not connect to the idea of social-class hierarchy and the accoutrements of class. Their executives do not have special dining rooms, parking spaces, executive washrooms, and so on; they do not send their kids away to elite schools to mix with other very rich kids. Instead, they live in the same communities as the workers. Their lifestyle does not vary that much from that of the wage earners who work for the company. While Japanese executives earn much more than average workers, they do not earn nearly as much as their counterparts in this country. We will get back to this point in a moment.

Then there is the problem of explaining what happened in Russia, and other countries that were formerly part of the Soviet bloc, to cause a reversal in life expectancy. The decline in life expectancy started in 1990 but abated by the end of that decade (Field, Kotz, and Bukhman 1999). In 1991, life expectancy in Russia was 63.4, but it fell to 59.8 by 1996 (*Health, United States, 2001*, table 27). Because the reversal in the trend toward increasing life expectancy is an exception to the established pattern, that phenomenon has received a considerable amount of attention (Bobadilla, Costello, and Mitchell 1997; Wnuk-Lipinski and Illsley 1990). By 2006, life expectancy had risen to 65.6 and per capita income stood at $5,770. There is a great deal of evidence both formal and informal that links the decline in life expectancy to a tremendous increase in alcoholism, organized crime, and street crime, all of which sociologists consider to be indicators of "social disorganization." It is worth noting that the rate of death from cancer remained stable during this period while the rate of death from causes that are more closely related to alcohol consumption and social stress increased (Leon et al. 1997). This indicates that the change in the mortality rate cannot be attributed to measurement error, but is a real and disturbing finding that needs to be explained.

While most observers agree that the increase in risky behaviors, including a high rate of alcoholism, is important, they argue that risky behavior is an intermediate factor and not at the heart of what needs to be explained (Rose 2000). Accordingly, researchers have focused their attention on the events that took place during this period to cause an increase in risky health behaviors.

The single most significant change that occurred in the Soviet Union was the decline of communism, which began to falter during the 1970s and proceeded to fall faster than anyone expected during the 1980s. This is the period that coincides with the slowdown in the rate at which life expectancy had been increasing (Field, Kotz, and Bukhman 1999; Wilkinson 1996, 121–30). The explanation goes like this—when communism lost its legitimacy, people could no longer depend on their society to provide them with the means of survival. Any protest led to use of military power to crush resistance. What people saw being valued was obedience, loyalty, and mediocrity. The only place left to turn was the family, which helps to explain why single persons, particularly single men, had and continue to have higher death rates than married persons. Consistent with trends in other countries, death rates were found to vary according to socioeconomic status. The decrease in life expectancy has been steepest amongst those in the lowest educational groups, indicating that the negative consequences that are associated with social disorganization are not equally distributed across social classes (Leon and Shkolnikov 1998).

Returning to more familiar territory, there is the problem of explaining why the United States and Britain, both rich and highly developed countries, have a lower life expectancy than other highly developed countries, many not nearly as rich. Consistent with what applies in other countries, social inequality provides a powerful explanation. The United States and Britain accept considerably more socioeconomic inequality than other highly developed countries. Using the ratio of the average CEO's compensation to the pay received by the average worker in 2000 makes the point. The following is reported by *Business Week* (Reingold 2000): CEOs in the UK were making twenty-five times more and in the United States they were making thirty-one times more than the average worker. This is in contrast to nineteen times more in Italy; sixteen times more in France; eleven times more in Germany; and ten times more in Japan. (These are figures for all CEOs, which is not the same as the figures discussed in the last chapter when we looked at the ratio between the pay of the average production worker and only those CEOs who are associated with Fortune 500 companies. For that reason, the ratios were far higher.) These ratios are difficult to ignore when we try to understand why Japan has consistently maintained one of the highest life expectancy rates in the world and why life expectancy in the United States and the UK is lower than it is in some other highly industrialized countries.

The extent to which inequality affects life expectancy came into particularly sharp focus during the decade of the 1980s. As you know, life expectancy increased steadily throughout the twentieth century in all highly industrialized countries. The fact that the increase in life expectancy plateaued in Britain and in the United States during the 1980s means that something was happening to cause that. The major change that occurred in both countries was that the disparity in income began widening at an unprecedented pace (Wilkinson 1996, 94–100).

This was not due to chance. What happened in both countries was that the leadership of the government shifted from the more liberal to the more conservative political party. This is when Ronald Reagan and Margaret Thatcher began heading their respective governments. Both promised to alter the course of their respective country's economic policy. The logic behind the changes embraced by both, which resulted in increased economic inequality in the two countries, was clearly articulated by Reagan. He argued that society would benefit if the rich got to keep more of their money. Allowing wealthy persons to keep more of their income by lowering their taxes would cause them to invest those extra dollars. They would do so wisely because it would be in their self-interest to do so, which he did not need to explain in much more detail—because we all know economic self-interest is a major motivating factor in this country. He assured us that his agenda would bring about economic expansion, which, in turn, would produce more jobs, thereby benefiting all those lower down on the economic scale. This strategy became known as the "trickle down" economic theory. Conservative politicians in the United States continue to promote the very same set of ideas, but now object to the "trickle down" label.

Americans were quick to accept the logic behind Reagan's proposal. However, as we can see in retrospect, what this policy actually produced comes closer to "trickle down mortality" both here and in Britain. The growth in inequality had the effect of increasing the mortality rate, which resulted in a slowdown in the long-term trend toward increasing life expectancy hitting a plateau during the1980s.

The commonly accepted interpretation of the international data linking inequality and health is that countries that enjoy the longest life expectancy also have the lowest levels of income inequality (Machenbach 2006). Denmark and Sweden, for example, are often used to illustrate the beneficial social effects of policies designed to reduce inequality and the advantage this has for life expectancy of their populations (Dahl et al. 2006). Further evidence comes from John Komols, who tracks shifts in height across countries. He is finding that European men's height is outstripping American men's height (Hundley 2008). Men in the Netherlands and Scandinavian countries are now the tallest. What is even more interesting is Komols's assertion that he found men's height to be virtually perfectly correlated with life expectancy and that this correlation is closely related to equity in the distribution of national wealth.

The data on the impact of inequality on health are so strong that researchers have been able to establish a ratio of inequality that predicts to an increase or decrease in life expectancy. Based on cross-country comparisons focusing on the proportion of income received by the bottom 50 percent of the population (calculated using the Gini coefficient) researchers have found that even a small increase (7 percent) in the share of income going to the bottom half of the population increases life expectancy for the population as a whole by two years (Wilkinson 1996, 107; Kunst and Machenbach 1994; Gramlich, Kasten, and Sammartino 1993). This calculation forms the basis of the Robin Hood Index argument—giving a greater share of income to the bottom half of the population increases the life expectancy of the country as a whole.

The level of inequality has continued to increase in the United States since then. By one calculation, the United States could achieve a 7 percent reduction in mortality by bringing the level of inequality down to the level that prevailed in England during the Thatcher administration (Kawachi, Wilkinson, and Kennedy 1999, xxx).

Infant mortality turns out to be even more sensitive to income inequality than adult health. In a study of infant mortality in twenty-six developed countries, researchers found infant mortality to be directly associated with income inequality (Hales et al. 1999). The same researchers also compared the relationship between the infant mortality rate and income in over one hundred less-developed countries to infant mortality and income in developed countries. They determined that an increase in the income level of all households reduces infant mortality in poor countries. However, in rich countries, lowering income inequality reduces infant mortality. This conclusion is consistent with the assessment reached by another researcher, who examined infant mortality rates in seventy countries. He came up with the startling conclusion that the higher the share of the income that goes to the richest 5 percent, the higher the infant mortality rate for the country as a whole (Waldman 1992, 1287). That finding should act like a flashing red light with regard to the kinds of policies we have been pursuing in the effort to reduce infant mortality in this country. We will address policy more directly in the next chapter.

Work and Its Effects on Health Inequalities

As you know from our review of the results of the Whitehall studies, work matters a great deal when it comes to explaining why some people are healthier and live longer than others. The question that researchers continue to struggle with is how much is associated with *direct* as opposed to *indirect* effects. In other words, how much is due to such direct or practical aspects as higher income, better working conditions, more benefits like insurance, time off, pension plan, and so on, versus how much is due to indirect effects. Indirect effects include all those intangible rewards such as sense of control over work, challenging work, greater job security, and opportunity for upward mobility. As we saw in the Whitehall studies, a lower level of control over work combined with less challenge is associated with higher levels of mortality. Other studies consistently report similar findings. For example, in one case, when researchers compared the level of strain experienced by manual workers versus white collar workers, they found that the relationship between low decision latitude and high demands explains a major share of the excess risk for mortality experienced by manual workers (Hallqvist et al. 1998). Although middle managers confront different pressures and constraints, the relationship between the two factors is the same—it is the manifestation of high effort and low reward that is responsible for negative health outcomes (Peter and Siegrist 1997).

The classic illustration of the situation in which someone applies intensive effort over a sustained period of time without commensurate reward is known as "John Henryism" (Riska 2004). According to legend, John Henry was an African American man who worked laying railroad tracks during the latter half of the nineteenth century. When challenged, he agreed to compare his strength against that of a mechanized drill, the challenge being drilling through the side of a mountain. He won the bet. However, it took so much effort that he died shortly after he completed this feat. In short, working to prove that one is highly competent may require more exertion and stress than a person can handle.

One particularly thorough review of the literature on health and work revealed which features associated with work are linked to mortality (Pavalko,

Elder, and Clipp 1993). The review points out, however, that research generally focuses on the current job and current health behaviors. It turns out that when the researchers focused on "career" as opposed to job, they found that work has an even bigger impact on health over the long term. People whose work lives show a pattern of upward progression enjoy better health. Those who move laterally from one job to another are at higher risk of mortality. The researchers determined that such factors as stress and lifestyle did not explain the variation. In fact, the researchers concluded that intellectual challenge and flexibility were the most important factors (Pavalko, Elder, and Clipp 1993, 376). That is of course highly consistent with the Whitehall study results.

The evidence that social class and health are closely linked sometimes comes from research that did not start out with the intent of investigating that relationship. One particularly striking example of this comes from a study that begins from a medical model view of health from which to test the relationship between using aspirin on a daily basis and the reduction of risk of cardiovascular mortality. Physicians served as the study population (Angell 1993). The most interesting finding was not that aspirin does have some protective effects. It was that the mortality rate for the physicians in the study was a mere 12 percent of that of men of the same age in the general population. True, it is not possible to say with certainty that this finding can be interpreted to mean that their social class, as indicated by their relatively high income and occupational status, fully explained their low mortality rate. Yet, the physician researchers could not identify any other variables, including medical care and health behavior, that could provide a better explanation. There is no question that they were not prepared to find that social class provided the best explanation.

Community or Place of Residence

Everyone agrees that the *environment* one lives in or grows up in matters. The problem is that it is not always clear what someone has in mind when they refer to environment. Do they mean the home environment, the neighborhood environment, something related to the environment of the whole town, county, or something even bigger than that? Then there is the question of physical environment versus social environment. The following body of research focuses on the impact on health of living in a particular geographic location, that is, community or neighborhood, with special emphasis on the social environment (Mellor and Milyo 2001; Subramanian, Kawachi, and Kennedy 2001).

Some years ago researchers began noticing that poor people at similar levels of income did not die at the same rate from one community to the next (Polednak 1991). The data seemed to indicate that poor people in cities with a small impoverished community were at a lower risk of dying than poor people in cities with a large impoverished community. Now that was a surprising finding that needed to be explained. Maybe it isn't income inequality after all. Maybe it is something about community. Admittedly, this is a thorny question to get at.

As we saw earlier when we focused on international differences in life expectancy, having a higher mean or average income level did not necessarily predict to a higher life expectancy. Can the same be said of income differences between states and cities within the same country? The answer is yes. As was true in the case of life expectancy in China in comparison to the United States, the explanation lies not in *absolute level of income* but *relative income* and how it is distributed, that is, the level of socioeconomic inequality.

Researchers who compare mortality rates across states consistently find that greater income inequality by state is associated with increased mortality rates within the states that tolerate greater economic inequality (Lochner et al. 2001; Waitzman and Smith 1998a). The same conclusions are drawn by those who use county-level data (McLaughlin and Stokes 2002). A recent review of U.S. mortality statistics from 1961 to 1999 revealed ". . . a steady increase in mortality among the worst-off segment of the population . . ." during the 1983–1999 period (Ezzati et al. 2008, e66 0557). Remember this is the period during which conservative economic policies resulted in a steady increase in economic inequality. The increase in mortality among females was greater than for males. The explanation, according to the researchers, is largely attributable to an increase in the rate of chronic diseases which was, in turn, related to smoking, increased rate of obesity, and high blood pressure.

What is most intriguing is that it is not just those at lower income levels who are at greater risk of dying with increasing inequality. Everyone in the area is at greater risk (Lynch et al. 1998). In short, income inequality has a negative effect on the mortality rate of everyone living in the area. We will explore why this is so at a couple of levels both concrete (i.e., there is likely to be more violent crime) and subtle (feeling that one does not belong and is socially isolated from one's neighbors).

While we still do not have the complete answer, the question of what it is about living in an impoverished community that results in an increased risk of mortality has been receiving an overwhelming amount of attention. The question has forced scholars to clarify what they mean when they talk about "poor" communities. Three themes have repeatedly come up in discussions regarding poor communities. Geographic location is one. The others involve time, or the persistence of poverty, and finally, behavior—more specifically, deviant behavior.

The attention the issue of variation in mortality by community was receiving produced a consensus on the definition of "how poor" a community has to be to be considered impoverished. The generally accepted standard that has been used for some years in identifying poverty communities is that 40 percent of the population falls under the poverty line (Jargowsky and Bane 1990, 20). No one questions the strength of the association between living in an area characterized by a 40 percent poverty rate and high mortality and morbidity rates (Shaw et al. 2000; Guest, Almgren, and Hussey 1998; Waitzman and Smith 1998b). What is much harder to explain is the finding that the association persists even after individual income, education, and occupation are all eliminated as possible sources of variation (Diez-Roux et al. 2001; House et al. 2000). One practical effect may be the lack of access to medical care in the community (Soobader and LeClere 1999). How a community organizes its approach to caring for the indigent varies across communities, which has a direct effect on the health of the residents (Cunningham and Kemper, 1998). Researchers have been finding similar outcomes even at considerably lower community poverty rates, so this stream of research promises to continue producing results. It is clear that the relationship between community of residence and health is complex.

Focusing on the pathways linking individual health and community of residence has helped to clarify the connection (Robert 1999). A summary of existing research indicates that one pathway defines the opportunities and limitations on opportunity available in the community, that is, education, jobs, and the socioeconomic resources others in the community can contribute. That has a direct impact on the socioeconomic status of residents and that is what affects their health. Another pathway has a more direct impact on health, which occurs apart from individual socioeconomic status because it affects everyone in the area. This occurs where the social environment is threatening—fear prevents walking and getting to know neighbors; the physical environment is unhealthy—higher levels of air pollution; and the service environment is inadequate—less adequate fire, police, and sanitation services. Thus, while community socioeconomic context and individual socioeconomic status affect each other, they also have separate pathways that link them to health.

The answer to the question of what it is about living in an impoverished area that matters may seem obvious on the surface. It is however important to identify the factors that have the greatest explanatory power to address those factors. To illustrate, a study comparing mortality data across forty-nine states revealed that premature mortality was greatest in rural counties in the Southeast and Southwest (Mansfield et al. 1999). The researchers expected to find that access to medical care matters and they found that it did. However, an even more powerful predictor of increased levels of county mortality turned out to be the proportion of female-headed households. Other strong predictors were race, education, and chronic unemployment (National Center for Health Statistics 2001). While this research tells us which factors are most closely associated with increased risk of mortality and morbidity, it does not tell us what it is about those factors, combined with living in an area where there is a concentration of poor people, that increases risk.

Remember the seven health habits that John Knowles identified as basic to the maintenance of good health that we discussed in the chapter on health behavior? Ten years after Knowles announced those seven habits, scholars who continued to study the health status of Alameda County residents began reporting that it was socioeconomic differences of communities in the area that were most closely connected to variations in mortality. However, they also said that they could not determine exactly what it was about living in a poor community that was primarily responsible. They reported that differences persisted even after they controlled for a large list of factors including such central factors as health behavior and access to health care. In other words, medical care and health habits could not explain why poorer areas had higher mortality levels. The researchers finally concluded that the sociophysical environment in which people reside, which is characterized by concrete, tangible factors such as poor housing, high crime rates, higher levels of environmental contaminants, lack of transportation, and so forth, is detrimental to health (Haan, Kaplan, and Camacho 1987).

While variation in health and income distribution by county and by state has been readily available for some time, the same has not been true of data by city. Data collected by health departments in cities across the country had simply not been compiled and compared. That changed when the Chicago Board of Health organized a conference to address the health needs of large urban areas in 1993. The result was a study of twenty health indicators, from heart disease rates to AIDS, low infant birth weight, through homicide for forty-six U.S. cities with populations of three hundred and fifty thousand or more (Benbow, Wang, and Whitman 1998). The profile of cities this study revealed is too extensive to report in detail here. We will focus on the findings the researchers said they found to be most surprising or significant. They found that in twenty-seven cities, AIDS killed more people than homicide and infant mortality combined. This is significant given the attention that crime and crime prevention receives. The fact that more people died from AIDS than gunshot wounds in Chicago led the researchers to make the following observation: "AIDS is more deadly than bullets." In summarizing their findings, they stated that "premature mortality is the best single proxy for reflecting differences in the health status." "Years of life lost," which reflects how many years the average person lives versus persons in any particular racial/ethnic category, is a measure that has been gaining the attention of health researchers in recent years. That the health of urban residents has not gotten better is confirmed by the 2007 Big Cities Health Inventory, which indicates that the nation's largest cities had a combined mortality rate in 2004 that was 20 percent higher than the national rate (National Association of County & City Health Officials 2007).

This is an important statement in light of the Healthy Cities movement being sponsored by WHO. WHO is striving to improve people's lives in urban areas by raising awareness, mobilizing community participation, and developing the roles of local government throughout the world. It admits that it is still struggling to define health and measures of health as it proceeds with this agenda (Kinzer 2000). Why WHO has targeted urban areas as requiring special attention becomes clearer as we consider the data presented in the following section.

The Special Case of Segregated Poor, Black Communities

There is an enormous amount of evidence to substantiate the observation that living in a poor, black community increases mortality risk (House et al. 2000; Jackson et al. 2000; Geronimus et al. 1996; Williams and Collins 1995; Massey and Denton 1993). The question is—what is it about the intersection between community of residence and race that produces this effect? Let's begin searching for the answer to this question by considering the data on infant mortality, which are particularly striking. As you recall, black infant mortality is substantially higher than white infant mortality. However, black infant mortality is not universally high. The rate varies by community. In one study, a comparison of infant mortality rates across thirty-eight large metropolitan areas in this country revealed that the greater the level of segregation, that is, the more concentrated the black population in a geographic area in addition to concentration of poverty, the higher the infant mortality. In communities with low levels of segregation, there were smaller black–white variations in infant mortality despite a high level of poverty (Polednak 1991). Why this is so is an interesting question. Various interpretations are under consideration. Let's examine what those who have given most attention to the question have to say.

The underlying problem that an increasing number of researchers have become interested in addressing has to do with the effects of an accelerating rate of racial segregation in combination with economic segregation (Jargowsky 1996a, 1996b; Massey 1996; Massey and Denton 1993). The researchers who focus on these issues say that the two trends have the effect of increasing isolation, which exacerbates whatever problems are associated with poverty and race. As the middle-class members of the community leave, the concentration of poverty becomes more intense. That leads to a downward spiral. More property becomes dilapidated as property owners leave and only the poorest renters remain. Stores are abandoned because the owners cannot make enough money to keep them up. That causes unemployment to increase because employers and the jobs they can offer move elsewhere. The people who remain find it harder to get basic goods and services. As the number of unemployed adults, especially men, becomes more apparent, the youth have less reason to believe that their fate will be any different. Young people, especially young men, find it harder to find social support in such a depressed environment, which explains, in part, why they turn to gangs. They do so knowing very well that gang membership increases their risk of death before they reach age twenty-one. But they also have no reason to think that they will be able to find a good job. So why bother going to school? Why take care of your health if you don't expect to live very long anyway? Why avoid getting high now, if there is no future? Such an attitude describes the "underclass" who are the "truly disadvantaged" that William Julius Wilson has written about (1993, 1987).

Poor minority children are particularly vulnerable to the disadvantages of growing up in a poor, segregated neighborhood (Acevedo-Garcia et al. 2008). Using 2000 census data, researchers have found that a typical poor white child lives in a neighborhood where the poverty rate is 13.6 percent; a typical poor black child lives in a neighborhood where the poverty rate is 30 percent; a typical poor Latino child lives in a neighborhood where the poverty rate is 26 percent. Black children (17 percent) and Latino children (20 percent) are more than twelve times as likely as white children to be poor and live in a poor neighborhood, putting them into "double jeopardy." The authors say that minority children and white children are growing up in two different worlds. They argue that even the poorest white children are more likely to grow up in neighborhoods rich in opportunity with good schools, safe streets, and healthy environments. By contrast, poor minority children face: (1) limited economic advancement because of poor education, limited job opportunities, and a poor return on housing investment; (2) exposure to violent crime, environmental hazards, poor municipal services, and a lack of grocery stores and healthy food options; and (3) segregated health-care settings with poorer health care.

There is little disagreement about the deleterious effects of residential segregation for blacks, whether for adults or children. One indicator of the health consequences is the prevalence of hypertension among African Americans. Nancy Kreiger uses what is becoming known as an "ecosocial" perspective to explain it (Kreiger 2001). She identifies six multilevel pathways.

1. economic and social deprivation, which is associated with living in neighborhoods without good supermarkets, which is linked, in turn, to eating cheap, high-fat foods; economic deprivation increases the risk of being born preterm, which is linked to underdevelopment of kidneys and increasing likelihood of salt retention (a factor linked to high blood pressure for some people).
2. toxic substances and hazardous conditions, which increases exposure to lead paint and soil contamination from car exhausts due to proximity of streets and freeways, leading to renal damage.
3. socially inflicted trauma, which provokes fear and anger, triggering the "flight-or-fight" response and the damage that causes.
4. targeted marketing of commodities such as high alcohol-content beverages, which are used to reduce feelings of distress; excess alcohol consumption elevates risk of hypertension.
5. inadequate health care, specifically poor detection and clinical management of hypertension.
6. resistance to racial oppression; hypertension is amenable to individual and community efforts to counter racism and enhance dignity.

It is worth noting that evidence of the negative health effects associated with ethnic/racial segregation is less clear in the case of Hispanics (Lee and Ferraro 2007). It appears that it is more disadvantageous to low-income Puerto Ricans than it is to Mexicans. The prevailing hypothesis to explain this is that the high degree of social contact that occurs in Mexican American communities is promoting the flow of information about health resources and other forms of social support. What this tells us is that more research that differentiates health effects across Hispanic subgroups is needed.

Some researchers argue that the feelings of hopelessness and powerlessness that are so prevalent in impoverished black communities are directly responsible for increased health risk. These feelings are brought on by the realization on the part of persons living in such neighborhoods that they cannot do anything to improve their living conditions, which include high crime rates, vandalism, graffiti, drugs, and so on (Ross, Mirowsky, and Pribesh 2001). This reality and the negative feelings it engenders are directly linked to mistrust in other residents who cannot be counted on to be supportive. In fact, there is reason to expect neighbors to be self-interested and dishonest, which, in turn, prevents those who would like to do so from forming positive social relationships based on trust. All of this, in combination, ultimately results in an amplification of mistrust with all the negative consequences that lack of social support has for health.

The literature on impoverished communities makes it perfectly clear that people growing up in impoverished communities have a slim chance of getting out. There is little question that they have had a poor early education because students in areas of poverty are invariably far behind in academic achievement compared to their peers who live and go to schools in areas that do not have poverty (Jencks and Mayer 1990). Inadequate education means they have little chance of climbing onto even the bottom rung of a ladder that will allow them to move to a better job. For a start, there are very few businesses in poor neighborhoods to provide the first rung on the ladder. It is true that they might be able to find a minimum-wage job in another neighborhood, especially during a period of low unemployment, as was true during the late 1990s. However, such jobs do not provide a ladder for upward mobility. They are dead-end jobs that do not pay enough to support a family and offer very few benefits, such as health insurance. Although, as we all have been discovering over the last couple of years, even that option is less available at a time when the economy is shrinking rather than expanding.

Other researchers take the position that problems associated with *urbanization* may explain a great deal more than *social disorganization*. In other words, the real problem is urban decay as indicated by increasing homelessness, doubling-up in deteriorating housing, decline of social health and welfare services in the community, and so on. The evidence for this is that poor whites who live in deteriorating urban areas also face a higher risk of mortality than whites nationwide (Geronimus 1999).

What is troubling to many researchers is that an examination of the leading causes of death for adults reported in poor, black neighborhoods certainly indicates that there is excess mortality due to social disorganization and related causes of death such as HIV and homicide. However, although those rates are exceptionally high across the country, the leading causes of death among blacks of all ages are chronic, stress-related diseases, namely, heart disease and cancer. (This is not the same as saying that AIDS accounts for the highest rate of *premature* death discussed above [Benbow, Wang, and Whitman 1998].)

You may have become aware of an inherent contradiction in this body of literature. If inequality is detrimental to health, then why does living in a community where poor minorities are less concentrated bring health advantages? After all, doesn't having closer contact with those who are more advantaged make a person's disadvantaged status more readily apparent? Haven't we been saying all along that relative deprivation is what makes people feel bad and it is that which has detrimental psychosocial consequences? The explanation is that a person's sense of his or her own worth is largely influenced by the person's sense of belonging and connectedness both to the larger society and immediate community in which he or she lives. That brings up the topic of *social capital*, which we touch on again later in this chapter and discuss more extensively in the following chapter. Before we do that, let us return to a range of community problems directly linked to social inequality.

Spillover Effects

We all know that there is more crime in poor neighborhoods. Economic inequality is obviously a factor. Let's examine the relationship between inequality and crime more systematically.

We all know where the "bad" neighborhoods are in our cities. Looking at such neighborhoods from an historical perspective reveals an interesting fact. It appears that it is the neighborhoods themselves that are unsafe—regardless of who lives there. That observation was made in 1942 by two researchers, Shaw and McKay, who studied juvenile delinquency records in twenty-one U.S. cities over a period of several decades (Wilkinson, Kawachi, and Kennedy 1999). The researchers concluded that it was the inability of the community to impose common values and enforce them that was associated with delinquency. The problem has been conceptualized since then as social disorganization, which we have touched on before. It is interesting to see how researchers interested in health inequalities are applying this concept currently.

In a major study comparing homicide rates to state rates of income inequality, researchers determined that violent crime is indeed closely related to income inequality (Wilkinson, Kawachi, and Kennedy 1999). The researchers found that a greater degree of income inequality by state was consistent with a higher rate of homicide, aggravated assault, and robbery, but not rape in that state (Kawachi, Kennedy, and Wilkinson 1999). What was surprising to the researchers was finding a lack of any relationship between inequality and property crime. In fact, the researchers note that if anything, larceny and motor vehicle theft are more common in areas where median income is higher. They also found that the relationship between income inequality and firearm violent crime remained strong even after adjusting for poverty and availability of firearms (Kennedy et al. 1999).

Remember the discussion of homicide rates and the variables that we identified as relevant in chapter 4, namely age, sex, and race? Let's look at homicide rates through the lens we are employing in this chapter—social inequality. Homicide rates rose during the 1980s, but began declining as of 1993. Researchers who approach this topic from a public health and epidemiology perspective report findings consistent with those coming out of criminal justice research. All agree that age is the strongest predictor of criminal activity. In other words, the homicide rate has been declining because the proportion of young men in the population has been declining. Because young men are the most likely to be involved in violent crime, a decline in the number of young men tends to be perfectly correlated with a decline in homicide rates.

A more specific explanation for the rise and decline of youth homicide rates revolves around the sudden rise in the demand for crack cocaine during the 1980s, which led to deadly turf wars (the following is based on Rosenfield [2002]). The crack epidemic peaked around 1990, which is when the rate of youth homicide began to decline as well. However, these trends do not explain the decline in the adult homicide rate. The list of factors being explored and debated to explain the decline in the adult homicide rate includes the following: legalization of abortion in the 1970s (fewer unwanted babies who would have been more likely to turn to crime in the 1990s), prison expansion (about 1.3 million inmates are being deterred from crime), stricter firearm policies, smarter policing, and finally, an improved economy and expanded employment opportunities.

That said, the research carried out by health researchers targets a somewhat different set of explanatory variables (Cubbin, Pickle, and Fingerhut 2000; Fingerhut, Ingram and Feldman 1998). Researchers who include data on inequality in their research say that the level of *urbanization* for both white and black men is the second most important factor. They conclude that income disparity, rather than low median income, that is, poverty per se, is associated with high homicide rates for both black and white men. They also report finding substantially higher homicide rates for black men in areas with high percentages of female-headed households.

The percentage of female-headed households in a community is increasingly being reported as a particularly powerful predictive indicator of excess mortality in general, not only high homicide. The same researchers say that there are probably a number of unaccounted for factors that would explain the significance of finding that a high proportion of female-headed households matters. They go on to say that those factors are all closely related to racial segregation and social deprivation, including higher levels of poverty, social isolation, inadequate housing, and so on. It is worth noting that there is consensus in sociology of the family literature on the benefits that the presence of another adult in the household is highly beneficial. Having a grandmother live in the household and share the load of childrearing ameliorates but does not overcome the negative effects generally attributed to female-headed households. It does help to provide psychological support needed to maintain discipline and potentially raises household income.

Discussing crime in the context of health is becoming more common because the public health community has begun arguing that violent crime leading to injury and death should be addressed by society through means other than law enforcement alone. Indeed, epidemiologists are using the same approach to violence as the analytical tools they use in identifying patterns of illness and death related to other causes. The researchers who have been studying the social effects of economic inequality have also been finding that areas with high crime rates tend to exhibit excess mortality rates from all causes (Kawachi, Kennedy, and Wilkinson 1999, 719). They conclude that "crime and population health share the same social origins." Accordingly, they say that crime is "a mirror of the quality of the social environment."

At a more concrete level, poor people live in communities that are near highways and in apartments that are poorly maintained. Associated with this is a factor that might explain the variation in crime rates—the level of prenatal and childhood exposure to lead. It seems that people in poor neighborhoods are more likely to be exposed to lead, which leads to brain damage, and a high blood level of lead is highly correlated with risk of arrest, especially for violent crime (Wright et al. 2008).

An increasing number of researchers have been saying that poor health and high mortality levels are associated with the lack of social cohesion within a community. We touched on ideas related to this topic briefly already in discussing economic and racial segregation. The concept that has emerged to encompass the array of factors that may be involved is *social capital*. Social capital is defined as trust and willingness to come together to address common concerns, which is manifested in civic engagement or involvement in community affairs. This is typically measured by membership in civic and other associations and groups that bring people together around shared interests (Kennedy et al. 1999), which we will discuss in greater detail in the next chapter. For now let's wind up this portion of the discussion by returning briefly to the relationship of social and economic inequality to age, sex, and race.

Notes on Age, Sex, and Race

Age has not been considered in relationship to inequality by researchers except to note that income drops for many people as they grow older, particularly women, which has an obvious effect on their ability to maintain their accustomed standard of living. Some researchers are critical of the way age has been treated by researchers, saying that researchers are defining age "as a variable to control rather than a concept to be understood in social terms" (Denton and Walters 1999, 1233). Aging is sometimes associated with a declining sense of valued self-identity, together with progressive encounters with discrimination, which may explain why aging might have a more extensive negative impact on health than previous research has credited.

Research on aging points to structural factors associated with education and income as the primary determinants of better health and greater longevity. However, there is clear evidence that there are effects that can be identified at every stage in life. A particularly topical illustration captures the idea. In the case of males, aging has more negative effects for those with less education and lower-status occupations as indicated, for example, by the increased risk of deterioration of sexual function (Aytac et al. 2000). For older women there are disadvantages in being in a lower-income category, working part-time or not at all rather than full-time, and having the sense that little social support is available. Not only are employed women healthier when they are younger, but participation in the labor force has beneficial effects on health over time (Ross and Bird 1994). In short, the evidence is consistent with regard to aging. Structural factors, which are not so easily altered, turn out to be more important determinants of health status than behavioral and lifestyle factors (Sacker et al. 2001; Denton and Walters 1999).

Researchers keep trying to identify exactly what it is about working that produces health benefits over the long run (Marmot and Shipley 1996). The question has received special attention as it applies to women and work because women have traditionally had the option of staying out of the labor market. In a study of the effects of work on women in Britain, researchers found that women reported more negative work characteristics than men, but those in full-time employment report fewer negative characteristics of work than those employed part-time (Matthews et al. 1998). Employed women reported having little opportunity to learn, greater monotony combined with too fast a pace of work, and less flexibility of breaks. Women who stayed home reported even less opportunity for learning and substantially greater monotony than paid workers. While there was a clear gradient in self-reported health that correlated with work characteristics, the gradient was consistent with the socioeconomic status of the women even apart from their jobs.

When researchers compare women's health using U.S. state-level indicators of inequality, the results are even more enlightening. In one study, researchers used four composite indices to compare women's status across states including: political participation, economic autonomy, employment and earnings, and reproductive rights (Kawachi et al. 1999). They found higher political participation and a smaller wage gap between men and women to be strongly associated with lower female mortality and morbidity. The researchers stated that they were not surprised to find that women's status indices were also highly correlated with male mortality rates. They interpreted this to mean that structural factors common to both men and women were responsible for the health outcomes exhibited by both sexes.

That interpretation is supported by a study of voting participation at the state level among both males and females (Blakely, Kennedy, and Kawachi 2001). In this case, researchers found political participation, as measured by voter turnout, to be associated with self-rated health, which is, in turn, correlated with household income. The lower the voter turnout, the lower the average self-rated health ratings within the state. The explanation is that the gap between rich and poor leads to a polarization of interests, which results in reduced spending on social goods that benefit all, such as education and health care. That has the effect of diminishing social trust in the ability of the wider society to address problems. That further limits the development of the sense of belonging to the larger society. We will examine these observations in more detail in the next chapter.

Structural factors are particularly important in creating the pathways that lead to increased mortality and morbidity rates when the variable at issue is race. More specifically, let us consider the evidence that connects the effects of racial discrimination directed at African Americans first at the collective level and then at the individual level to health. The results of a national survey conducted in thirty-nine states indicate that there is a clear correlation between the percentage of residents who hold negative attitudes toward African Americans and the mortality rate of African Americans (Kennedy et al. 1999). States in which a higher proportion of residents reported negative attitudes toward African Americans also exhibited higher mortality rates for whites, although considerably lower than the rates reported for African Americans. The researchers say that racial "disrespect" is indicative of a lack of trust between races, which translates into structural barriers with detrimental economic consequences as those attitudes play out in decisions related to hiring and firing. Needless to say, this is likely to have various negative effects on the community, such as higher rates of poverty, social disorganization, crime, and so forth. How much change in attitudes there has been is not clear. The fact that the country elected an African American to the highest office in the land indicates that negative attitudes about African Americans have dropped significantly. Whether this constitutes evidence of a permanent change remains to be seen.

Returning to consideration of the effects of discrimination at the individual level, let us once again consider the question of why African Americans have higher rates of hypertension than other groups. It is widely accepted that there is a strong link between stress and elevated blood pressure rates. Extending this observation, researchers find that there is a clear connection between increased blood pressure and self-reported experiences of discrimination or unfair treatment (Kreiger and Sidney 1996). In one study that included 1,480 black women, 1,157 black men, 1,307 white women, and 1,171 white men, nearly 80 percent reported having experienced unfair treatment. However, blood pressure was higher among the black men and women who reported having experienced no racial discrimination in contrast to those who did report such experiences. Social class mediated this somewhat. Working-class blacks had the highest blood-pressure levels. By contrast, professional-level black men and women, who reported experiencing unfair treatment and discrimination and doing something about it, had comparatively low blood pressure. The interpretation is that those who suppress anger and hostility are at higher risk of hypertension. In fact, the researchers conclude by saying that such feelings plus internalization of negative social attitudes in combination with limited socioeconomic resources go a long way in explaining the production of poor health among blacks (Clark et al. 1999; Kreiger and Sidney 1996).

When you consider these findings in light of the shift in social attitudes in this country regarding who is to be blamed for the disadvantaged status of African Americans, it is not hard to see why African American mortality and morbidity rates are not declining. As we saw in chapter 5, there has been a significant increase between 1963 and 1995 in the proportion of white Americans who say that African Americans who do not succeed have no one to blame but themselves (Schuman and Krysan 1999). As I keep repeating, this may be changing given the willingness of Americans to elect an African American to the highest office in the land. We have to wait and see.

Summary and Conclusions

The views of Michael Marmot, the epidemiologist who brought the relationship between inequality and health to the forefront through his work on Whitehall, are of special significance to this discussion. In assessing the scholarly findings that grounded his work, he says that a great deal more research is needed before we can understand the relationship between inequality and health.

> We do not know the extent to which social circumstances influence disease pathways through exposure to physical, chemical and biologic agents, or through the mind. My own view is that the mind is a crucial gateway through which social influences affect physiology to cause disease. The mind may work through effects on health-related behavior, such as smoking, eating, drinking, physical activity, or risk taking, or it may act through effects of neuroendocrine or immune mechanisms.
>
> In essence, there is no question that all of these factors play a role and are important. It is just that we still do not know enough about the pathways that connect all the factors to produce disease and death. (Marmot 2001, 135)

Having said that, we also know that we must work with what we have and go on to consider social policy with regard to variations in health, morbidity, and mortality. Obviously, the first question we must address is whether what we have discovered is sufficiently worrisome to require a social response. Only then can we go on to outline what policy initiatives we would like to see advanced and those we would like to see contained or reversed.

CHAPTER TWELVE

~

Policy

The first chapter of this book opened with a statement about how many stories we see in the public media related to health and how challenging it is to sift out what is new and important versus what confirms prevailing understandings. We proceeded to examine a wide range of research results that scholars were presenting us with. To be precise, we set out to discover why some people end up having long and healthy lives, while others suffer ill health and premature death. More specifically, we said we would be focusing on attempts to explain the persistence of significant health disparities.

The question at this point is—how successful have we been? In my view, the evidence on the factors that influence our health status is becoming far clearer than it was even a few years ago. Before we go on to consider policy interventions designed to improve the health status of people in this country based on what we have learned in preceding chapters, let us review some basic facts.

- Age and Sex. With each passing year, most Americans have been living a little longer, but not as long as persons in many other highly industrialized societies. More distressing is finding that life expectancy for some people, namely those with less income and education, has plateaued; it has stopped increasing. We also learned that the most dangerous year of life occurs between birth and year one; that the safest years are between five and fifteen; and that women live longer than men, but that they do so with a higher level of chronic illness. Because we have only been focusing on women's health more directly during the last couple of decades, we have not yet been able to identify the full range of factors responsible for the differences between women's and men's health.

- Race and Poverty. We organize health statistics by age, sex, and race or ethnicity. Both those who collect the statistics and the researchers who analyze them agree that racial/ethnic categorization is based on superficial rather than biological differences. The rationale for continuing to use race as a differentiating factor is that this is the way it has been done all along and it would be a great loss to drop these designations since that would make all the data we have collected to date useless for assessing trends. Given that most scientists continue to believe that race or ethnicity reflects superficial physical characteristics, race or ethnicity should not make a difference in health outcomes. Yet we find very large differences, which is the primary reason why we cannot ignore race and ethnicity, and why we continue to try to identify the reasons behind the differences. Increasingly the consensus is that the main reason that mortality and morbidity rates vary by race is the higher level of social disadvantage faced by blacks. Rather than abandoning race and ethnicity as variables, the reverse has occurred. We now have statistics on a greater number of racial and ethnic categories. This has resulted in more information, but has not helped to explain more fully the reasons behind variations in morbidity and mortality. Instead, it introduced new questions. To illustrate, we need to explain why the Hispanic mortality and morbidity rates are substantially lower than those of blacks, given that the poverty rate for the two categories is similar. Thus far, no one has come up with a complete explanation. The fact that variation, indeed significant variation, exists across racial and/or ethnic mortality rates has caused researchers to expand their search for factors that would account for the variation. Accordingly, they have been devoting greater attention to behavior and lifestyle.
- Health Behavior and Lifestyle. We all know that lifestyle is closely related to morbidity and mortality. But what has become much clearer over the last couple of decades is that behavior detrimental to health is neither randomly distributed across the population nor linked as closely to race and ethnicity as the conventional wisdom would have us believe. We repeatedly find that people with less income and education are the ones who are more likely to engage in behavior that is detrimental to health regardless of race and ethnic background. That

presents us with yet another challenging question, namely, what is it about having less income and education that produces unhealthy behavior? In most cases, it cannot be lack of information. Everyone in this country knows that smoking is bad for one's health; that eating foods high in fat and becoming severely overweight is bad for one's health; that engaging in little or no exercise is bad for one's health, and so on. It is not entirely clear why people with more education and income do not engage in negative health behaviors and people with less education and income do. Part of the answer is less money to buy more expensive, healthier foods, but it is only a partial answer. The literature on health behavior does not really attempt to answer the question. The newly emergent body of work on population health goes much further in providing answers. Before turning to those answers, let us review how much of the variation in health status can be garnered from the three other variables we examined—medical care, genetics, and stress.

- Medical Care. Not having medical care when it is needed is clearly associated with increased mortality and morbidity. Yet it is very clear that having access to health-care services is not enough to eliminate variations in morbidity and mortality. We need look no further than the United Kingdom, where the government has been providing health care to all its citizens for the last six decades. Researchers in Britain have noted the existence of a clear gradient in mortality associated with social class, in spite of the fact that everyone has access to medical care, in reports on the health status of the population issued periodically throughout the twentieth century. Obviously, medical care matters to the health of the individual who needs it. Researchers consistently find that those who do not have access to health-care services have worse health than those who do. What is more difficult to explain is the variation in health status among people who have access to medical care which, in this country, includes those who are insured, that is, those who have private insurance, veterans, and those on Medicaid and Medicare. In each of these populations, those with less income and education tend to be sicker and die at an earlier age. It is impossible to ignore the fact that a high proportion of those with access to health-care services also tend to have higher incomes, more education, and jobs that offer more security in addition to a range of other intrinsic and extrinsic benefits. This has led an increasing number of researchers to conclude that the wide range of benefits that go with higher socioeconomic status explains more about variations in health status than access to medical care.

- Genetics. We have been hearing a great deal about the progress geneti-cists have been making in unlocking the secrets of the genetic code and how that promises to bring vast improvements in health care. A closer look indicates that genetic science is making huge advances, but that the process of translating genetic science into medical treatment is moving at a much slower pace. Even when impressive advances in diagnostic techniques are achieved, new and effective treatments do not accompany those advances. The current interest in developing drugs that target far more precisely diseases identified through genetic testing, holds the greatest promise. At the same time, the single most valuable lesson that the recent breakthroughs in genetic science have taught us is that genes are highly susceptible to environmental influ-ences. Indeed, many geneticists are saying that, for now, focusing on social environmental factors constitutes a far more promising approach for improving health than counting on genetic tests and treatments. That seems to bring us back to behavior, which we know varies with income and education.

- Stress. No one would deny that stress matters. Yet, there are few fac-tors affecting health status that are as nebulous as stress. Measuring it is difficult enough. Identifying intervention mechanisms designed to lower stress levels is even more uncertain. Recent research based on animal studies reveals why it is so difficult. That body of research indicates that personality matters, social connectedness matters, and social status—which is relative to the context in which one operates on a daily basis—matters. When we consider whether these findings might apply to human beings, what becomes clear is that individuals, whether they are baboons or people, cannot readily alter any of these factors. It is very difficult to alter one's personality after it has been shaped during the early formative years. There is no assurance that one can arrange to have friends and relatives who have the emotional and practical resources to be supportive. And it is basically impossible to alter, at least on an individual basis, the institutional structures cre-ated by the society in which people carry out their lives. In short, some people come into the world with advantages at all of these levels that reduce the chances of encountering stress with any regularity. It is the level of unavoidable stress that one experiences on a regular basis that accumulates to undermine physical health over time. Researchers point out that those who are socially disadvantaged are likely to encounter more stress, on a more consistent basis, than those who have a greater range of resources to deal with stressful situations when they occur.

- Inequality. A review of all the variables that affect morbidity and mortality indicates that social class must be a more important factor than anyone realized, which led more researchers to turn their attention to health implications associated with social inequality. This, in turn, has led an even larger number of scholars to become convinced that the association between social inequality and poor health is consistent and powerful. Researchers have been repeatedly finding that it is not absolute income or wealth but the relative degree of socioeconomic advantage or disadvantage that matters. This observation was unexpected but has been hard to ignore. We see it holding up regardless of whether the population being studied is a community, a state, or a whole society.

What is new is not the recognition that relative disadvantage matters, but that it matters in this context. Amartya Sen, the Nobel Prize–winning economist, has devoted a great deal of attention to examining the nature of economic inequality in general and relative inequality in particular. He says that the essence of equality and ultimately social justice is the freedom to achieve, which translates into the capability to function in society. Inequality is associated with the difficulty that a person experiences in "converting 'primary goods' into actual freedoms to achieve" (Sen 1992, 148). He defines relative inequality as follows:

> *relative* deprivation in terms of *incomes* can yield *absolute* deprivation in terms of capabilities. Being relatively poor in a rich country can be a great capability handicap, even when one's absolute income is high in terms of world standards. In a generally opulent country, more income is needed to buy enough commodities to achieve the *same social functioning*. (Sen 1999, 89) (Italics in the original.)

No one would deny that risk factors such as hypertension and health behaviors such as diet, exercise, and access to medical care are the proximate causes of disease. However, we now have over well thirty years of data ". . . documenting the consistent and inverse relationship between socioeconomic status and measures of both morbidity and mortality across time, across countries, and across the life course" (Herd, Schoeni, and House 2008, 7). This has led a growing number of researchers to posit that socioeconomic position is not simply a proxy for all the other factors that predict poor health, such as smoking, lack of exercise, obesity, even access to health care. They argue that an individual's wherewithal to avoid disease and death is more directly linked to and "shaped by resources of knowledge, money, power, prestige, and beneficial social connections" (Link and Phelan 2002, 730). Yet, we continue to expend resources and energy in an effort to identify mechanisms that will change individual behaviors, as if socioeconomic status were not a significant consideration. This has had the effect of obscuring efforts to address the "fundamental causes" that account for an individual's decision to engage in damaging behavior (Herd, Schoeni, and House 2008; Link and Phelan 1995, 2000, 2002; House et al. 2000; Lantz, et al. 2001; Adler and Matthews 1994).

Social Class and Social Inequality

There have been a number of other striking revelations connected to the relationship between social inequality and health that bear repeating. Social inequality is generally defined in terms of three basic components: income, education, and occupation. More often than not, researchers devote primary attention to either income or education rather than a combination of indicators in any one study.

Starting with income, the relationship between income and health manifests itself "in three ways: the gross national product of countries, the income of individuals, and the income inequalities among rich nations and among geographic areas" (Marmot 2003, 31; 1998). A high level of consensus can be found in the international comparative literature regarding the relationship between income and life expectancy. Per capita income is directly correlated with life expectancy in the poorest countries. However, the two are not nearly as closely correlated in developed countries. In developed countries, it is the level of economic inequality in a country that is highly correlated with variation in mortality. Indeed, the slowing down of the rate of decline in mortality that occurred in the United States and England during the decade of the 1980s parallels the period during which economic inequality began to increase at a rate that had not been seen since the early decades of the twentieth century. The same thing has occurred again in the United States over the first decade of the twenty-first century.

According to a growing number of researchers, education is a better predictor of life expectancy and mortality than income (Marmot 2003). Income and education together are even better than either education or income considered independently. Using the two indicators in combination explains more than any other variable generally employed to explain variations in health including race, health behavior, and access to medical care. The fact that health behaviors and lifestyle are closely associated with education and income indicates that shifts in education and income can be expected to have a direct effect on behavior. This is significant because efforts to alter individual behavior patterns have been very discouraging.

As you know, education and income are used as indicators of social class in this country because the United States does not collect data using social class as a differentiating variable. Americans had not taken an interest in the relationship between social class and health until relatively recently—after the research being carried out in England began to be more widely disseminated. The fact that the differential between the lowest classes and the highest classes in England was increasing over several decades in the later part of the twentieth century is largely responsible for the intense effort aimed at explaining that development as well as the sudden interest in the relationship between health and social inequality in this country. The Whitehall studies of English civil servants, which encompass all three dimensions of social class—education, income, and occupation—have been especially important in identifying the factors that are associated with the existence of variations in morbidity and mortality by social class.

Moving from Conclusions to Policy Implications

Let us shift, at this point, from the link between the conclusions based on the review of findings specifically related to the variables we examined in previous chapters to the implications that this body of knowledge as a whole has for health policy in this country. I will assume that you agree that the health differences among people in the United States are large, in fact large enough to require a purposeful response and to warrant moving on to consider how society might address such differences.

We begin by addressing the most basic question that has stood behind all the findings we have been considering: where should we direct our efforts and resources to improve the health of our society? To date, health policy in this country has focused on the individual's responsibility for his or her own health. Public health policy has emphasized health education, that is, convincing people to change their lifestyle—to get more exercise, stop smoking, eat less fatty food, lose weight, and so on. Persuading people to seek medical care sooner, even working toward facilitating increased access to medical care has been high on the health policy agenda. Some in the medical and health research communities have taken this perspective a step further. They admit that changing people's behavior is difficult. Accordingly, they argue we would be better off putting our faith and resources in medical and genetic research. Americans do not seem ready to wait until that happens, but we also do not seem to have a better solution that we can all embrace.

The major alternative to a policy agenda aimed at changing individual behavior is accepting the idea that variations in morbidity and mortality are best explained by socioeconomic inequality as opposed to individual behaviors. That conclusion logically requires one to recognize that reducing economic inequality will have a much bigger impact on the health of the population than changing the behavior of individuals one at a time. That approach comes hard to Americans.

Policy that focuses on altering the choices made by individuals is consistent with the core values of American culture. The American cultural value system holds that we all have plenty of opportunity not only to better our health, but to succeed in other endeavors (read that as "get rich"), and it is up to each of us to make that effort. Consistent with this set of beliefs is the idea that those who don't succeed in having good health and long life have no one to blame but themselves. The only justification for not achieving these things is that one's health problems are due to a genetic flaw, over which a person has no control. That, of course, explains why talk about genetic factors is so prevalent.

Some sociologists say putting the focus on individuals and the choices they make amounts to "victim blaming." This explains why sociologists who invoke this concept in outlining the power of culture to provide people with a set of beliefs to account for lack of good health and lack of financial success have generally been labeled as radicals whose ideas should be ignored. However, things have changed over the last decade or so. An increasing number of health researchers are saying that victims are being blamed inappropriately and they are backing up what they say with convincing evidence. (To name a few: Siegrist and Marmot [2006]; Kawachi and Kennedy [2002]; Berkman et al. [2000].)

Upstream Versus Downstream Efforts

Critics of the American health system have consistently said that the way we have been responding to morbidity and mortality is to do everything we can for individuals after they are already sick. Or, to use an analogy that is now well integrated into the public health and epidemiology literature—once they have traveled "downstream." The source of the imagery associated with "upstream" versus "downstream" intervention comes from a story told by a doctor to a sociologist, Irving Zola, who passed it on to another sociologist, John McKinlay. McKinlay built on this imagery to lay out the following analysis of the problem then went on to consider policy solutions. (The following is based on McKinlay [1974].)

Imagine the following scenario. The doctor telling the story says his work seems like a rescue operation near the shores of a fast-running river. He keeps having to jump in to save people who are drowning. As soon as he revives one person, he hears another yelling for help and must jump in again and rescue that person. He is so busy rescuing people that he cannot go upstream to see who is pushing them all in. As I am sure you will agree, the story has lost none of its impact to capture one's attention even after the passage of many decades since it first appeared.

After relating this story, McKinlay proceeded to argue in the same article that policy makers should strive to curb the activities of the "manufacturers of illness." He despaired in noting that the downstream efforts of practitioners have little chance of overcoming the efforts of the profit-making corporations located upstream, which are able to devote enormous resources designed to convince us to engage in behaviors that are detrimental to our health. In short, he took the position that the rates of morbidity and mortality in this country are neither accidental nor inexplicable. He said that they were due in large part to behaviors closely linked to the cultural values we espouse. Smoking was linked to such values as masculinity, "being cool," and sexy, more so then than now—even as the cigarette companies try to find images that will capture the attention of a new generation of smokers. (You may remember the cigarette companies' past successes attributed to the Marlboro man and the Virginia Slims woman billboards.) Parental love has consistently been tied to permitting children to consume highly sweetened foods, soda, candy, cookies, and so on. In fact, according to McKinlay, the food industry bears enormous responsibility for the high rate of morbidity in this country. It has manipulated our tastes in an effort to convince us to choose synthetic, highly processed, fatty foods, and decrease our consumption of fresh fruit and vegetables.

This makes sense from the food industry's perspective because it is much cheaper to make products look and taste like the real thing through use of additives and preservatives than it is to grow and transport the real thing before it loses its freshness. The effect is reduction of nutrients, which are then replaced in the form of chemical additives. When people succumb to high-powered advertising that promises high levels of satisfaction and enjoyment, and become obese, develop diabetes and heart disease, and so on, the sociocultural response is to scorn them and attribute their ills to individual weakness and culpability.

Observations by another sociologist, George Ritzer, are worth calling upon to extend McKinlay's criticisms. Ritzer warns us about the effects of the ongoing McDonaldization of America (Ritzer 2000). He points out that fast-food ads emphasize quantity rather than quality. The ads encourage us to buy enormous portions, which we must consume to feel satisfied because the food is tasteless even if it is fatty and full of calories, which has obvious implications for our health.

Returning to McKinlay, while he clearly blames large corporations for the part they play in manufacturing illness, he also does not let health-care providers, that is, doctors, off the hook. He says that physicians contribute to a cultural belief system that blames individuals for their poor health. By treating individuals one at a time at the downstream end of the process, without considering why so many are succumbing to illness, health-care providers are ignoring the upstream causes of ill health. In short, he concludes that focusing efforts upstream would do a great deal more to benefit health than increasing funding for research and health care at the downstream end. Many of the most highly respected epidemiologists have been saying exactly the same thing (Rose 1992).

Holding tobacco companies responsible for causing smoking-related illnesses is exactly the kind of thing that McKinlay wanted to see effected when he first identified the upstream source of our ill health in 1974. As a matter of fact, the courts have held tobacco companies liable for their role in hiding information about the consequences of smoking. When state attorney generals argued that the enormous amount of money they were asking for was needed to compensate states for expenditures for care of persons with smoking-related diseases, the courts found in their favor. Unfortunately such bonanzas have a way of dissipating when they fall into the hands of politicians. The funds have been used to pave highways, to support pet projects favored by local politicians, and as tax rebates designed to earn favor with voters.

An analysis of how states distributed tobacco settlement funds is very revealing (Gross et al. 2002). The average settlement received by states was $28.35 per person living in the state. The average amount states actually spent in 2001 was $3.49, with a range of spending from $0.10 to $15.47. The rate of smoking by state residents did not determine spending. States like Massachusetts and Hawaii, which have smoking rates well below 20 percent, spent over $10.00 per person. By contrast, Nevada spent $0.59 even though well over 30 percent of its population smokes.

So how bad can it be to spend tobacco settlement funds on other projects that have some benefit for the state? How bad is it to share the windfall with state residents through a tax rebate? I know of one couple in Illinois who applied their entire rebate to buying cartons of cigarettes. (In Illinois, the settlement was $9.1 billion to be distributed over twenty-five years, or around $350 million a year.) The wife was already suffering from emphysema but refused to quit smoking. What would you say about this situation? Would you say that it is her choice and that she, or she and her husband, who was the one who went to buy the cigarettes, should take responsibility for what happens? Or would you say that making this monetary windfall available to someone with an addiction was a mistake and the money would have been better applied to statewide smoking prevention efforts or other pressing needs such as extending health insurance to the uninsured—perhaps even using it in ways that would reduce social inequality and advance health at the same time?

More recently, McKinlay has turned his attention to researchers who, he says, should also not be let off the hook. To make his point, he uses an old joke about a fellow who drops his keys in a parking lot on a dark night. The man goes to search for them under a nearby bright street light. When asked why he is looking there instead of where he dropped the keys he says, "but this is where the light is" (McKinlay 2001). This story, he says, captures exactly the approach used by those researchers who focus on identifying the risk factors associated with particular diseases.

He goes on to say that the results of recent research focusing on risky behavior have been disappointing for a couple of reasons. For one, the risk factors associated with many diseases are already well known. New risk factors are not likely to be discovered. Second, interventions designed to prevent or modify any particular risk factor do not produce measurable changes. He says that focusing on social determinants of health would be far more productive, but that is an arena that scientists trained to look "inside of the skin" are not comfortable exploring. He puts it this way:

> Moving upstream to the social determinants of health takes many public health practitioners into territories with which they are not familiar, for which many are not trained and which are not appropriately funded. And there are philosophical and political obstacles [i.e., searching for keys in the dark]. (McKinlay 2001, 5)

He ends by saying that public health is a political activity that requires looking more closely at the sociopolitical determinants of health. Limiting the research question to the search for risk factors, which leads to advocating prevention and promoting changing individual risk behaviors, is to focus on "epiphenomena."

Indeed, research on health behaviors, even when it is carried out by highly respected medical researchers, can overlook important interpretations that can be found right next to the "bright street light" that McKinlay refers to. A study carried out by respected researchers, who shall go unnamed, from a respected medical center provides an apt example. The study compared the effects of exercise and diet to the use of pharmaceuticals in treating diabetes. The results of the study attracted considerable media attention in response to the finding that the persons in the control group, who received no medication and relied solely on diet and exercise, were surprisingly more successful in controlling their diabetes than the group taking medications. What I found interesting, but which was mentioned only in passing by the researchers during media interviews, has to do with the arrangements surrounding the exercise regimen.

It seems that the members of the control group enrolled in this experiment were expected to meet regularly and to exercise as a group. The participants came together knowing that they shared a life-threatening problem, fully appreciating how difficult it would be to overcome that problem. I would argue that the members of this group offered each other the kind of support that visiting a doctor once in a while for monitoring and obtaining a new prescription does not provide. They shared recipes and encouraged each other to persist when exercising got tedious. It seems to me that the degree of support the group was providing to the individuals involved goes well beyond what so many support groups purport to offer. For reasons that we can only speculate about, the circumstances in which this group of experimental subjects found themselves caused them to form a close-knit friendship group. That, I submit, is at the heart of what brought about major lifestyle and behavioral changes. It is not hard to imagine that fellow enrollees were there to encourage each other to persist in the face of discouraging results and to celebrate each other's successes when they achieved hard-won results. In short, someone, in fact many people, suddenly cared whether they did or did not change their behavior and improve their health.

I am not suggesting that support groups are the single most effective solution. I am suggesting that, in this case, the circumstances were right. Joining together to address a shared problem had a powerful effect. There is no assurance that such a dynamic will emerge just because someone is assigned to a support group. However, when a close-knit group does form, it obviously has significant health benefits. The social benefit that comes from being involved in a highly supportive group is a topic that is stimulating a good deal of interest. We will return to it in a moment when we turn to the topic of *social capital*.

The research on social networks was largely inspired by the growing rec-ognition that the opposite, that is, *social isolation*, has a negative impact on one aspect of health—a person's stress level. As we saw in chapter 9, social psychologists have long argued that women's membership in social networks helped them cope with stress and blamed the lack of close-knit friendships among men for their higher stress levels. However, these assessments con-tinued to be debated since the question of whether stress levels were being accurately measured had not really been settled. That also allowed some crit-ics to argue that women's readiness to talk about their stress was overrated as a health benefit.

All the attention that has been directed at promoting the value of so-cial networks over the years inspired Lisa Berkman and Maria Melchior to seek clarification a few years ago (Berkman and Melchior 2006). The two researchers tell us that there is no guarantee that belonging to a network will be advantageous. On the positive side, belonging to a large network can strengthen immunity to catching a cold (Kawachi and Kennedy 2002, 127). And, as Berkman and Melchior found and we discussed in greater detail in chapter 6, people tend to quit smoking in clusters. However, as we saw in the same chapter, in the case of obesity, membership in a close-knit friendship network may be health damaging since obesity seems to be "contagious." Berkman and Melchior also point out that poor people are more likely to experience social isolation than the nonpoor. They say that social isolation exacerbates the increased risk of early onset of disease that the poor are more likely to experience it for a number of reasons. In the end, it appears that there may be room for more research on how either membership in a social network or social isolation operate to influence health in general and health behavior in particular.

The Political Economy and Population Health

Researchers, most notably economists, and more specifically left-leaning political economists, take a broader view of what sociologists call victim blaming. They consider it to be a consequence of "neoliberal" thinking, which is what many would recognize as conservative political thinking. (The following is based on Shakow and Irwin [1999]). Neoliberalism is defined as an economic theory that asserts that the market, when allowed to operate unfettered, is the most efficient and effective mechanism for distributing society's resources through the choices made by individuals. Proponents of neoliberal economic theory argue that "liberating" the economy from market restrictions and fostering free choice among the range of options offered by the market is not only essential, it constitutes the "basic unit of economic be-havior and social existence." Referring to the "free market" and "free market reform" certainly connotes broader images of freedom and liberty that are so highly valued by Americans. According to the critics of neoliberal policies, however, free markets are managed according to rules set down in complex legislation and commercial arrangements that impose severe constraints on individual choice, which hardly makes individual choice "free."

Those who advocate the neoliberalism approach to structuring economic policy maintain that the market should regulate society rather than the reverse. When society attempts to regulate the market, it interferes with what they say is a "natural process." Opponents point out that this natural process is largely responsible for the existence of poverty and go on to point out that the neoliberal model does not acknowledge that the poor do not have the same range of choices as the nonpoor. When confronted with this accusation, proponents of neoliberalism do not deny the existence of suffer-ing among the poor. They say, however, that what happens to the poor is an unavoidable side effect of a process that is self-evidently beneficial to society as a whole. That makes the suffering of the poor predictable. Following the syllogism from beginning to end—it is predictable precisely because of the personal choices the poor are making. Therefore, it is not a matter for social intervention.

The recommendations issued by the IOM report on racial and ethnic dis-parities are interesting in this regard because market intervention in health sector organizational arrangements is exactly what the IOM is advocating (Smedley, Stith, and Nelson 2002). The recommendations address a very broad range of issues with special attention directed to changes in health-care arrangements, including the following:

- strengthening legal, regulatory, and policy interventions to correct for fragmentation in health-care delivery
- increasing the proportion of underrepresented minorities among health professionals
- addressing health-system arrangements that contribute to poor quality of care
- implementing patient education and empowerment
- integrating cross-cultural education into the training of health profes-sionals
- improving data collection and monitoring
- conducting further research to identify sources of disparity

The population health body of research does not focus on particular health-care system changes. It does, however, take the position that blaming individuals for the unfavorable circumstances they find themselves in is not only unreasonable—it actually exacerbates the problem. The work of the scholars whose research we have been reviewing in the last two chapters indicates that individuals are not equipped to overcome socioeconomic inequality, which brings with it certain predictable consequences. It is precisely those consequences that come full circle to produce positive health effects for individuals of high socioeconomic status and negative health effects for those of low status.

The important point to be made about socioeconomic status is that it is entrenched in a multitude of psychosocial and structural factors that are very difficult to transcend through individual effort. Structural barriers include discrimination on the basis of age, sex, and race, which restricts access to various social resources such as education, employment opportunities, housing, medical care, and so on. Confronting such barriers and not being able to overcome them has a wearing effect that operates at the psychological level. That can produce a lowered sense of self-worth, lead to lower levels of social interaction, and ultimately cause detrimental psychological effects that intensify with increasing social isolation (Berkman and Glass 2000).

That brings us back to the question that we considered in the last chapter but did not answer, namely—why poor people who live in less-segregated communities exhibit lower mortality rates than those who live in highly segregated communities. It must be that living alongside others who are successful has positive effects that are both structural and psychosocial, just as living alongside others who are unsuccessful has negative effects. Why this is so becomes clearer when we focus more directly on *social capital*, as we do in the discussion that follows.

Social Trust, Social Cohesion, and Social Capital

Discussion regarding an appropriate population-health policy response to the variation in mortality rates introduces such topics as *social trust* and *social cohesion*, both of which are linked to *social capital*. What social capital means is best understood in contrast to related concepts.

> *Physical capital* consists of buildings, machinery, and any other material structures that are intended for some productive use. The term is used in contrast to *human capital*, which includes skills, education, and health; [and] *social*

capital, such as networks of trust that facilitate cooperation and collective action. (Gershman and Irwin 2000, 430n25)

Social capital is a concept that has been appearing with greater frequency
in literature dealing with health issues (Kawachi and Kennedy 1997a). According to one recent count, a search of the PubMed Internet site reveals
27,500 articles when one references "social capital and health" and a Google
search produces over nine million hits (Kawachi, Subramanian, and Kim
2008).

The researchers most closely associated with the study of health inequalities take the position that improving the health of the population requires
increasing social trust and social cohesion which, in combination, contribute
to enhancing social capital. They say that it is possible to adopt policies
aimed at accomplishing this via programs designed to benefit people at a
very practical level, by promoting activities that bring people together in the
community to participate in activities that produce mutual benefit. That,
they say, would lead to important benefits at the psychosocial level; and in
combination, the two sets of improvements would benefit the health of the
population as a whole (Marmot and Wilkinson 1999).

Some practical advice on how this might be achieved comes from John
McKnight, who tells us about a community that found a way to "decom-
modify" health by:

transferring [government] funds budgeted for medical care into activities that
involve community action to change the sickening elements in the local environment. The funds' transfer reflects their movement from client to citizen,
from commodity to community. (McKnight 1995, 67)

McKnight says that the basic problem that people, especially those in poor
communities, confront is that they must struggle "against a vision of health as
the product of specialized technique dominated by a complex control system"
(McKnight 1995, 67). He relates a story about a poor neighborhood in Chicago where the leaders of a local community organization decided to try to
help people achieve better health by taking greater control over the problem
and ended up "politicizing health care." To become better informed about
community health-care needs, they approached one of the local hospitals
to see what diseases were bringing people to the hospital. What they found
was not what they had expected. The list did include drug-related problems,
alcoholism, and violence. But it also included automobile accidents and dog
bites. They went after the dog bites first and succeeded in rounding up most

of the wild dogs in the area, virtually eliminating that problem. With that achievement to give them encouragement, they decided to tackle automobile accidents. They determined that new traffic lights would help, which meant getting the city to address the problem. That worked too. A number of other successes followed, which brought more people from the community together, instilled pride based on tangible accomplishments, and released creative energies to initiate new community projects—all building social capital plus enhancing health.

While the essence of the argument regarding the relationship between social capital and social inequality is firm, identifying specific pathways that lead to better health is what researchers have been striving to pinpoint (Marmot 2003; Cattell 2001). The question that continues to challenge researchers is the following. What is more important—is it being able to buy more goods to improve living conditions? Or is it that income is really a marker for greater control over life circumstances, particularly the greater chance to participate in social activities that are rewarding? In short, is the "Fundamental Causes" theory explanation correct?

The problem is that the concepts are so broad that identifying an objective measure of the relationship between health and social inequality is complicated. That is, of course, what allows those whose worldview stands in opposition to this line of reasoning to argue that the link has not been convincingly established. Those who are committed to the validity of the association between health inequality and socioeconomic inequality respond by compiling more evidence and attracting more allies, who keep finding new dimensions to study. There are also some interesting scattered pieces of evidence based on studies carried out by people who come to similar conclusions but begin from very different starting points.

The Roseto story illustrates what social capital is and how it operates in a particularly vivid fashion (Bruhn and Wolf 1979; Richard Wilkinson is to be credited with bringing the Roseto story to the attention of health researchers in his 1996 book). Roseto, a small town in Pennsylvania, was notable for its exceptionally low rate of heart disease as compared to other towns in the same region. The cardiologist who made this observation during the first decades of the century inspired a couple of researchers several decades later to track what these people were doing to give them the advantage. It turns out that there was nothing special about their health-behavior patterns. The researchers found that the main thing that distinguished this town from neighboring towns was the quality of social interaction among the residents. Not only was no one excluded from participating in the town's activities, all the residents exhibited a sense of social equality in the way they lived their lives. There were virtually no indicators of social class difference among first-generation settlers, who all came from the same small town in Italy. The houses, cars, and all the other things they owned did not serve to indicate social differentiation. As the next generation grew to maturity, signs of differentiation became more apparent. This is also when the rate of heart disease started to rise, eventually matching the rate in surrounding communities. Genetics was obviously not involved. The conclusion reached by the investigators was that the social capital that characterized this community as a whole during its early development is what offered its population protection against heart disease.

One way to understand why the Roseto story was, and still is, considered so special is that ideas about variations in health were tied for so long to the belief that our well-being depends on material *consumption* rather than *social aspects* of life. As one of the leading proponents of the link between health and socioeconomic inequality, Richard Wilkinson has had a great deal to say about the nature of the evidence involved (Wilkinson 2001). Reacting to assessments about what motivates people to act the way they do made by renowned economists, he says:

> consumption is powered by concern over relative social status, it may not be too much of an exaggeration to suggest that the individual desire for more income is largely a desire for improved social position. (Wilkinson 1999, 496)

Most Americans would agree. We call it "keeping up with the Joneses." Except that we not only try to keep up, we try to better the Joneses. As a matter of fact, we can see the cultural message that keeping up with the Joneses is a good thing to do being conveyed in a variety of contexts. The message is not so different from the one that comes through when people voice the familiar platitude that "it is not winning or losing that counts, it is playing the game." We all know that it is winning that counts.

So what is wrong with that? Ichiro Kawachi and Bruce Kennedy argue that economists tell us that we, as Americans, are striving to insure our happiness by doing what economists call "maximizing utility." However, because we never seem to get there, we keep trying to achieve happiness using this approach. In recent years, we have been actively encouraged to "maximize consumption" by our elected officials in Washington, D.C. Whether this was supposed to lead to increased satisfaction and/or happiness, or that we were being told that it would reflect our loyalty to the country and in an effort to help promote its economic well-being, is not entirely clear. What is particularly distressing about the message is finding that the products that Americans consume are increasingly not a matter of need. They are "positional goods" that are purchased to achieve self-esteem. In Kawachi and Kennedy's assessment, "the growth of our consumer culture conceals a deep underlying pathology, namely the widening rift between the haves and the have-nots" (Kawachi and Kennedy 2002, 21).

This is consistent with Wilkinson's observations:

> Just as high status is built—by definition—at the expense of others who are rendered low status, so the relatively deprived can regain some shreds of the sense of self-worth taken from them by treating the most vulnerable as their inferiors—by discrimination and violence against them. (Wilkinson 1999, 496)

Support for the consequences of these statements is not hard to find. There is strong evidence to indicate that violence and discrimination are greatest where socioeconomic inequality is most extreme, which is, in turn, linked to higher levels of hostility (Marmot 2000). While interpreting what is cause and what is effect is not easy, the consistency of the relationship across such indices is hard to ignore. At the same time, the evidence of psychosocial benefit associated with the sense of belonging, trust, and confidence that one's social network can be counted on for support is overwhelming and also very hard to ignore. It is difficult to see how trust and confidence could be sustained in the face of socioeconomic inequality and discrimination (Kreiger 2001 and 2000). Discussion regarding the foundations that have to be there for trust in persons other than one's family and closest friends to evolve has been mounting. Trust and confidence in the society at large is nurtured through social engagement, participation in clubs and associations, socializing with work mates, and so on (Veenstra 2000).

This is exactly the opposite of the trend toward "bowling alone," an idea that has attracted a great deal of attention over the last decade (Putnam 2000). What's wrong with bowling alone? According to Putnam, who coined the concept, it indicates that we are no longer participating in shared activities that in the past provided us with a sense of belonging to something beyond our immediate family. We no longer think our participation in a variety of activities will make any difference. We are witnessing a rising sense of alienation and declining sense of confidence in our neighbors. There is evidence to indicate that our confidence in social institutions declined steadily since the 1960s (Budrys 1997, 42). With decline in trust in the social arrangements that shape how we carry out our day-to-day activities, there is no longer any reason to work for anything beyond our own self-interest.

An especially graphic illustration of the point comes from Gary La Free's assessment of crime rates over time (La Free 1998). He is particularly interested in examining the reasons behind the tremendous difference between the rate of violent crime involving young black men compared to young white men. As you recall, the graph in chapter 4 indicated that the death rate for homicide among young African American men was in sharp contrast to that of the other three demographic categories (white men and women and black women). La Free argues that the African American involvement in violent crime parallels the decline of trust in the political institutions in this country on the part of African Americans. That is consistent with their loss of trust in America's economic institutions. He makes sure that we understand that crime rate trends also parallel income inequality trends (La Free 1998, 130). Finally, the rise of female-headed households parallels rising crime rates, indicating the significance of loss of legitimacy in the family as the third of the three basic social institutions linked to these trends—political, economic, and family. La Free says that the simultaneous decline of these three social institutions explains why the crime rate among poor, young African American males is as high as it is.

Not surprisingly, there is strong evidence to indicate that a higher level of trust is correlated with a higher level of socioeconomic status (Kawachi and Kennedy 2002). The evidence comes from the General Social Survey conducted by the National Opinion Research Center, which has asked a question about trust almost every year since 1972. Survey respondents are asked to agree or disagree with the following two statements: "You can generally trust other people" and "You cannot be too careful about trusting other people." The results correlated with the social class of the respondents indicate that the level of "distrust" is related to social class. Those in the lower class consistently report the lowest level of trust in others. For the first decade during which the survey was conducted, the level of trust could be seen increasing with social-class level among working- and middle-class respondents and dropping down again for upper-class respondents. That pattern changed during the 1980s when those in the upper class began reporting an increased level of trust. Remember, the 1980s is the decade during which the rich suddenly got richer while the poor started falling further behind. Perhaps even more disturbing is finding that as of the late 1990s, we are seeing a decline in the percentage of respondents across all social classes who are willing to trust others.

State-level comparisons reveal that a lower level of interpersonal trust is associated with a higher level of income inequality (Kawachi, Wilkinson, and Kennedy 1999). That is consistent with the finding that states with high income inequality are less likely to be interested in creating strong safety nets for more vulnerable members, which results in lower levels of public welfare.

There are those who say that there will always be some people who have more money and who feel they fully deserve it and who are not interested in sharing it with those who have less. That is just the way it is in this society and every other society. Those who treat inequality as an indicator of social well-being do not dispute this fact. What they do say is that it is the degree of inequality that matters.

The connection between the declining level of confidence in social institutions, declining degree of trust in our neighbors, and social inequality is reflected in the rising concern about the need for campaign reform. The issue is that the biggest political donors have become more flagrant in their efforts to gain political advantages. To be crass about it, they are buying legislation that will work to their advantage and to the disadvantage of the rest of us. We are repeatedly confronted with stories about corporations that are involved in shaping national policy and greatly benefiting from it—on pharmaceutical pricing, energy policy, reconstruction of Iraq. The stories have convinced many Americans that this is how government works and there is little they can do about it. In short, the basic concern is that economic inequality undermines democracy as those with more at stake participate in the democratic process and those with little at stake not only stop participating in the political arena but become alienated from civic participation in general.

When people feel disenfranchised and disconnected, they have little to lose by not voting. Taking that observation a step further—they have little to lose in violating various other social norms and expectations that those who do vote want upheld. The practical effects of the connection between social inequality and political participation can be found in the reduction of spending on social goods, which translates into a declining emphasis on developing social capital. That is, of course, detrimental to population health. The evidence is clear—low voter participation, as measured by voter turnout, is directly associated with poor self-rated health (Blakely, Kennedy, and Kawachi 2001).

Expanding Applications:
Neoliberalism and the Global Economy

Curiously, policy makers working in the foreign-policy arena, in contrast to their counterparts involved in domestic policy, are apparently readier to accept the policy implications pointed to in the population health literature.

That is especially true in the United States. The recognition of the significance of the link between foreign policy and health has led to what some are calling a paradigm change (Bunyavanich and Walkup 2001). The change is meant to herald the growing recognition that health must be considered in developing foreign policy for reasons of "narrow self-interest, enlightened self-interest, and humanitarian interests" (Kassalow 2001). *Self-interest* requires that the United States protect its citizens from the spread of infectious diseases, which do not respect political borders. *Enlightened self-interest* requires those responsible for determining U.S. foreign policy to recognize that health status and political stability are closely linked. We will get back to *humanitarian interest* later in this discussion. Meanwhile, the fact that a growing number of highly influential parties concur with these assessments is worth noting. These include the CIA (Whiteside 2001), Organization for Economic Cooperation and Development (Faure 2000), Council on Foreign Relations and Milbank Memorial Fund (Kassalow 2001), and the Institute of Medicine (1997), to name a few such organizations. It is worth noting that Congress allocated $466 million to address international HIV/AIDS efforts in 2000 in response to the determination that HIV/AIDS is a threat to national security; Congress went on to request the Government Accounting Office to assess UN efforts to deal with what is a recognized global epidemic (GAO-01-625 2001). As an aside, the fact that the Gates Foundation has allocated far more to dealing with the international AIDS epidemic than the U.S. government raises some interesting questions about the interpretation of urgency of the matter. However, we cannot address that question adequately here.

Let us turn instead to a review of the disquieting findings in the State Failure Task Force Report, which ends up raising some pressing questions (Esty et al. 1998). This body of research was funded by the CIA's Directorate of Intelligence. Its purpose is to identify the variables that are associated with political instability in countries throughout the world so that agencies such as the CIA can be better prepared for such eventualities. The authors of the report take pains to tell us that the report represents their views and not those of the CIA. However, the document has been widely quoted by policy analysts, including those associated with various government agencies, who have reason to be interested in predicting international political instability. The report contains a comprehensive analysis of factors that are predictive of political instability, based on an analysis of 113 cases of state failure in contrast to 339 control cases where state failure did not occur. The authors of the report identified thirty-one factors that distinguish instances of political failure from those in which failure had not occurred. The authors determined that the three best indicators are level of democracy, openness to international trade, and infant mortality. With regard to infant mortality, they have this to say:

> Like the canary in a coal mine, whose death indicates serious health risks to miners, infant mortality serves as a powerful indicator of more broadly deleterious living conditions. . . . Infant mortality plays a key role in the global model not because infant deaths *per se* are a causal factor, but because infant mortality is the single-most-efficient variable for reflecting a country's overall quality of material life. (Esty et al. 1998, 2)

Those who express concern about the relationship between international development and health seem to be leaning toward giving more serious consideration to Amartya Sen's observations on this topic. Sen questions why mortality rate should not be treated as an indicator of a country's economic success, and by extension, an indicator of the risk of political instability (Sen 1998).

It is worth noting that the growing recognition that health status is closely related to the conditions, social and physical, in which people live, signals a radical shift in thinking in some English-speaking countries. It does not come as news to policy analysts in Latin America. The concept of "social medicine," which Latin Americans employ in addressing the social determinants of health (in contrast to "public health," which they consider to be closer to public sanitation) has been used in Latin American countries since the beginning of the twentieth century (Waitzkin et al. 2001).

In a statement that aims to identify processes that contribute to creating and preserving international health inequalities, David Coburn argues that "globalization" is at the root of the problem (Coburn 2000). The position taken by Joseph Stiglitz, the Nobel Prize–winning economist, not only confirms this assessment, but offers evidence showing that the problems associated with globalization are due to the policies imposed by the International Monetary Fund (IMF) on countries seeking loans (Stiglitz 2002). He argues that IMF policies are guided by an ideological commitment to a textbook economic model that it applies in a cookie-cutter-like approach, ignoring such basics as lack of access to information on which to base consumer choice decisions. According to Stiglitz, the IMF's policies work to reward creditors while punishing the majority of the people in the country being "helped."

While Coburn and Stiglitz say it somewhat differently, their basic messages are the same. They argue that globalization is advocated by those who are committed to the integration of economic, political, and cultural beliefs that are grounded in the high value placed on free markets. The essence of the argument is that globalization is being sponsored by those who favor the combination of market-dominated economic goals and neoliberal political goals. This is responsible for the increasing level of economic inequality within and between countries.

The connection between political and economic ideologies at the international level has further, largely unacknowledged domestic consequences. It creates a chain response that has had a powerful detrimental effect on domestic social policy. The policies enacted in England and the United States during the 1980s and again during the early years of the twenty-first century illustrate the point. They reflect reduced investment in the kinds of social benefits that increase social capital within the country, such as education, medical care, community development, and so forth. That leads, in turn, to declining social trust, civic participation, and family integrity, together with increasing rates of crime, delinquency, and violence.

If you are still not convinced that globalization and domestic policy are related, consider the economic power that global or transnational corporations have accumulated over the last century. Of the world's one hundred largest economies, forty-nine are countries and fifty-one are corporations (Gershman and Irwin 2000, 36). Moreover, corporations tend to dominate the top of that list—of the top sixty economies, forty-three are corporations (Millen and Holtz 2000, 181). The corporations obviously have a profound effect on the people living in the countries in which they operate through the practices they adopt and promote—their environmental policies, treatment of agricultural and factory workers, support of despotic regimes, and so forth. It does not take much imagination to see how such practices spill over so that all of us must bear the consequences.

Isolationists, whether they espouse a neoliberal domestic perspective or not, have until very recently expressed little interest in how globalization was proceeding. They argue that we should focus on solving our own problems and let other countries, including poor countries, solve theirs. They say that it is simply not America's problem. However, that is exactly the point of view that those who talk about the global economy want the rest of us to understand (Kim et al. 1999). The critics of globalization and neoliberalism say that the global economy is very much America's problem if the poor in the world blame us for their plight. The argument ceased to be theoretical, abstract, and of interest only to policy makers as of September 11, 2001, in the face of the violent attack on New York. At the time, Americans were surprised to discover that people in poor countries are encouraged to think that rich countries are to blame for the circumstances in which poor countries find themselves. Americans also learned that the radicals who are committed to sponsoring economic and political instability in their own countries and terrorism in rich countries are regarded as heroes at home. A lot has happened since 9/11, most notably the wars this country has been conducting in Afghanistan and Iraq, the effect of which makes these observations far less surprising, if not far less controversial.

Some people in this country, as well as people across the world, understand that self-interest is not to be dismissed given the new political reality: that we find ourselves the most powerful nation in the world with world-leadership responsibilities. Many also think that this new status should have brought with it an increased level of humanitarian responsibility. However, a sizeable contingent of Americans do not favor greater involvement in such an agenda because they believe that the United States already spends a great deal on foreign aid and should not consider spending more. Yet, according to the Organisation for Economic Cooperation and Development (OECD), Japan, France, and Germany spent more than the United States in 1996 in real dollars. The United States spent a smaller proportion of its gross national product (GNP) on foreign aid than the twenty other member countries (about 1 percent) (IOM 1999, 20). When asked about it, Americans, both Republicans and Democrats, say they do support foreign assistance provided it goes to needy people and not political allies of rich and powerful corporate interests (IOM 1999, 19).

If you are beginning to think that this discussion has moved too far from health and now comes much closer to radical political, economic, and social science than any science related to health, I invite you to consider a statement made by one of the fathers of biomedical research, Rudolph Virchow. His work on cell theory during the middle of the nineteenth century laid the groundwork for the development of research on pathological disease processes. Virchow made the following oft-quoted observation: "Medicine is a social science, and politics is nothing but medicine on a large scale." He backed up his commitment to this statement by entering politics with the aim of ameliorating the social conditions that he reasoned were largely responsible for the devastating outbreak of typhus in an area that is now part of Germany where he was living. Virchow was simply ahead of his time. His message is very similar to the ones articulated earlier in this discussion by McKnight, who focuses on poor communities in Chicago, and Waitzkin, who tells us how South Americans address community health issues.

Following in this tradition is research that examines the relationship between political philosophy and population health. A recent international study of the relationship between the values espoused by the political party in power and the extent of socioeconomic inequality in the country indicates that there is a clear relationship. Using an OECD database that tracks socioeconomic trends in twenty-four highly developed countries, analysts found a direct relationship between political party in power and health inequalities (Navarro and Shi 2001). The more socially and politically liberal the government policy is, the healthier the members of that society are. ("Liberal," in this case, stands in direct opposition to the political and economic philosophy embraced by neoliberals.)

Thus, we have now come full circle. The polarization of interests, as indicated by the division of social-class interests, has the further effect of diminishing social trust as well as social capital both within countries and between countries. We end with the conclusion that this is what ultimately affects the health of the population as a whole, regardless of the size of the population involved, whether we focus on cities, states, or whole countries.

The answer to the question of how social inequality is related to health inequality and why that matters should be eminently clear by now. Health inequalities are a manifestation of broader social inequalities. In the end there is a wide spectrum of reasons for caring. If not for reasons having to do with humanitarian values, then there is a long list of practical, instrumental reasons since social inequality has extensive spillover effects. The quality of life of everyone in the society is affected by the spillover that occurs when some people feel they are restricted from sharing in the benefits of the society in which they live.

If that is not sufficiently convincing, let us consider reasons that might impress those whose primary interests revolve around their pocketbooks. The reason that Americans do not favor extending health insurance to the poor is that they are convinced the poor do not use medical-care services appropriately. They do not seek treatment early enough, and when things get bad enough they go to the emergency room and run up high costs. Actually, it is worse than that. Americans might be far more willing to extend Medicaid to a greater proportion of the poor if they were made aware of the following two facts: (1) the uninsured are 30 to 50 percent more likely to be hospitalized for an avoidable condition, and (2) the average cost of an avoidable hospitalization in 2002 was estimated to be about $3,300 (Hadley 2002). The costs have risen since then because we have been employing more sophisticated, and costly, technology on a more regular basis.

Higher economic disparity has a range of negative consequences for business as well (Kawachi and Kennedy 2002). A high level of a society's economic inequality is reflected in the cost of workforce turnover and instability, which has a negative impact on national productivity. Kawachi and Kennedy make a number of additional troubling observations that have consequences at the individual level; for example, they note that competitive consumption reduces free time, which is damaging to family and community relationships; and that the ratio of credit-card debt to family income is a stronger predictor of poor health than family income.

Then there is the effect of poor health on earnings. Changing a person's health status from fair/poor to good/excellent is estimated to increase annual earnings by about 10 to 30 percent (Henry Kaiser Family Foundation 2002). The potential benefits include increased tax revenues, reduction of disability payments, increased labor-force participation of caregivers who currently tend to disabled members of the family, reduction of expenditures for public insurance programs, such as Medicare and Medicaid—all of which would contribute to economic growth.

That still leaves unresolved the question of how we might get policy makers to respond to this kind of information. In the end, I leave that assignment to you. The only thing I would warn you against is throwing in the towel and saying that nothing will change or that the kinds of changes that the preceding discussion requires are too difficult. If no one takes the first step in advocating change, there will certainly be no change. If a few people begin to think that the potential benefits are certain to outweigh the difficulties involved in making changes, which admittedly will require a certain amount of sacrifice on our part, others might join in. You can't expect people to climb on, if there is no bandwagon for them to climb on to.

THE LIBRARY
TOWER HAMLETS COLLEGE
POPLAR HIGH STREET
LONDON E14 0AF
Tel: 0207 510 7763

References

Abraido-Lanza, Ana, Bruce Dohrenwend, Daisy Ng-Mak, and J. Blake Turner. 1999. The Latino mortality paradox: A test of the "salmon bias" and healthy migrant hypotheses. *American Journal of Public Health* 89 (October): 1543–48.

Acevedo-Garcia, Dolores, Theresa Osypuk, Nancy McArdle, and David Williams. 2008. Toward a policy-relevant analysis of geographic and racial/ethnic disparities in child health. *Health Affairs* 27:321–33.

Adler, Nancy, and Karen Matthews. 1994. Health psychology: Why do some people get sick and some stay well? *Annual Review of Psychology* 45:229–59.

Agency for Healthcare and Quality Excellence. 2001. *Excellent centers to eliminate ethnic/racial disparities (EXCEED)* 01-P021. May.

Agency for Healthcare Research and Quality. 2005a. *2005 National healthcare disparities report.*

Agency for Healthcare Research and Quality. 2005b. Economic and health costs of diabetes. *AHRQ* 05-0013.

Alonzo, Angelo. 2000. The experience of chronic illness and post-traumatic stress disorder: The consequences of cumulative adversity. *Social Science and Medicine* 50 (10): 1477–84.

Altman, Stuart, Uwe Reinhardt, and Alexandra Shields. 1998. *The future of the U.S. healthcare system: Who will care for the poor and uninsured?* Chicago: Health Administration Press.

American Academy of Neurology. 2008. Larger belly in mid-life increases risk of dementia. Press release. March 18.

American Cancer Society. 2008. Cancer facts and figures, 2009. http://www.cancer.org/docroot/home/index.asp.

American Heart Association. 2008. Heart and stroke death rates steadily decline; risks still too high. *AHA News*. Press release. January 22.

Angell, Marcia. 1993. Privilege and health—What is the connection? *New England Journal of Medicine* 329 (July): 126–27.

Angier, Natalie. 2007. Its poor reputation aside, our fat is doing us a favor. *New York Times*. August 7.

Arber, Sara, and Jay Ginn. 1993. Gender and inequalities in health in later life. *Social Science and Medicine* 36 (1): 33–46.

Asch, Steven, Eve Kerr, Joan Keesey, John Adams, Claude Setodji, Shaista Malik, and Elizabeth McGlynn. 2006. Who is at greatest risk for receiving poor-quality health care? *New England Journal of Medicine* 354:1147–56.

Aytac, Isik, Andre Arujo, Catherine Johannes, Ken Kleinman, and John McKinlay. 2000. Socioeconomic factors and incidence of erectile dysfunction: Findings of the longitudinal Massachusetts male aging study. *Social Science and Medicine* 51 (5): 771–78.

Bach, Peter, Laura Cramer, Joan Warren, and Colin Begg. 1999. Racial differences in the treatment of early-stage lung cancer. *New England Journal of Medicine* 341 (October): 1198–205.

Backlund, Eric, Paul Sorlie, and Norman Johnson. 1999. A comparison of the relationships of education and income with mortality: The national longitudinal mortality study. *Social Science and Medicine* 49 (10): 1373–84.

Baird, P. A. 1994. The role of genetics in population health. In *Why are some people healthy and others not?* ed. Robert Evans, Morris Barer, and Theodore Marmor. New York: Aldine.

Bakalar, Nicholas. 2005. Child's asthma linked to grandmother's habit. *New York Times*. April 12.

Bakalar, Nicholas. 2008. Skipping cereal and eggs and packing on pounds. *New York Times*. March 25.

Bakalar, Nicholas. 2009. Sex ratio seen to vary by latitude. *New York Times*. April 21.

Baker, David, Joseph Sudano, Jeffrey Albert, Elaine Borawski, and Avi Dor. 2001. Lack of health insurance and decline in overall health in late middle age. *New England Journal of Medicine* 345 (October): 1106–12.

Balfour, Jennifer, and George Kaplan. 2002. Neighborhood environment and loss of physical function of older adults: Evidence from the Alameda County study. *American Journal of Epidemiology* 155 (March): 507–15.

Baltrus, Peter, John Lynch, Susan Everson-Rose, Trivellore Raghunathan, and George Kaplan. 2005. Race/ethnicity, life-course socioeconomic position, and body weight trajectories over 34 years: The Alameda County study. *American Journal of Public Health* 95:1595–1601.

Banks, James, Michael Marmot, Zoe Oldfield, and James Smith. 2006. Disease and disadvantage in the United States and in England. *Journal of the American Medical Association* 295 (May): 2037–45.

Barker, D. J. P., C. Osmond, J. Golding, D. Kuh, and M. E. J. Wadsworth. 1989. Growth in utero, blood pressure in childhood and adult life, and mortality from cardiovascular disease. *British Medical Journal* 298 (March): 564–67.

Barrett, John. 1981. Intra-uterine experience and its long-term outcome. In *Foundations of psychosomatics*, ed. Margaret Christie and Peter Mellet. Chichester, UK: John Wiley & Sons.

Barsky, Arthur. 1988. The paradox of health. *New England Journal of Medicine* 318 (February): 414–18.

Bartley, Mel, and Ian Plewis. 1997. Does health-selective mobility account for socioeconomic differences in health? Evidence from England and Wales, 1971 to 1991. *Journal of Health and Social Behavior* 38 (September): 376–86.

Beckett, Megan. 2000. Converging health inequalities in later life—An artifact of mortality selection? *Journal of Health and Social Behavior* 41 (March): 106–19.

Begg, Colin. 2001. The search for cancer risk factors: When can we stop looking? *American Journal of Public Health* 91 (March): 360–64.

Benbow, Nanette, Yue Wang, and Steven Whitman. 1998. The big cities health inventory, 1997. *Journal of Community Health* 23 (December): 471–89.

Berkman, Lisa, and Thomas Glass. 2000. Social integration, social network, social support, and health. In *Social epidemiology*, ed. Lisa Berkman and Ichiro Kawachi. Oxford, UK: Oxford University Press.

Berkman, Lisa, Thomas Glass, Ian Brissette, and Teresa Seeman. 2000. From social integration to health: Durkheim in the new millennium. *Social Science and Medicine* 51 (January): 99–104.

Berkman, Lisa, and Maria Melchior. 2006. The shape of things to come: How social policy impacts social integration and family structure to produce population health. In *Social Inequality in Health*, ed. Johannes Siegrist and Michael Marmot. Oxford, UK: Oxford University Press.

Bhopal, Raj, and Liam Donaldson. 1998. White, European, Western, Caucasian, or what? Inappropriate labeling in research on race, ethnicity, and health. *American Journal of Public Health* 88 (September): 1303–07.

Bierman, Arlene, Thomas Bubolz, Elliott Fisher, and John Wasson. 1999. How well does a single question about health predict the financial health of Medicare-managed care plans? *Effective Clinical Practice* 2 (2): 56–62.

Blackwell, Debra, Mark Hayward, and Eileen Crimmins. 2001. Does childhood health affect chronic morbidity in later life? *Social Science and Medicine* 52 (8): 1269–84.

Blair, Steven, Harold Kohl, Ralph Paffenbarger, Debra Clark, Kenneth Cooper, and Larry Gibbons. 1989. Physical fitness and all cause mortality. *Journal of the American Medical Association* 262 (November): 2395–2401.

Blakely, Tony, Bruce Kennedy, and Ichiro Kawachi. 2001. Socioeconomic inequality in voting participation and self-rated health. *American Journal of Public Health* 91 (January): 99–104.

Blane, David, George Davey Smith, and Mel Bartley. 1993. Social selection: What does it contribute to social class differences in health? *Sociology of Health and Illness* 15 (1): 1–15.

Bobadilla, Jose Luis, Christine Costello, and Faith Mitchell. 1997. *Premature death in the new independent states.* Washington, DC: National Academy Press.

Bosma, Hans, Carola Schrijvers, and Johan Machenbach.1999. Socioeconomic inequalities in mortality and importance of perceived control: Cohort study. *British Medical Journal* 319 (December): 1469–70.

Breeze, Elizabeth, Astrid Fletcher, David Leon, Michael Marmot, Robert Clarke, and Martin Shipley. 2001. Do socioeconomic disadvantages persist into old age? Self-reported morbidity in a 29-year follow-up of the Whitehall study. *American Journal of Public Health* 91 (February): 277–83.

Brook, Robert, John Ware, William Rogers, Emmett Keeler, Allyson Davies, Cathy Donald, George Goldberg, Kathleen Lohr, Patricia Masthay, and Joseph Newhouse. 1983. Does free care improve adults' health? *New England Journal of Medicine* 309 (December): 1426–34.

Brownlee, Shannon. 2007. *Overtreated.* New York: Bloomsbury.

Bruder, C. E., A. Piotrowski, A. A. Gjisbers, R. Andersson, S. Erickson, T. D. de Stahl, U. Menzel, J. Sandgren, D. von Tell, A. Poplawski, M. Crowley, C. Crasto, E. C. Partridge, H. Tiwari, D. B. Allison, J. Komorowski, G. J. van Ommen, D. I. Boomsma, N. L. Pedersen, J. T. den Dunnen, K. Wirdefeldt, and J. P. Dumanski. 2008. Phenotypically concordant and discordant monozygotic twins display different DNA copy-number-variation profiles. *American Journal of Human Genetics* 82 (March): 763–71.

Bruhn, John, and Stewart Wolf. 1979. *The Roseto story.* Norman: University of Oklahoma Press.

Buchanan, Allen, Dan Brock, Normal Daniels, and Daniel Wikler. 2000. *From chance to choice, genetics and justice.* Cambridge, UK: Cambridge University Press.

Budrys, Grace. 1986. *Planning for the nation's health.* Westport, CT: Greenwood.

Budrys, Grace. 1997. *When doctors join unions.* Ithaca, NY: Cornell University Press.

Budrys, Grace. 2005. *Our unsystematic health care system.* 2nd ed. Lanham, MD: Rowman & Littlefield.

Bunker, John, Howard Frazier, and Frederick Mosteller. 1994. Improving health: Measuring effects of medical care. *Milbank Quarterly* 72 (2): 225–58.

Bunyavanich, Supinda, and Ruth Walkup. 2001. U.S. public health leaders shift toward a new paradigm of global health. *American Journal of Public Health* 91 (October): 1556–58.

Bureau of Labor Statistics. 1978. The Consumer Price Index: Concepts and content over the years. Washington, DC: U.S. Department of Labor.

Byrd, W. M., and L. A. Clayton. 2000. *An American health dilemma: A medical history of African Americans and the problem of race: Beginnings to 1900,* vol. 1. New York: Routledge.

Byrd, W. M., and L. A. Clayton. 2002. *An American health dilemma: Race, medicine, health care in the United States 1900–2000*, vol. 2. New York: Routledge.

Calle, Eurgenia, Carmen Rodriquez, Kimberly Walker-Thurmond, and Michael Thun. 2003. Overweight, obesity, and mortality from cancer in a prospectively studied cohort of U.S. adults. *New England Journal of Medicine* 348:1625–38.

Cancer death rate decline doubling. 2007. *Science Daily*. October 15.

Capitano, Jack, and Marina Emborg. 2008. Contributions of non-human primates to neuroscience research. *Lancet* 371 (March): 1126–35.

Caraballo, Ralph, Gary Giovino, Terry Pechacek, Paul Mowery, Patricia Richter, Warren Strauss, Donald Sharp, Michael Erickson, James Pirkle, and Kurt Maurer. 1998. Racial and ethnic differences in serum cotinine levels of cigarette smokers. *Journal of the American Medical Association* 280 (July): 135–39.

Caspi, Avshalom, Joseph McClay, Terrie Moffitt, Jonathan Mill, Judy Martin, Ian Craig, Alan Taylor, and Richie Poulton. 2002. Role of genotype in the cycle of violence in maltreated children. *Science* 297 (August): 851–54.

Cattell, Vicky. 2001. Poor people, poor places, and poor health: The mediating role of social networks and social capital. *Social Science and Medicine* 51 (1): 139–50.

CDC. 2006. Fact sheet, tobacco-related mortality. Atlanta: Office on Smoking and Health.

Chandola, Tarani, Annie Britton, Eric Brunner, Harry Hemingway, Marek Malik, Meera Kumari, Ellena Badrick, Mika Kivimaki, and Michael Marmot. 2008. Work stress and coronary health disease: What are the mechanisms? *European Heart Journal*. January 23.

Chano, Tokukiro, Shiro Ikegawa, Keiichi Kontani, Hidetoshi Okabe, Nicola Bladini, and Yukikozu Saeki. 2002. Identification of RB1CC1, a novel human gene that can induce RBI in various human cells. *Oncogene* 21 (February): 1295–98.

Chibnall, John, Joseph Jeral, and Michael Cerullo. 2001. Experiments on distant intercessory prayer: God, science, and the lesson of Massah (commentary). *Archives of Internal Medicine* 161 (November): 2529–38.

Christakis, Nicholas, and James Fowler. 2007. The spread of obesity in a large social network over 32 years. *New England Journal of Medicine* 357 (July): 370–79.

Christakis, Nicholas, and James Fowler. 2008. The collective dynamics of smoking in a large social network. *New England Journal of Medicine* 358 (July): 2249–58.

Clancy, Carolyn, and Charlea Massion. 1992. American women's health care. *Journal of the American Medical Association* 268 (October): 1918.

Clark, Rodney, Norman Anderson, Venessa Clark, and David Williams. 1999. Racism as a stressor for African Americans, a biopsychological model. *American Psychologist* 54 (10): 805–16.

Clarke, Adele, and Virginia Olesen. 1998. *Revisioning women, health and healing*. New York: Routledge.

Cleck, Jessica, and Julie Blendy. 2008. Making a bad thing worse: Adverse effects of stress on drug addiction. *Journal of Clinical Investigation* 2:454–61.

Coburn, David. 2000. Income inequality, social cohesion and health status of populations: The role of neo-liberalism. *Social Science and Medicine* 51 (1): 139–50.

Cohen, Cynthia, Sondra Wheeler, David Scott, Barbara Edwards, and Patricia Lusk. 2000. Prayer as therapy. *Hastings Center Report* 30 (May/June): 40–48.

Collins, Judith, and Nancy Sharpe. 1994. Women and the health care system. In *Women's health, a primary care clinical guide*, ed. Ellis Youngkin and Marcia Davis. Norwalk, CT: Appleton and Lange.

Committee on Bioethics, American Academy of Pediatrics. 2001. Ethical issues with genetic testing in pediatrics. *Pediatrics* 107 (June): 1451–55.

Connor, Steve. 2006. Genetic breakthrough that reveals the difference between humans. *The Independent*. November 23. http//www.independent.co.uk.

Consumers Union of U.S., Inc. 1998. Can spirituality uplift your health? *Consumers Reports on Health* 30 (June): 7–8.

Cook, Edwin, Margaret Christie, Soni Gartshore, Robert Stern, and Peter Venables. 1981. After the executive monkey. In *Foundations of psychosomatics*, ed. Margaret Christie and Peter Mellet. Chichester, UK: John Wiley & Sons.

Cooper-Patrick, Lisa, Joseph Gallo, Junius Gonzales, Hong Thi Vu, Neil Powe, Christine Nelson, and Daniel Ford. 1999. Race, gender, and partnership in the patient-physician relationship. *Journal of the American Medical Association* 282 (August): 583–89.

Critchley, Julia, and Simon Capewell. 2003. Mortality risk reduction associated with smoking cessation in patients with coronary heart disease: A systematic review. *Journal of the American Heart Association* 290:86–97.

Cubbin, Catherine, Linda Pickle, and Lois Fingerhut. 2000. Social context and geographic patterns of homicide among U.S. black and white males. *American Journal of Public Health* 90 (April): 579–87.

Cunningham, Peter, and Peter Kemper. 1998. Ability to obtain medical care for the uninsured. *Journal of the American Medical Association* 280 (September): 921–27.

Cunningham-Burley, Sarah, and Mary Boulton. 2000. The social context of the new genetics. In *Handbook of social studies in health and medicine*, ed. Gary Albrecht, Ray Fitzpatrick, and Susan Scrimshaw. London: Sage.

Dahl, Espen, John Fritzell, Eero Lahelma, Pekka Martikainen, Anton Kunst, and Johan Machenbach. 2006. Welfare state regimes and health inequalities. In *Social inequality in health*, ed. Johannes Siegrist and Michael Marmot. Oxford, UK: Oxford University Press.

Damasio, Antonio. 2005. Brain trust. *Nature* 435:571–72.

Davey Smith, G., M. J. Shipley, and G. Rose. 1990. Magnitude and causes of socioeconomic differentials in mortality: Further evidence from the Whitehall study. *Journal of Epidemiology and Community Health* 44:265–70.

Davidson, Jonathan. 2001. Recognition and treatment of posttraumatic stress disorder. *Journal of the American Medical Association* 286 (August): 584–88.

Davis, Devra, Michelle Gottlieb, and Julie Stampnitsky. 1998. Reduced ratio of male to female births in several industrial countries. *Journal of the American Medical Association* 279 (April): 1018–23.

Deaton, Angus. 2002. Policy implications of the gradient of health and wealth. *Health Affairs* 21 (March/April): 13–30.

Demakis, John. 2002. Preface to variation in health care. *Medical Care* 40 (1, supplement): 1–2.

DeNoon, Daniel. 2008. Heart, stroke deaths decline in U.S. WebMD. January 22. http://www.cbsnews.com/.

Denton, Margaret, and Vivienne Walters. 1999. Gender differences in structural and behavioral determinants of health: An analysis of the social production of health. *Social Science and Medicine* 48 (9): 1221–35.

Department of Health and Human Services. 1985. Report of the secretary's task force on black and minority health. Atlanta.

Des Jarlais, Don. 2000. Prospects for a public health perspective on psychoactive drug use. *American Journal of Public Health* 90 (March): 335–37.

Diez-Roux, Ana, Sharon Merkin, Donna Arnett, Lloyd Chambless, Mark Massing, Javier Nieto, Paul Sorlie, Moyses Szklo, Herman Tyroler, and Robert Watson. 2001. Neighborhood of residence and incidence of coronary heart disease. *New England Journal of Medicine* 345 (July): 99–106.

Diez-Roux, Ana, Mary Northridge, Alfredo Morabia, Mary Bassett, and Steven Shea. 1999. Prevalence and social correlations of cardiovascular disease risk factors in Harlem. *American Journal of Public Health* 89 (March): 302–307.

Dimsdale, Joel. 2008. Psychological stress and cardiovascular disease. *Journal of the American College of Cardiology* (13): 1237–46.

Domhoff, G. William. 2006. Wealth, income, and power. http://sociology.ucsc.edu/whorulesamerican/power/wealth.html.

Doyal, Lesley. 1995. What makes women sick? New Brunswick, NJ: Rutgers University Press.

Ecob, Russell, and George Davey Smith. 1999. Income and health: What is the nature of the relationship? *Social Science and Medicine* 48 (March): 693–705.

Elliott, Victoria Stagg. 2007. Gene found that affects links to food intake and weight. *American Medical News* (May): 32–33.

Elo, Irma, and Samuel Preston. 1996. Educational differentials in mortality: United States, 1979–1985. *Social Science and Medicine* 42 (1): 47–57.

Emanuel, Ezekial. 2008. The cost-coverage trade-off. *Journal of the American Medical Association* 299 (February): 947–49.

Epstein, Arnold, Robert Stern, and Joel Weissman. 1990. Do the poor cost more? A multihospital study of patients' socioeconomic status and use of hospital resources. *New England Journal of Medicine* 322 (April 19): 1122–28.

Escarce, Jose, Kenneth Epstein, David Colby, and Stanford Schwartz. 1993. Racial differences in the elderly's use of medical procedures and diagnostic tests. *American Journal of Public Health* 83 (July): 948–54.

Estes, Carroll, and Karen Linkins. 2000. Critical perspectives and aging. In *Handbook of social studies of health and medicine*, ed. Gary Albrecht, Ray Fitzpatrick, and Susan Scrimshaw. London: Sage.

Esty, Daniel, Jack Goldstone, Ted Robert Gurr, Barbara Harff, Marc Levy, Geoffrey Dabelko, Pamela Surko, and Alan Unger. 1998. *State failure task force report: Phase II findings.* McLean, VA: Science Applications International Corporation.

Ezzati, Majid, Ari Friedman, Sandeep Kulkarni, and Christopher Murray. 2008. The reversal of fortunes: Trends in country mortality and cross-country mortality disparities in the United States. *PLoS Medicine* 5:e66 0557–e66 0568.

Fairfield, Kathleen, and Robert Fletcher. 2002. Vitamins for chronic disease prevention in adults: Scientific review. *Journal of the American Medical Association* 287 (June): 3116–26.

FamiliesUSA. 2007. Wrong direction: One out of three Americans are uninsured. September.

FamiliesUSA. 2009. Americans at risk: One in three uninsured. March.

Farmer, Paul. 2001. The major infectious diseases in the world—To treat or not to treat? *New England Journal of Medicine* 345 (July): 208–209.

Faure, Jean-Claude. 2000. *Development cooperation 1999 report.* Paris: Organisation for Economic Co-operation and Development.

Feinglass, Joe, Suru Lin, Jason Thompson, Joseph Sudano, Dorothy Dunlop, Jing Song, and David Baker. 2007. Baseline health, socioeconomic status, and 10-year mortality among older middle-aged Americans: Findings from the health and retirement study, 1992–2002. *Journal of Gerontology: Social Sciences* 62B:S209-S217.

Feldman, Jacob, Diane Makuc, Joel Kleinman, and Joan Cornoni-Huntley. 1989. National Trends in Educational Differentials in Mortality. *American Journal of Epidemiology* 129 (5): 919–33.

Ferraro, Kenneth, and Cynthia Albrecht-Jensen. 1991. Does religion influence adult health? *Journal for the Scientific Study of Religion* 30 (2): 193–202.

Ferraro, Kenneth, and Melissa Farmer. 1996. Double jeopardy to health hypothesis for African Americans: Analysis and critique. *Journal of Health and Social Behavior* 37 (March): 27–43.

Ferraro, Kenneth, and Tariqah Nuriddin. 2006. Psychological distress and mortality: Are women more vulnerable? *Journal of Health and Social Behavior* 47 (September): 227–41.

Ferraro, Kenneth, and Ya-ping Su. 2000. Physician-evaluated and self-reported morbidity for predicting disability. *American Journal of Public Health* 90 (January): 103–108.

Field, Mark, David Kotz, and Gene Bukhman. 1999. Neoliberal economic policy, "state desertion," and the Russian health crisis. In *Dying for growth*, ed. Jim Yong Kim, Joyce Millen, Alec Irwin, and John Gershman. Monroe, ME: Common Courage Press.

Filmer, Deon, and Lant Pritchett. 1999. The impact of public spending on health: Does money matter? *Social Science and Medicine* 49 (10): 1309–23.

Fingerhut, Lois, Deborah Ingram, and Jacob Feldman. 1998. Homicide rates among U.S. teenagers and young adults. *Journal of the American Medical Association* 280 (August): 423–27.

Finkelstein, Eric, Ian Fiebelkorn, and Guijing Wang. 2003. National medical spending attributable to overweight and obesity: How much, and who's paying? *Health Affairs* (May): W3-219–226.

Fiscella, Kevin, and Peter Franks. 2000. Quality, outcomes and satisfaction, individual income, income inequality, health and mortality: What are the relationships? *Health Services Research* 35(April, Part II): 305–18.

Flegal, Katherine, Barry Graubard, David Williamson, and Mitchell Gail. 2007. Cause-specific excess deaths associated with underweight, overweight, and obesity. *Journal of the American Medical Association* 298 (November): 2028–37.

Fletcher, Gerald, Gary Balady, Steven Blair, James Blumenthal, Carl Caspersen, Bernard Choitman, Stephen Epstein, Erika Froelicher, Victor Froelicher, Ileana Pina, and Michael Pollack. 1996. Statement on exercise: Benefits and recommendations for physical activity programs for all Americans. *Circulation* 94 (August): 857–62.

Francis, Charles. 1997. Research in coronary heart disease in blacks: Issues and challenges. *Journal of Health Care for the Poor and Underserved* 8 (3): 250–69.

Freeman, Harold, and Richard Payne. 2000. Racial injustice in health care. *New England Journal of Medicine* 342 (April): 1045–47.

Fuchs, Victor. 1974. *Who shall live*. New York: Basic Books.

Fullilove, Mindy. 1998. Comment: Abandoning "race" as a variable in public health research—An idea whose time has come. *American Journal of Public Health* 88 (September): 1297–98.

Fung, Teresa, Stephanie Chiuve, Marjorie McCullough, Kathryn Rexrode, Giancarlo Logroscino, and Frank Hu. 2008. Adherence to DASH-style diet and the risk of coronary heart disease and stroke in women. *Archives of Internal Medicine* 168 (7): 713–20.

Furumoto-Dawson, Alice, Sarah Gehlert, Dana Sohmer, Olufunmilayo Olopade, and Tina Sacks. 2007. Early-life conditions and mechanisms of population health vulnerabilities. *Health Affairs* 26 (September): 1238–48.

Ganz, Michael. 2000. The relationship between external threats and smoking in central Harlem, New York. *American Journal of Public Health* 90 (March): 367–71.

GAO (United States General Accounting Office). 2000. *Women's health: NIH has increased its efforts to include women in research*. Washington, DC (GAO-HEHS-00-96).

GAO (United States General Accounting Office). 2001a. *Health insurance: Characteristics and trends in the uninsured population*. Washington, DC (GAO-01-507T).

GAO (United States General Accounting Office). 2001b. *Global health: Joint U.N. programme on HIV/AIDS needs to strengthen country-level efforts and measure results*. Washington, DC (GAO-01-625).

GAO (United States General Accountability Office). 2003. *CDC's April 2002 report on smoking: Estimates of selected consequences of cigarette smoking were reasonable*. Washington, DC (GAO-03-942R).

GAO (United States General Accountability Office). 2006. *Childhood obesity: Factors affecting physical activity*. Washington, DC (GAO-07-260R).

Gaskin, Darrell, Christine Spencer, Patrick Richard, Gerard Anderson, Neil Powe, and Thomas LaVeist. 2008. Do hospitals provide lower-quality care to minorities than to whites? *Health Affairs* 27 (March/April): 518–27.

Geiger, H. Jack. 1996. Race and health care—An American dilemma? *New England Journal of Medicine* 335 (September): 815–16.

Geronimus, Arline. 1999. Economic inequality and social differentials in mortality. *Economic Policy Review* 5 (September): 23–36.

Geronimus, Arline, John Bound, Timothy Waidman, Marianne Hillemeier, and Patricia Burns. 1996. Excess mortality among blacks and whites in the United States. *New England Journal of Medicine* 335 (November): 1552–58.

Gershman, John, and Alec Irwin. 2000. Getting a grip on the global economy. In *Dying for growth*, ed. Jim Yong Kim, Joyce Millen, Alec Irwin, and John Gershman. Monroe, ME: Common Courage Press.

Gianelli, Diane M. 1998. Fatal gene therapy plan stirs fears over long-term safety. *American Medical News* (October): 10–11.

Glendinning, David. 2005. IOM: New agency needed to simplify pay-for-performance measurement. *American Medical News* (December): 1–2.

Golden, Sherita. 2007. A review of the evidence for a neuroendocrine link between stress, depression and diabetes mellitus. *Current Diabetes Review* (4): 252–59.

Goodman, Elizabeth. 1999. The role of socioeconomic status gradients in explaining differences in U.S. adolescents' health. *American Journal of Public Health* 89 (October): 1522–28.

Gorman, Bridget, and Jen'Nan Ghazal Read. 2006. Gender disparities in adult health: An examination of three measures of morbidity. *Journal of Health and Social Behavior* (47): 95–110.

Gornick, Marian, Paul Eggers, Thomas Reilly, Renee Mentech, Leslye Fitterman, Lawrence Kucken, and Bruce Vladek. 1996. Effects of race and income on mortality and use of services among Medicare beneficiaries. *New England Journal of Medicine* 335 (September): 791–99.

Gramlich, Edward, Richard Kasten, and Frank Sammartino. 1993. Growing inequality in the 1980s: The role of federal taxes and cash transfers. In *Uneven tides, rising inequality in America*, ed. Sheldon Danziger and Peter Gottschalk. New York: Russell Sage Foundation.

Greenfield, Thomas, Lorraine Midanik, and John Rogers. 2000. A 10-year national trend of alcohol consumption, 1984–1995: Is the period of declining drinking over? *American Journal of Public Health* 90 (January): 47–52.

Gregg, Edward, and Jack Guralnick. 2007. Is disability obesity's price of longevity? *Journal of the American Medical Association* 298 (November): 2066–67.

Gross, Cary, Benny Soffer, Peter Bach, Rahul Rajkumar, and Howard Forman. 2002. State expenditures for tobacco-control programs and the tobacco settlement. *New England Journal of Medicine* 347 (October): 1080–86.

Guest, Avery, Gunnar Almgren, and Jon Hussey. 1998. The ecology of race and socioeconomic distress: Infant and working-age mortality in Chicago. *Demography* 35 (1): 23–34.

Haan, Mary, George Kaplan, and Terry Camacho. 1987. Poverty and health, prospective evidence from the Alameda County study. *American Journal of Epidemiology* 125 (6): 989–98.

Haas, J. S., and L. Goldman. 1994. Acutely injured patients with trauma in Massachusetts: Differences in care and mortality, by insurance status. *American Journal of Public Health* 84 (October): 1605–1608.

Haddock, Keith, Walker Poston, and Jennifer Taylor. 2003. Smoking and health outcomes after percutaneous coronary intervention. *American Heart Journal* 145:652–57.

Hadley, Jack. 2002. Sicker and poorer: The consequences of being uninsured. Washington, DC: The Kaiser Commission on Medicaid and the Uninsured.

Hadley, Jack. 2008. Insurance coverage, medical care use, and short-term health changes following an unintentional injury or the onset of a chronic condition. *Journal of the American Medical Association* 297 (March): 1073–84.

Hadley, Jack, and John Holahan. 2003. How much medical care do the uninsured use, and who. *Health Affairs.* February 12.

Haiman, Christopher, Daniel Stram, Lynne Wilkens, Malcolm Pike, Laurence Kolonel, Brian Henderson, and Loic Le Marchand. 2006. Ethnic and racial differences in the smoking-related risk of lung cancer. *New England Journal of Medicine* 354 (January): 333–42.

Hales, Simon, Phillipa Howden-Chapman, Clare Salmond, Alistair Woodward, and Johan Machenbach. 1999. National infant mortality rates in relation to gross national product and distribution of income. *Lancet* 354 (December): 2047.

Hallqvist, Johan, Finn Diderichesen, Tores Theorell, Christina Reuterwall, Anders Ahlbom, and SHEEP Study Group. 1998. Is the effect of job strain on myocardial infarction risk due to interaction between high psychological demands and low decision latitude? Results from Stockholm Heart and Epidemiology Program (SHEEP). *Social Science and Medicine* 46 (11): 1405–15.

Hansen, Dave. 2008. After 13 years, Congress OKs genetic bias ban. *American Medical News* (May): 1–4.

Hanson, Barbara. 1995. See "genetic" read inexplicable: The social construction of blame. Paper presented at the Canadian Sociology and Anthropology Association meetings, Montreal.

Harmon, Amy. 2008. Gene map becomes a luxury item. *New York Times.* March 4.

Harrigan, Deborah, Jane Sprague Zones, Nancy Worcester, and Maxine Jo Grad. 1997. Research to improve women's health. In *Women's health,* ed. Sheryl Burt Ruzek, Virginia Olesen, and Adele Clarke. Columbus: Ohio State University Press.

Harvard School of Public Health. 2005. Harvard researchers gather more evidence implicating menthol in health disparities between while and black smokers. Press release. August 18.

Hayward, Mark, Eileen Crimmins, Toni Miles, and Yu Yang. 2000. The significance of socioeconomic status in explaining the racial gap in chronic health conditions. *American Sociological Review* 65 (December): 910–30.

Hayward, Mark, and Melonie Heron. 1999. Racial inequality in active life among adult Americans. *Demography* 36 (February): 77–91.

Health, United States. This annual publication is produced by the Centers for Disease Control and Prevention (CDC), National Center for Health Statistics. Sources for all data cited can be found at www.cdc.gov/nchs/hus.htm.

Healy, Bernadine. 1995. *A new prescription for women's health*. New York: Viking.

Henry Kaiser Family Foundation. 2002. Sicker and poorer: The consequences of being uninsured. A review of the research on the relationship between health insurance, health, work, income and education. Publication #4004. Washington, DC.

Herd, Pamela, Robert Schoeni, and James House. 2008. Upstream solutions: Does the supplemental income program reduce disability in the elderly? *Milbank Quarterly* 86:5–45.

Herman, Allen. 1996. Toward a conceptualization of race in epidemiological research. *Ethnicity Digest* 6:7–20.

Himmelstein, David, Elizabeth Warren, Deborah Thorne, and Steffie Woolhandler. 2005. Illness and injury as contributors to bankruptcy. *Health Affairs*. February 2. W5-63-71. http//www.healthaffairs.org.

Hollingsworth, J. Rogers. 1981. Inequality in levels of health in England and Wales, 1891–1971. *Journal of Health and Social Behavior* 22 (September): 269–83.

Holmes, T. H., and R. H. Rahe. 1967. The social readjustment rating scale. *Journal of Psychosomatic Research* 11 (August): 213–18.

Holtzman, Jeremy, Khal Saleh, and Robert Kane. 2002. Gender differences in functional status and pain in a Medicare population undergoing elective surgery. *Medical Care* 40 (6): 461–70.

Hoover, Robert. 2000. Cancer—Nature, nurture, or both. *New England Journal of Medicine* 343 (July): 135–36.

House, James, James Lepkowski, David Williams, Richard Mero, Paula Lantz, Stephanie Robert, and Jieming Chen. 2000. Excess mortality among urban residents: How much, for whom, and why? *American Journal of Public Health* 90 (December): 1898–1904.

Hundley, Tom. 2008. The tall and short of it. *Chicago Tribune*. May 28.

Idler, Ellen. 1995. Religion, health and nonphysical senses of self. *Social Forces* 74 (December): 683–704.

Institute of Medicine. 1997. *America's vital interest in global health*. Washington, DC: National Academies Press.

Institute of Medicine. 1999. *To err is human*. Washington, DC: National Academies Press.

Institute of Medicine. 2001. *Coverage matters*. Washington, DC: National Academies Press.

Institute of Medicine. 2002a. *Care without coverage: Too little, too late*. Washington, DC: National Academies Press.

Institute of Medicine. 2002b. *The future of the public's health in the 21st century*. Washington, DC: National Academies Press.

Institute of Medicine. 2003. U.S. loses up to $130 billion annually as a result of poor health, early death due to lack of insurance. Press release. June 17. Washington, DC: National Academies Press.

Institute of Medicine. 2004. *Consequences of uninsurance*. Washington, DC: National Academies Press.

Institute of Medicine. 2005. Addressing racial and ethnic health care disparities: Where do we go from here? http//www.national-academies.org.

Jackson, Sharon, Roger Anderson, Norman Jackson, and Paul Sorlie. 2000. The relation of residential segregation to all-cause mortality: A study in black and white. *American Journal of Public Health* 90 (April): 615–17.

Jargowsky, Paul. 1996a. *Poverty and place: Ghettos, barrios, and the American segregation in the city*. New York: Russell Sage Foundation.

Jargowsky, Paul. 1996b. Take the money and run: Economic U.S. metropolitan areas. *American Sociological Review* 61 (December): 984–98.

Jargowsky, Paul, and Mary Jo Bane. 1990. Ghetto poverty: Basic questions. In *Inner-city poverty in the United States*, ed. Laurence Lynn and Michael McGeary. Washington, DC: National Academy Press.

Jencks, Christopher, and Susan Mayer. 1990. The social consequences of growing up poor in a poor neighborhood. In *Inner-city poverty in the United States*, ed. Laurence Lynn and Michael McGeary. Washington, DC: National Academy Press.

Jones, Steve. 2000. *Genetics in medicine: Real promises, unreal expectations*. New York: Milbank Memorial Fund.

Kaiser Commission on Medicaid and the Uninsured. 2007. The uninsured, a primer: Key facts about Americans without health insurance. The Henry J. Kaiser Family Foundation. (October): 1–39.

Kaiser Family Foundation. 2005. Growth in uninsured Americans outpacing spending on the health care safety net. Press release. November 4.

Kaiser Family Foundation. 2006. Employer health benefits.

Kaiser Family Foundation. 2008. No asset tests required under Medicaid for pregnant women. January.

Karter, Andrew, Jeannie Gazzaniga, Richard Cohen, and Michel Casperet. 1998. Ischemic health disease and stroke mortality in African-American, Hispanic, and non-Hispanic white men and women, 1985–1991. *Western Journal of Medicine* 169 (September): 139–45.

Kasper, Judith. 2000. Health care and barriers to health care. In *Handbook of social studies in health and medicine*, ed. Gary Albrecht, Ray Fitzpatrick, and Susan Scrimshaw. London: Sage.

Kassalow, Jordan. 2001. Why health is important to U.S. foreign policy. *Council on Foreign Relations* (April 19).

Kaufert, Patricia. 2000. Health policy and the new genetics. *Social Science and Medicine* 51 (6): 821–29.

Kawachi, Ichiro, and Bruce Kennedy. 1997a. Health and social cohesion: Why care about income inequality? *British Medical Journal* 314 (April): 1037–40.

Kawachi, Ichiro, and Bruce Kennedy. 1997b. The relationship of income inequality to mortality: Does the choice of the indicator matter? *Social Science and Medicine* 45 (7): 1121–27.

Kawachi, Ichiro, and Bruce Kennedy. 2002. *The health of nations: Why inequality is harmful to your health.* New York: The New Press.

Kawachi, Ichiro, Bruce Kennedy, and Roberta Glass. 1999. Social capital and self-rated health: A contextual analysis. *American Journal of Public Health* 89 (August): 1187–93.

Kawachi, Ichiro, Bruce Kennedy, and Richard Wilkinson. 1999. Crime: Social disorganization and relative deprivation. *Social Science and Medicine* 48 (6): 719–31.

Kawachi, Ichiro, S. V. Subramanian, and Daniel Kim. 2008. Social capital and health. In *Social capital and health,* ed. Ichiro Kawachi, S. V. Subramanian, and Daniel Kim. New York: Springer.

Kawachi, Ichiro, Richard Wilkinson, and Bruce Kennedy. 1999. *The society and population health reader,* vol. 1. New York: The New Press.

Keehan, Sean, Andrea Sisko, Chritopher Truffler, Sheila Smith, Cathy Cowan, John Poisal, M. Kent Clemens, and the National Health Expenditure Accounts Projection Team. 2008. Health spending projections through 2017: The baby-boom generation is coming to Medicare. *Health Affairs* (February):145–55.

Keister, Lisa. 2000. *Wealth in America.* New York: Cambridge University Press.

Kelly, Susan, and Rebecca Miles-Doan. 1997. Social inequality and injuries: Do morbidity patterns differ from mortality? *Social Science and Medicine* 44 (1): 63–70.

Kennedy, Bruce, Ichiro Kawachi, Deborah Prothrow-Stith, Kimberly Lochner, and Vanita Gupta. 1999. Social capital, income inequality, and firearm violent crime. In *The society and population health reader,* vol. 1, ed. Ichiro Kawachi, Bruce Kennedy, and Richard Wilkinson. New York: The New Press.

Khashan, Ali, Kathryn Abel, Roseanne McNamee, Marianne Pedersen, Roger Webb, Philip Baker, Louise Kenny, and Preben Mortensen. 2008. Higher risk of offspring schizophrenia following antenatal maternal exposure to severe adverse life effects. *Archives of General Psychiatry* 2:146–52.

Kiefe, Catarina, O. Dale Williams, Cora Lewis, Jeroan Allison, Padmini Sekar, and Lynne Wagenkneckt. 2001. Ten-year changes in smoking among young adults: Are racial differences explained by socioeconomic factors in the CARDIA study? *American Journal of Public Health* 91 (February): 213–18.

Kim, Jim Yon, Joyce Millen, Alec Irwin, and John Gershman. 1999. *Dying for growth.* Monroe, ME: Common Courage Press.

Kim, Kwangkee, and Philip Moody.1992. More resources, better health? A cross-national perspective. *Social Science and Medicine* 34 (8): 837–42.

Kimbro, Rachel, Sharon Bzostek, Noreen Goldman, and German Rodriguez. 2008. Race, ethnicity, and the education gradient in health. *Health Affairs* 27 (March/April): 361–72.

King, Michael, Peter Speck, and Angela Thomas. 1994. Spiritual and religious beliefs in acute illness—Is this a feasible area for study? *Social Science and Medicine* 38 (4): 631–36.

King, Talmadge, and Paul Brunetta.1999. Racial disparity in rates of surgery for lung cancer. *New England Journal of Medicine* 16 (October): 1231–33.

Kinzer, Marina. 2000. Health cities: A guide to the literature. *Public Health Reports* 115 (March): 279–89.

Kitagawa, Evelyn, and Philip Hauser. 1973. *Differential mortality in the United States. A study in socioeconomic epidemiology.* Cambridge, MA: Harvard University Press.

Kittner, Steve, Lon White, Katalin Losonczy, Philip Wolf, and J. Richard Hebel. 1990. Black-white differences in stroke incidence in a national sample. *Journal of the American Medical Association* 264 (September): 1267–70.

Kjerulff, K. H., K. D. Frick, J. A. Rhoades, and C. S. Hollenbeak. 2007. The cost of being a woman: A national study of health care utilization and expenditures for female-specific conditions. *Women's Health Issues* (January/February): 13–21.

Knowles, John.1977. *Doing better, feeling worse.* New York: Norton.

Koenig, Harold, Michael McCullough, and David Larson. 2001. *Handbook of religion and health.* Oxford, UK: Oxford University Press.

Kohn, Linda, Janet Corrigan, and Molla Donaldson, eds. 1999. *To err is human: Building a safer health system.* Institute of Medicine. Washington, DC: National Academies Press.

Kolata, Gina. 2007. Genes take charge, and diets fall by the wayside. *New York Times.* May 8.

Konrad, Thomas, Daniel Howard, Lloyd Edwards, Anastasia Ivanova, and Timothy Carey. 2005. Physician-patient racial concordance, continuity of care, and patterns of care for hypertension. *American Journal of Public Health* 95 (December): 2186–90.

Kreiger, Nancy. 2000. Discrimination and health. In *Social epidemiology,* ed. Lisa Berkman and Ichiro Kawachi. Oxford, UK: Oxford University Press.

Kreiger, Nancy. 2001. Theories for social epidemiology in the 21st century: An ecosocial perspective. *International Journal of Epidemiology* 30:668–77.

Kreiger, Nancy, and Stephen Sidney. 1996. Racial discrimination and blood pressure: The CARDIA study of young black and white adults. *American Journal of Public Health* 86 (October): 1370–78.

Krugman, Paul. 2007. *The conscience of a liberal.* New York: Norton.

Kuh, D. J. L., and M. E. J. Wadsworth. 1993. Physical health status at 36 years in British national birth cohort. *Social Science and Medicine* 37 (7): 905–16.

Kunst, Anton, and Johan Machenbach. 1994. The size of mortality differences associated with educational level in nine industrialized countries. *American Journal of Public Health* 84 (June): 932–37.

La Free, Gary. 1998. *Losing legitimacy.* Boulder, CO: Westview Press.

Landers, Susan. 2002. Tobacco fund only a fraction of health care costs of smoking. *American Medical News*. May 6.

Landers, Susan. 2004. Vitamin D found to boost health, if people get enough. *American Medical News*. April 5.

Landers, Susan. 2008. Down Syndrome is the target of ambitious NIH research initiatives. *American Medical News* (February): 20–21.

Lane, Sandra, and Donald Cibula. 2000. Gender and health. In *Handbook of social studies in health and medicine*, ed. Gary Albrecht, Ray Fitzpatrick, and Susan Scrimshaw. London: Sage.

Lannin, Donald, Holly Matthews, Jim Mitchell, Melvin Swanson, Frances Swanson, and Maxine Edwards. 1998. Influence of socioeconomic and cultural factors on racial differences in late-stage presentation of breast cancer. *Journal of the American Medical Association* 279 (June): 1801–1807.

Lantz, Paula, James House, James Leplowski, David Williams, Richard Mero, and Jieming Chen. 1998. Socioeconomic factors, health behaviors, and mortality. *Journal of the American Medical Association* 279 (June): 1703–1708.

Lantz, Paula, John Lynch, James House, James Lepowski, Richard Mero, Marc Musick, and David Williams. 2001. Socioeconomic disparities in health change in a longitudinal study of U.S. adults: The role of health-risk behaviors. *Social Science and Medicine* 53 (1): 29–40.

LaVeist, Thomas. 1994. Beyond dummy variables and sample selection: What health services researchers ought to know about race as a variable. *Health Services Research* 29 (April): 1–16.

LaVeist, Thomas, and Lydia Isaac. 2008. Examples of racial disparities in health care. Robert Wood Johnson Foundation. February.

Lee, Crystal Man Ying, Rachel Huxley, Rachel Wildman, and Mark Woodward. 2008. Indices of abdominal obesity are better discriminators of cardiovascular risk factors than BMI: A meta-analysis. *Journal of Clinical Epidemiology* 61 (7): 646–53.

Lee, I-Min, Chung-cheng Hsieh, and Ralph Paffenbarger. 1995. Exercise intensity and longevity in men: The Harvard alumni study. *Journal of the American Medical Association* 273 (April): 1179–84.

Lee, I-Min, Kathryn Rexrode, Nancy Cook, JoAnn Manson, and Judie Buring. 2001. Physical activity and coronary heart disease. *Journal of the American Medical Association* 285 (April): 1179–84.

Lee, Min-Ah, and Kenneth Ferraro. 2007. Neighborhood residential segregation and physical health among Hispanic Americans: Good, bad, or benign? *Journal of Health and Social Behavior* 48 (June): 131–48.

Lee, Sei, K. Lindquist, and K. E. Covinsky. 2007. The relationship between self-rated health and mortality in older black and white Americans. *Journal of the American Geriatric Society* 55: 1624–29.

Leibovici, Leonard. 2001. Effects of remote, retroactive intercessory prayer on outcomes in patients with bloodstream infection: Randomized controlled trial. *British Medical Journal* 323 (December 22): 1450–51.

Leon, David, Laurent Chenet, Vladimir Shkolnikov, Judith Shapiro, Galina Ra-khmanova, Sergie Vassin, and Martin McKee. 1997. Huge variation in Russian mortality rates 1984–1994: Artefact, alcohol, or what? *Lancet* 350 (August): 383–88.

Leon, David, and Vladimir Shkolnikov. 1998. Social stress and the Russian mortality crisis. *Journal of the American Medical Association* 279 (March): 790–91.

Levin, Jeffrey. 1994. Religion and health: Is there an association, is it valid, and is it causal? *Social Science and Medicine* 38 (11): 1475–82.

Levitan, Emily, Amy Yang, Alicija Wolk, and Murray Mittleman. 2009. Adiposity and incidence of health failure hospitalization and mortality: A population-based prospective study. *Circulation*. April 7. http//www.circ.ahajouranls.org.

Levy, D. E., and E. Meara. 2006. The effect of the 1998 agreement on prenatal smoking. *Journal of Health Economics* 25:276–94.

Levy, Judith, Richard Stephens, and Duane McBride. 2000. *Emergent issues in the field of drug abuse*. Stamford, CT: JAI Press.

Li, Ming D., Lou Xiang-Yang, Randolph Dupont, Nancy William, and Robert Elston. 2006. A genomewide search finds major susceptibility loci for nicotine dependence on Chromosome 10 in African Americans. *American Journal of Human Genetics* 79:745–51.

Lille-Blanton, Marsha, and Catherine Hoffman. 2005. The role of health insurance coverage in reducing racial/ethnic disparities in health care. *Health Affairs* 24 (March/April): 398–408.

Link, Bruce, and Jo Phelan. 1995. Social conditions as fundamental causes of disease. *Journal of Health and Social Behavior* 35 (extra issue): 80–94.

Link, Bruce, and Jo Phelan. 2000. Evaluating the fundamental cause explanation for social disparities in health. In *Handbook of medical sociology*, ed. Chloe Bird, Peter Conrad, and Allen Fremont. Upper Saddle River, NJ: Prentice Hall.

Link, Bruce, and Jo Phelan. 2002. McKeown and the idea that social conditions are fundamental causes of disease. *American Journal of Public Health* 92 (May): 730–32.

Lochner, Kim, Elsie Pamuk, Diane Makuc, Bruce Kennedy, and Ichiro Kawachi. 2001. State-level income inequality and individual mortality risk: A prospective multilevel study. *American Journal of Public Health* 91 (March): 385–91.

Lorber, Judith. 1997. *Gender and the social construction of illness*. Thousand Oaks, CA: Sage.

Lynch, John. 2000. Income inequality and health: Expanding the debate. *Social Science and Medicine* 51 (7): 1001–05.

Lynch, John, George Kaplan, Elsie Pamuk, Richard Cohen, Katherine Heck, Jennifer Balfour, and Irene Yen. 1998. Income inequality and mortality in metropolitan areas of the United States. *American Journal of Public Health* 88 (July): 1974–80.

Lynch, J. W., G. A. Kaplan, and J. T. Salonen. 1997. Why do poor people behave poorly? Variation in adult health behaviors and psychosocial characteristics by stages of the socioeconomic lifecourse. *Social Science and Medicine* 44 (6): 809–19.

Lynch, John, George Kaplan, and Sarah Shema. 1997. Cumulative impact of sustained economic hardship on physical, cognitive, psychological, and social functioning. *New England Journal of Medicine* 337 (December): 1889–95.

Machenbach, Johan. 2006. Socio-economic inequalities in health in Western Europe: From description to explanation to intervention. In *Social inequality in health*, ed. Johannes Siegrist and Michael Marmot. Oxford, UK: Oxford University Press.

Macintyre, Sally. 1993. Gender differences in the perceptions of common cold symptoms. *Social Science and Medicine* 36 (1): 15–20.

Macintyre, Sally, Graeme Ford, and Kate Hunt. 1999. Do women "over-report" morbidity? Men's and women's responses to structured prompting on a standard question on long-standing illness. *Social Science and Medicine* 48 (1): 89–98.

MacKenzie, Thomas, Carl Bartecchi, and Robert Schrier. 1994. The human costs of tobacco use. *New England Journal of Medicine* 330 (April): 975–80.

Mansfield, Christopher, James Wilson, Edward Kobrinki, and Jim Mitchell. 1999. Premature mortality in the United States: The roles of geographic area, socioeconomic status, household type, and availability of medical care. *American Journal of Public Health* 89 (June): 893–98.

Markel, Howard, and Sam Potts. 2009. American epidemics: A brief history. *New York Times*. May 3.

Marmot, Michael. 1998. Improvement of social environment to improve health. *Lancet* 351 (January): 57–60.

Marmot, Michael. 2000. Inequalities in health: Causes and policy implications. In *The society and population health reader, vol. 2. A state and community perspective*, ed. Alvin Tarlov and Robert St. Peter. New York: The New Press.

Marmot, Michael. 2001. Inequalities in health. *New England Journal of Medicine* 345 (July): 134–36.

Marmot, M. G. 2003. Understanding social inequalities in health. *Perspectives in Biology and Medicine* 46 (Summer): S9–S23.

Marmot, Michael, Carol Ryff, Larry Bumpass, Martin Shipley, and Nadine Marks. 1997. Social inequalities in health: Next questions and converging evidence. *Social Science and Medicine* 44 (6): 901–10.

Marmot, M. G., and Martin Shipley. 1996. Do socioeconomic differences in mortality persist after retirement? Twenty-five-year follow-up of civil servants from the first Whitehall study. *British Medical Journal* 313 (November): 1177–80.

Marmot, M. G., and George Davey Smith. 1989. Why are the Japanese living longer? *British Medical Journal* 299 (December): 1547–51.

Marmot, M. G., George Davey Smith, Stephen Stansfeld, Chandra Patel, Fiona North, Jenny Head, Ian White, Eric Brunner, and Amanda Feeney. 1991. Health inequalities among British civil servants: The Whitehall II study. *Lancet* 337 (June): 1387–93.

Marmot, Michael, and Richard Wilkinson. 1999. *Social determinants of health*. Oxford, UK: Oxford University Press.

Massey, Douglas. 1996. The age of extremes: Concentrated affluence and poverty in the twenty-first century. *Demography* 33 (November): 395–412.

Massey, Douglas, and Nancy Denton. 1993. *American apartheid, segregation and the making of the underclass*. Cambridge, MA: Harvard University Press.

Matthews, Sharon, Clyde Hertzman, Aleck Ostry, and Chris Power. 1998. Gender work roles and psychosocial work characteristics as determinants of health. *Social Science and Medicine* 46 (January): 1417–24.

Matthews, T. J., and B. E. Hamilton. 2005. Toward trend analysis of the sex ratio at birth in the United States. *National Vital Statistics Report* 53 (20): 1–18.

Maxey, Randall, and Richard Allen Williams. 2007. Second-class medicine: Implications of evidence-based medicine for improving minority access to the correct pharmaceutical therapy. In *Eliminating healthcare disparities in America*, ed. Richard Allen Williams. Totowa, NJ: Humana Press.

McCord, Colin, and Harold Freeman. 1990. Excess mortality in Harlem. *New England Journal of Medicine* 322 (January): 173–77.

McDonough, Peggy, Greg Duncan, David Williams, and James House. 1997. Income dynamics and adult mortality in the United States, 1972 through 1989. *American Journal of Public Health* 87 (September): 1476–83.

McKeown, Thomas. 1976. *The role of medicine*. London: The Nuffield Provincial Hospitals Trust.

McKinlay, John. 1974. A case for refocusing upstream: The political economy of illness. In *Applying behavioral science to cardiovascular risk*. Washington, DC: American Heart Association.

McKinlay, John. 1996. Some contributions form the social system to gender inequalities in heart disease. *Journal of Health and Social Behavior* 37 (March): 1–26.

McKinlay, John. 2001. Looking for causes in all the wrong places. *Medical Sociology Newsletter* 37 (Spring): 1, 4–6.

McKinlay, John, and Sonja McKinlay. 1977. The questionable contribution of medical measures to the decline of mortality in the United States in the twentieth century. *Milbank Memorial Fund Quarterly* 55 (3): 405–28.

McKnight, John. 1995. *The careless society*. New York: Basic Books.

McLaughlin, Diane, and Shannon Stokes. 2002. Income inequality and mortality in U.S. counties: Does minority racial concentration matter? *American Journal of Public Health* 92 (January): 99–104.

Meara, Ellen, Seth Richards, and David Cutler. 2008. The gap gets bigger: Changes in mortality and life expectancy, by education, 1981–2000. *Health Affairs* 27 (January/February): 150–60.

Meerlo, Peter, Andrea Sgoifo, and Deborah Suchecki. 2008. Restricted and disrupted sleep: effects on autonomic function, neuroendocrine stress systems and stress responsivity. *Sleep Medicine Review* 12 (June): 197–210.

Mellor, Jennifer, and Jeffrey Milyo. 2001. Reexamining the evidence of an ecological association between income and inequality and health. *Journal of Health Politics, Policy, and Law* 26 (June): 487–522.

Michels, Karin, and Anders Ekbom. 2004. Caloric restriction and incidence of breast cancer. *Journal of the American Medical Association* 291 (March): 1226–30.

Millen, Joyce, and Timothy Holtz. 2000. Dying for growth, part I: Transnational corporations and the health of the poor. In *Dying for growth*, ed. Jim Yong Kim, Joyce Millen, Alec Irwin, and John Gershman. Monroe, ME: Common Courage Press.

Mirowsky, John, and Paul Nongzhuang Hu. 1996. Physical impairment and the diminishing effects of income. *Social Forces* 74 (March): 1073–96.

Mirowsky, John, and Catherine Ross. 2003. *Social causes of psychological distress*, 2nd ed. Hawthorne, NY: Aldine de Gruyter.

Morch, Lina, Ditte Johansen, Lau Thygesen, Anne Tjonnel, Ellen Lokkegaard, Claudia Stahlberg, and Morten Gronbaek. 2007. Alcohol drinking, consumption patterns, and breast cancer among Danish nurses: A cohort study. *European Journal of Public Health* 17:624–29.

Mullan, Zoe. 2000. How much should we be drinking to minimize mortality? *Lancet* 355 (January): 123.

Mullen, Fitzhugh. 2004. Wrestling with variation: An interview with Jack Wennberg. *Health Affairs* 23 (October): 73–80.

Mustard, J. Fraser. 2000. Healthy societies: An overview. In *The society and population health reader, vol. 2: A state and community perspective*, ed. Alvin Tarlov and Robert St. Peter. New York: The New Press.

Nathanielsz, Peter. 2001. *The prenatal prescription*. New York: HarperCollins.

National Association of County & City Health Officials. 2007. *The 2007 big cities health inventory: The health of urban U.S.A.*

National Center for Health Statistics. 1996. Chartbook: Women's health. In *United States, 1995*. Hyattsville, MD: Public Health Service.

National Center for Health Statistics. 2001. Rural and urban chartbook. In *Health, United States, 2001*. Hyattsville, MD: Public Health Service.

National Institute on Drug Abuse. 2006. Black, white teens show differences in nicotine metabolism. Press release. January.

Navarro, Vincente. 1991. Race *or* class or race *and* class: Growing mortality differentials in the United States. *International Journal of Health Services* 21 (2): 229–35.

Navarro, Vincente, and Leiye Shi. 2001. The political context of social inequalities and health. *Social Science and Medicine* 52 (3): 481–91.

Nelson, Nancy. 2001. Draft human genome sequence yields several surprises. *Journal of the National Cancer Institute* 93 (April): 493.

Neugarten, Bernice, and Susan Reed. 1996. Social and psychological characteristics. In *Geriatric medicine*, ed. Christine Cassel, Harvey Cohen, Eric Larson, Diane Meier, Neil Resnick, Laurence Rubenstein, and Leif Sorenson. New York: Springer.

Newhouse, Joseph, Robert Brook, Naihua Duan, Emmett Keeler, Arleen Leibowitz, Willard Manning, M. Susan Marquis, Carl Morris, Charles Phelps, and John Rolph. 2008. Attrition in the RAND health insurance experiment: A response to Nyman. *Journal of Health Politics, Policy, and Law* 33 (2): 295–308.

Newhouse, Joseph, and the Insurance Experiment Group. 1993. *Free for all? Lessons from the RAND health insurance experiment.* Cambridge, MA: Harvard University Press.

Ng-Mak, Daisy, Bruce Dohrenwend, Ana Abraido-Lanza, and J. Blake Turner. 1999. A further analysis of race differences in the national longitudinal mortality study. *American Journal of Public Health* 89 (November): 1748–51.

Nieto, F. Javier. 1999. Cardiovascular disease and risk factor epidemiology: A look back at the epidemic of the 20th century. *American Journal of Public Health* 89 (March): 292–93.

NIH Consensus Panel on Physical Activity and Cardiovascular Health.1996. Physical activity and cardiovascular health. *Journal of the American Medical Association* 276 (July): 241–42.

Nyman, John. 2007. American health policy: Cracks in the foundation. *Journal of Health Politics, Policy, and Law* 32 (5): 759–83.

Nyman, John. 2008. Health plan switching and attrition bias in the RAND health insurance experiment. *Journal of Health Politics, Policy, and Law* 33 (2): 309–17.

O'Donnell, Katie, Ellena Badrick, Meera Kumari, and Andrew Steptoe. 2008. Psychological coping styles and cortisol over the day in healthy older adults. *Psychoneuroendocrinology* 33:601–11.

Omran, Abdel. 1971. The epidemiologic transition. *Milbank Memorial Fund Quarterly* 48:509–38.

Ong, Elisa, and Stanton Glantz. 2000. Tobacco industry efforts subverting agency for research on cancer's second-hand smoke study. *Lancet* 355 (April): 1253–59.

Oppenheimer, Gerald. 2001. Paradigm lost: Race, ethnicity, and the search for a new population taxonomy. *American Journal of Public Health* 91 (July): 1049–55.

O'Reilly, Kevin. 2006a. AMA to lead funding study to fight obesity. *American Medical News* (December): 37.

O'Reilly, Kevin. 2006b. Quality quandary. *American Medical News.* May 22/29. Chicago: American Medical Association.

Paffenbarger, Ralph, Robert Hyde, Alvin Wing, I-Min Lee, Dexter Jung, and James Kempert. 1993. The association of change in physician activity level and other lifestyle characteristics with mortality among men. *New England Journal of Medicine* 328 (February): 538–45.

Pappas, Gregory, Susan Queen, Wilbur Hadden, and Gail Fisher. 1993. The increasing disparity in mortality between socioeconomic groups in the United States, 1960 and 1986. *New England Journal of Medicine* 329 (July): 103–109.

Parkes, Gary, Trisha Greenhalgh, Mark Griffin, and Richard Dent. 2008. Effect of smoking quit rate of telling patients their lung age: The Step2quit randomized controlled trial. *British Medical Journal* 336 (March): 598–600.

Pate, Russel, Michael Pratt, Steven Blair, William Haskell, Caroline Mecera, Claude Bouchard, David Buchner, Walter Ettinger, Gregory Health, Abby King, Andrea Kriska, Arthur Leon, Bess Marcus, Jeremy Morris, Ralph Paffenbarger, Kevin Patick, Michael Pollack, James Rippe, James Sollis, and Jack Whitmore. 1995. Physical activity and public health. *Journal of the American Medical* Association 273 (February): 402–407.

Pavalko, Eliza, Glen Elder, and Elizabeth Clipp. 1993. Worklives and longevity: Insights from a life course perspective. *Journal of Health and Social Behavior* 34 (December): 363–80.

Pearlin, Leonard, and Carmi Schooler. 1978. The structure of coping. *Journal of Health and Social Behavior* 19 (June): 2–21.

Peck, Maria. 1994. The importance of childhood socio-economic group for adult health. *Social Science and Medicine* 39 (4): 553–62.

Peter, Richard, and Johannes Siegrist. 1997. Chronic work stress, sickness absence, and hypertension in middle managers: General or specific sociological explanations? *Social Science and Medicine* 45 (7): 1111–20.

Pickett, Kate, Shona Kelly, Eric Brunner, Tim Lobstein, and Richard Wilkinson. 2005. Wider income gaps, wider waistbands? An ecological study of obesity and income inequality. *Journal of Epidemiology and Community Health* 59:670–74.

Polednak, Anthony. 1991. Black-white differences in infant mortality in 38 standard metropolitan statistical areas. *American Journal of Public Health* 81 (November): 1480–82.

Pollack, Andrew. 2002. New era of consumer genetics raises hope and concerns. *New York Times*. October 1.

Power, Chris, and Diana Kuh. 2006. Life course development of unequal health. In *Social inequalities in health*, ed. Johannes Siegrist and Michael Marmot. Oxford, UK: Oxford University Press.

Powles, John. 1974. On the limitations of modern medicine. In *The challenges of community medicine*, ed. Robert Kane. New York: Springer.

Prentice, Ross, et al. 2006. Low-fat dietary pattern and risk of invasive breast cancer. *Journal of the American Medical Association* 295 (February): 629–42.

Putnam, Robert. 2000. *Bowling alone*. New York: Simon and Schuster.

Quellet-Morin, Isabella, Michel Bovin, Ginette Dionne, Sonia Lupien, Louise Arsenault, Ronald Barr, Daniel Perusse, and Richard Tremblay. 2008. Variations in heritability of cortisol reactivity to stress as a function of early familial adversity among 19-month-old twins. *Archives of General Psychiatry* 2:211–18.

RAND Corporation. 2007. RAND study finds people who are severly [sic] overweight grow faster than other obese Americans. Press release. April 9.

Reingold, Jennifer. 2000. Executive pay. *Business Week*. April 17. http://www.businessweek.com/.

Renehan, Andrew, Margaret Tyson, Matthias Egger, Richard Heller, and Marcel Zwarkeen. 2008. Body-mass index and incidence of cancer: A systematic review and meta-analysis of prospective observational studies. *Lancet* 371 (February): 569–78.

Reschovsky, James, and Ann O'Malley. 2008. Do primary physicians treating minority patients report problems delivering high-quality care? *Health Affairs* (April 22): 222–31.

Rice, Thomas, ed. 2003. The consequences of being uninsured. *Medical Care Research and Review* (Supplement to 60 [June]).

Rimpala, Arja, and Eero Pukkala. 1987. Cancers of affluence: Positive social class gradient and rising incidence in some cancer forms. *Social Science and Medicine* 24 (7): 601–606.

Riska, Elianne. 2004. *Masculinity and men's health: Coronary heart disease in medical practice and public discourse*. Lanham, MD: Rowman & Littlefield.

Ritzer, George. 2000. *The McDonaldization of society*. Thousand Oaks, CA: Pine Forge Press.

Robert, Stephanie. 1999. Socioeconomic position and health: The independent contribution of community context. *Annual Review of Sociology* 25:489–516.

Robert, Stephanie, and James House. 2000. Socioeconomic inequalities in health: An enduring sociological problem. In *Handbook of medical sociology*, ed. Chloe Bird, Peter Conrad, and Allen Fremont. Upper Saddle River, NJ: Prentice Hall.

Robeznieks, Andis. 2004. Report finds gaps in health care quality. *American Medical News*. October 18. Chicago: American Medical Association.

Roizen, Michael. 1999. *Real age: Are you as young as you can be?* New York: Cliff Street Books.

Rose, Geoffrey. 1992. *The strategy of preventive medicine*. Oxford, UK: Oxford University Press.

Rose, Richard. 2000. How much does social capital add to individual health? A survey study of Russians. *Social Science and Medicine* 51 (9): 1421–35.

Rosenblatt, Roger, and George Wright. 2000. The effect of the doctor-patient relationship on emergency department use among the elderly. *American Journal of Public Health* 90 (January): 97–102.

Rosenfield, Richard. 2002. Crime decline in context. *Contexts* 1 (Spring): 25–34.

Ross, Catherine. 2000. Walking, exercising, and smoking: Does neighborhood matter? *Social Science and Medicine* 51 (2): 265–74.

Ross, Catherine, and Chloe Bird. 1994. Sex stratification and health lifestyle: Consequences for men's and women's perceived health. *Journal of Health and Social Behavior* 35 (June): 161–78.

Ross, Catherine, John Mirowsky, and Shana Pribesh. 2001. Powerlessness and the amplifications of threat: Neighborhood disadvantage, disorder, and mistrust. *American Sociological Review* 66 (August): 569–91.

Ross, Catherine, and Chia-ling Wu.1995. The links between education and health. *American Sociological Review* 60 (October): 719–45.

Rothstein, William. 2001. The health of the nation. In *The nation's health*, ed. Philip Lee and Carroll Estes. Boston: Jones and Barlett.

Rubenstein, Sharon, and Benjamin Caballero. 2000. Is Miss America an undernourished role model? *Journal of the American Medical Association* 283 (March 22/29): 1569.

Ruccio, David. 2007. *Inequality, principles of microeconomics*. Washington, DC: Congressional Budget Office.

Ruzek, Sheryl, Adele Clarke, and Virginia Olesen. 1997. Social, biomedical, and feminist models of women's health. In *Women's health*, ed. Sheryl Ruzek, Virginia Olesen, and Adele Clarke. Columbus: Ohio State University Press.

Sacker, Amanda, Mel Bartley, David Firth, and Ray Fitzpatrick. 2001. Dimensions of social inequality in the health of women in England: Occupational, material and behavioural pathways. *Social Science and Medicine* 52 (5): 763–81.

Sapolsky, Robert. 1998. *Why zebras don't get ulcers*. New York: W. H. Freeman.

Sapolsky, Robert. 2004. *Why zebras don't get ulcers*. 2nd ed. New York: Henry Holt.

Satcher, David, George Fryer, Jessica McCann, Adewale Troutman, Steven Woolf, and George Rust. 2005. What if we were equal? A comparison of the black-white mortality gap in 1960 and 2000. *Health Affairs* 24 (March/April): 459–64.

Schoen, Cathy, Sara Collins, Jennifer Kriss, and Michelle Doty. 2008. How many adults are uninsured? Trends among U.S. adults, 2003 and 2007. *Health Affairs* (June): 298–309.

Schoen, Cathy, and Catherine DesRoches. 2000. Uninsured and unstably insured: The importance of continuous coverage. *Health Services Research* 35 (April, Part II): 187–206.

Schuman, Howard, and Maria Krysan. 1999. A historical note on whites' beliefs about racial inequality. *American Sociological Review* 64 (December): 847–55.

Schwartz, Robert. 2001. Racial profiling in medical research. *New England Journal of Medicine* 344 (May 4): 1392–93.

Seligman, Hilary, Andrew Bindman, Eric Vittinghoff, Alka Kanaya, and Margot Kushel. 2007. Food insecurity is associated with diabetes mellitus: Results from the National Examination and Nutrition Examination Survey (NHANES) 1999–2002. *Journal of General Internal Medicine* 22 (77): 1018–23.

Seligman, Martin. 1991. *Learned optimism*. New York: Pocket Books.

Sen, Amartya. 1992. *Inequality reexamined*. Cambridge, MA: Harvard University Press.

Sen, Amartya. 1998. Mortality as an indicator of economic success and failure. *The Economic Journal* 108 (January): 1–25.

Sen, Amartya. 1999. *Development as freedom*. New York: Alfred A. Knopf.

Shakow, Aaron, and Alec Irwin. 1999. Terms reconsidered: Decoding development discourse. In *Dying for growth*, ed. Jim Yong Kim, Joyce Millen, Alec Irwin, and John Gershman. Monroe, ME: Common Courage Press.

Shaw, Mary, David Gordon, Danny Dorling, Richard Mitchell, and George Davey Smith. 2000. Increasing mortality differentials by residential area level of poverty: Britain 1981–1997. *Social Science and Medicine* 51 (1): 151–53.

Sherkat, Darren, and Christopher Ellison. 1999. Recent developments in sociology of religion. *Annual Review of Sociology* 25:363–94.

Shi, Leiyu, and Barbara Starfield. 2001. The effect of primary care physician supply and income inequality on mortality among blacks and whites in U.S. metropolitan areas. *American Journal of Public Health* 91 (August): 1246–50.

Short, Pamela, and France Marie Weaver. 2008. Transitioning to Medicare before age sixty-five. *Health Affairs* (March 25): 175–84.

Siegrist Johannes, and Michael Marmot. 2006. Introduction. In *Social inequality in health*, ed. Johannes Siegrist and Michael Marmot. Oxford, UK: Oxford University Press.

Sikora, Andrew, and Michael Mulvihill. 2002. Trends in mortality due to legal intervention in the United States, 1979 through 1997. *American Journal of Public Health* 92 (May): 841–43.

Silverman, Robert. 2001. Unnatural selection. *Pediatrics* 107 (June): 1421–22.

Singh, Gopal, and Mohammad Siahpush. 2001. All-cause and cause-specific mortality of immigrants and native born in the United States. *American Journal of Public Health* 91 (March): 392–99.

Sloan, R., E. Bagiella, and T. Powell. 1999. Religion, spirituality, and medicine. *Lancet* 353 (February): 664–67.

Smaje, Chris. 2000. Race, ethnicity, and health. In *Handbook of medical sociology*, ed. Chloe Bird, Peter Conrad, and Allen Fremont. Upper Saddle River, NJ: Prentice-Hall.

Smedley, Brian, Adrienne Stith, and Alan Nelson. 2003. *Unequal treatment: Confronting racial and ethnic disparities in health care.* Washington, DC: National Academies Press.

Soobader, Mah-Jabeen, and Jelicia LeClere. 1999. Aggregation and the measurement of income inequality: Effects on morbidity. *Social Science and Medicine* 48 (6): 733–44.

Stapleton, Stephanie. 2007. Smoking quit rates stall as anti-tobacco funding declines. *American Medical News.* December.

Steptoe, A., and J. Wardle. 2005. Cardiovascular stress responsivity, body mass and abdominal adiposity. *International Journal of Obesity* 29:1329–37.

Steptoe, Andrew, and Gonneke Willemsen. 2004. The influence of low job control on ambulatory blood pressure and perceived stress over the working day in men and women from the Whitehall II cohort. *Journal of Hypertension* 22:915–20.

Stiglitz, Joseph. 2002. *Globalization and its discontents.* New York: Norton.

Stofan, John, Loretta DiPietro, Dorothy Davis, Harold Kohl, and Steven Blair. 1998. Physical activity patterns associated with cardiorespiratory fitness and reduced mortality: The aerobics center longitudinal study. *American Journal of Public Health* 88 (December): 1807–13.

Stoney, Catherine, Sheila West, Joel Hughes, Lisa Lentino, Montenique Finney, James Falko, and Linda Bausserman. 2002. Acute psychological stress reduces plasma triglyceride clearance. *Psychophysiology* 39:80–85.

Sturm, Roland. 2002. The effects of obesity, smoking, and drinking on medical problems and costs. *Health Affairs* 21 (March/April): 245–53.

Subramanian, S. V., Ichiro Kawachi, and Bruce Kennedy. 2001. Does the state you live in make a difference? Multilevel analysis of self-rated health in the U.S. *Social Science and Medicine* 53 (1): 9–19.

Sudano, Joseph, and David Baker. 2003. Intermittent lack of health insurance coverage and use of preventive services. *American Journal of Public Health* 93 (January): 13–137.

Sudano, Joseph, and David Baker. 2006. Explaining U.S. racial/ethnic disparities in health decline and mortality in late middle age: The roles of socioeconomic status, health behavior, and health insurance. *Social Science and Medicine* 62 (February): 909–22.

Tarlov, Alvin. 1996. Social determinants of health. In *Health and social organization*, ed. David Blane, Eric Brunner, and Richard Wilkinson. London: Routledge.

Taubes, Gary. 2002. What if it's all been a big fat lie? *New York Times Magazine*. July 7.

Taylor, Donald, Vic Hasselblad, Jane Henley, Michael Thun, and Frank Sloan. 2002. Benefits of smoking cessation for longevity. *American Journal of Public Health* 92 (June): 990–96.

The Roper Center for Public Opinion Research. 2001. 2000 General social survey. Storrs: University of Connecticut.

Thoits, Peggy. 1995. Stress, coping, and social support processes: Where are we? What next? *Journal of Health and Social Behavior* 35 (Extra Issue): 53–79.

Thoits, Peggy. 2006. Personal agency in the stress process. *Journal of Health and Social Behavior* 47 (December): 309–23.

Thomas, W. I. 1966 [1931]. The relations of research to the social process. In *W. I. Thomas on social organization and social personality*, ed. Morris Janowitz. Chicago: University of Chicago Press.

Thorgeirsson, T. E., et al. 2008. A variant associated with nicotine dependence, lung cancer, and peripheral arterial disease. *Nature* 452:638–42.

Tierney, John. 2008. Comfort food, for monkeys. *New York Times*. May 20.

Townsend, Peter, Nick Davidson, and Margaret Whitehead. 1992. *Inequalities in health*. London: Penguin Books.

United Press International. 2008. Poll sees women facing tougher campaign. Press release. March 19.

U.S. Preventive Services Task Force. 2005. Genetic risk assessment and BRCA mutation testing for breast and ovarian cancer susceptibility: Recommendation statement. *Annals of Internal Medicine* 143:355–61.

USA Today. 2001. Tobacco's death benefits. July 24.

Van Baal, Pieter, Johan Polder, G. Ardine de Wit, Rudolf Hoogenveen, Talitha Feenstra, Hendriek Boshuizen, Peter Engelfriet, and Werner Brouwer. 2008. Lifetime medical costs of obesity: Prevention no cure for increasing health expenditure. *PLoS Medicine* 5 (2): e29.

van Ryn, Michelle, and Jane Burke. 2000. The effect of patient race and socioeconomic status on physicians' perceptions of patients. *Social Science and Medicine* 50 (6): 813–28.

Veenstra, Gerry. 2000. Social capital, SES and health: An individual-level analysis. *Social Science and Medicine* 50 (5): 619–29.

Verbrugge, Lois. 1990. Pathways of health and death. In *Women, health and medicine in America*, ed. Rima Apple. New York: Garland Publishing.

Vernick, Jon, Lainie Rutkow, and Stephen Teret. 2007. Public health benefits of recent litigation against the tobacco industry. *Journal of the American Medical Association* 298 (July): 86–89.

Wachter, Robert. 2004. The end of the beginning: Patient safety five years after "To err is human." *Health Affairs*. November 30. W4-534-545. http://www.healthaffairs.org.

Waitzkin, Howard, Celia Iriart, Alfredo Estrada, and Silvia Lamadrid. 2001. Social medicine then and now: Lessons from Latin America. *American Journal of Public Health* 91 (October): 1592–1601.

Waitzman, Norman, and Ken Smith. 1998a. Separate but lethal: The effects of economic segregation on mortality in metropolitan America. *Milbank Quarterly* 76 (3): 341–73.

Waitzman, Norman, and Ken Smith. 1998b. Phantom of the area: Poverty-area residence and mortality in the United States. *American Journal of Public Health* 88 (June): 973–76.

Wakschlag, Lauren, Kate Pickett, Edwin Cook, Neal Benowitz, and Bennett Leventhal. 2002. Maternal smoking during pregnancy and severe antisocial behavior in offspring: A review. *American Journal of Public Health* 92 (June): 966–74.

Waldman, R. J. 1992. Income distribution and infant mortality. *Quarterly Journal of Economics* 107:1283–1302.

Waldron, Ingrid. 2001. What do we know about causes of sex differences in mortality? A review of the literature. In *The sociology of health and illness*, ed. Peter Conrad. New York: Worth.

Wallace, John, and Tyrone Forman. 1998. Religion's role in promoting health and reducing risk among American youth. *Health Education and Behavior* 25 (December): 721–41.

Wang, Thomas, Michael Pencina, Sarah Booth, Paul Jacques, Erik Ingelsson, Katherine Lanier, Emelia Benjamin, Ralph D'Agostino, Myles Wolf, and Ramachandran Vasan. 2008. Vitamin D deficiency and risk of cardiovascular disease. *Circulation*. January 7. http://www.circ.ahajournal.org.

Ware, John, and Cathy Donald Sherbourne. 1992. The MOS 36-item short-form health survey (SF-36), I. Conceptual framework and items selection. *Medical Care* 30 (6): 473–83.

Warner, David, and Mark Hayward. 2006. Early life origins of the race gap in men's mortality. *Journal of Health and Social Behavior* 47 (September): 209–26.

Weissman, Joel, Robert Stern, Stephen Fielding, and Arnold Epstein. 1991. Delayed access to health care: Risk factors, reasons, and consequences. *Annals of Internal Medicine* 114 (February): 325–31.

Weitzel, Jeffrey, and Laurence McCahill. 2001. The power of genetics to target surgical prevention. *New England Journal of Medicine* 344 (May): 1393–96.

West, Patrick. 1997. Health inequalities in the early years: Is there equalization in youth? *Social Science and Medicine* 44 (6): 833–58.

Whiteside, Alan. 2001. HIV/AIDS: A development crisis for Southern Africa. Listen to Africa Conference. Chicago. September 13.

Whittle, Jeff, Joseph Conigliaro, C. B. Good, and Richard Lofgren. 1993. Racial differences in the use of invasive cardiovascular procedures in the Department of Veterans Affairs medical system. *New England Journal of Medicine* 329 (August): 621–27.

WHO Report 2008. *Global tuberculosis control, surveillance, planning, financing.* Geneva, Switzerland: World Health Organization.

Wijdicks, Eelco. 2001. The diagnosis of brain death. *New England Journal of Medicine* 344 (April): 1215–21.

Wilkinson, Richard. 1986. Socio-economic differences in mortality: Interpreting the data on their size and trends. In *Class and health*, ed. Richard Wilkinson. London: Tavistock Publications.

Wilkinson, Richard. 1996. *Unhealthy societies: The afflictions of inequality.* London: Routledge.

Wilkinson, Richard. 1999. The culture of inequality. In *The society and population health reader*, vol. 1, ed. Ichiro Kawachi, Bruce Kennedy, and Richard Wilkinson. New York: The New Press.

Wilkinson, Richard. 2001. *Mind the gap.* New Haven, CT: Yale University Press.

Wilkinson, Richard, Ichiro Kawachi, and Bruce Kennedy. 1999. Mortality, the social environment, crime and violence. In *The society and population health reader*, vol. 1, ed. Ichiro Kawachi, Bruce Kennedy, and Richard Wilkinson. New York: The New Press.

Williams, David. 1994. The concept of race in *Health Services Research*: 1966 to 1990. *Health Services Research* 29 (August): 261–74.

Williams, David. 1996. Race/ethnicity and socioeconomic status: Measurement and methodological issues. *International Journal of Health Services* 26 (3): 483–505.

Williams, David, and Chiquita Collins. 1995. U.S. socioeconomic and racial differences in health: Patterns and explanations. *Annual Review of Sociology* 2:349–86.

Williams, Redford. 1998. Lower socioeconomic status and increased mortality, early childhood roots and the potential for successful interventions. *Journal of the American Medical Association* 279 (June): 1745–46.

Williams, Richard Allen. 2007. Historical perspectives of healthcare disparities: Is the past prologue? In *eliminating healthcare disparities in America*, ed. Richard Allen Williams. Totowa, NJ: Humana Press.

Willson, Andrea, Kim Shuey, and Glen Elder. 2007. Cumulative advantage processes as mechanisms of inequality in life course health. *American Journal of Sociology* 112 (6): 1886–1924.

Wilson, William Julius. 1987. *The truly disadvantaged: The inner city, the underclass, and public policy*. Chicago: University of Chicago Press.

Wilson, William Julius. 1993. The underclass: Issues, perspectives, and public policy. In *The ghetto underclass*, ed. William Julius Wilson. Newbury Park, CA: Sage.

Wnuk-Lipinski, Edmund, and Raymond Illsley. 1990. International comparative analysis: Main findings and conclusions. *Social Science and Medicine* 31 (8): 879–89.

Wolff, Edward. 1995. *Top heavy: A study of the increasing inequality of wealth in America*. New York: The Twentieth Century Fund Press.

Wolff, Edward. 2004. Changes in household wealth in the 1980s and 1990s in the U.S. Working Paper No. 407. Annandale-on-Hudson, NY: Levy Economics Institute.

Wolinsky, Frederic. 1980. *The sociology of health*. Boston: Little, Brown.

Wong, Mitchell, Ronald Andersen, Cathy Sherbourne, Ron Hays, and Martin Shapiro. 2001. Effects of cost-sharing on care seeking and health status: Results from the medical outcomes study. *American Journal of Public Health* 91 (November): 1889–94.

Wray, Linda, A. Regula Herzog, and Robert Wallace. 1998. The impact of education and heart attack on smoking cessation among middle-aged adults. *Journal of Health and Social Behavior* (December): 271–94.

Wright, John Paul, Kim Dietrich, M. Douglas Ris, Richard Hornung, Stephanie Wessel, Bruce Lanphear, Mona Ho, and Mary Rae. 2008. Association of prenatal and childhood blood lead concentrations with criminal arrests in early adulthood. *PLoS Medicine* 5 (5): e101; doi:10.371/journal pmed.0050101.

World Bank. 2001. World development indicators. www.worldbank.org.

Yates, Laurel, Luc Djousee, Tobias Kurth, Julie Buring, and J. Michael Gaziano. 2008. Exceptional longevity in men. *Archives of Internal Medicine* 168 (February): 284–90.

Yen, Irene, and George Kaplan. 1998. Poverty area residence and changes in physical activity level: Evidence from the Alameda County study. *American Journal of Public Health* 88 (November): 1709–12.

Young, Carlton, and Robert Gaston. 2000. Renal transplantation in black Americans. *New England Journal of Medicine* 343 (November): 1545–52.

Zhang, Shumin, I-Min Lee, JoAnn Manson, Nancy Cook, Walter Willett, and Julie Buring. 2007. Alcohol consumption and breast cancer risk in the women's health study. *American Journal of Epidemiology* 165:667–76.

Index

About the Author

Grace Budrys is professor of sociology at DePaul University. She is the author of *Our Unsystematic Healthcare System* (2nd edition, 2005). Her work focuses on health organizations and occupations, the structure of the health care system, and health disparities.